Clinical Case Studies for the Family Nurse Practitioner

Clinical Case Studies for the Family Nurse Practitioner

Leslie Neal-Boylan, PhD, CRRN, APRN-BC, FNP

Professor
Graduate Coordinator
Nursing Department
Southern Connecticut State University
New Haven, CT

WILEY-BLACKWELL

A John Wiley & Sons, Inc., Publication

This edition first published 2011 © 2011 by John Wiley & Sons, Inc.

Wiley-Blackwell is an imprint of John Wiley & Sons, formed by the merger of Wiley's global Scientific, Technical and Medical business with Blackwell Publishing.

Registered office: John Wiley & Sons Ltd, The Atrium, Southern Gate, Chichester, West Sussex, PO19 8SQ, UK

Editorial offices: 2121 State Avenue, Ames, Iowa 50014-8300, USA
The Atrium, Southern Gate, Chichester, West Sussex, PO19 8SQ, UK
9600 Garsington Road, Oxford, OX4 2DQ, UK

For details of our global editorial offices, for customer services and for information about how to apply for permission to reuse the copyright material in this book please see our website at www.wiley.com/wiley-blackwell.

Library of Congress Cataloging-in-Publication Data

Clinical case studies for the family nurse practitioner / [edited by] Leslie Neal-Boylan.
    p. ; cm.
  Includes bibliographical references and index.
  ISBN 978-0-8138-1144-4 (pbk. : alk. paper)
1. Family nursing–Case studies.   2. Nurse practitioners–Case studies.   I. Neal-Boylan, Leslie. [DNLM: 1. Family Nursing–Case Reports.   2. Nurse Practitioners–Case Reports.   3. Primary Care Nursing–Case Reports. WY 128]
  RT120.F34C55 2011
  616'.09–dc22

                                                                                          2011012018

A catalogue record for this book is available from the British Library.

Set in 10/12 pt Palatino by Toppan Best-set Premedia Limited
Printed and bound in Singapore by Fabulous Printers Pte Ltd

1   2011

Contents

Contributors

EDITOR

Leslie Neal-Boylan, PhD, CRRN, APRN-BC, FNP
Professor
Graduate Coordinator
Nursing Department
Southern Connecticut State University
New Haven, CT

CONTRIBUTORS

Ivy M. Alexander, PhD, APRN, ANP-BC, FAAN
Professor
Director–Adult, Family, Gerontological and Women's Health Primary Care Specialty
School of Nursing
Yale University
New Haven, CT

Nancy Cantey Banasiak, MSN, PNP-BC, APRN
Associate Professor
Pediatric Nurse Practitioner Specialty
School of Nursing
Yale University
New Haven, CT

Kathy J. Booker, PhD, RN
Professor, School of Nursing
Millikin University
Decatur, IL

Emily Croce, RN, MSN, CPNP
Pediatric Nurse Practitioner
Pediatric and Adolescent Dermatology
'Specially for Children
Dell Children's Medical Center of Central Texas
Austin, TX

Alison Moriarty Daley, MSN, APRN, PNP-BC
Associate Professor
Pediatric Nurse Practitioner Specialty
Master's Program
School of Nursing
Yale University
New Haven, CT

Tess Deshefy-Longhi, DNSc, RN
Visiting Assistant Professor
School of Nursing
Fairfield University
Fairfield, CT

Anna Faria, MSN, PNP-BC
Pediatric Nurse Practitioner
Southwest Community Health Center, Inc.
Bridgeport, CT

Tracey Fender, RN, MSN, CPNP
Sanson Pediatrics
Cottonwood, AZ

Anna Tielsch Goddard, CPNP-PC
Pediatric Nurse Practitioner
Children's Medical Center Dallas
Dallas, TX

Allison Grady, MSN, RN
Pediatric Nurse Practitioner
School of Nursing
Yale University
New Haven, CT

Elaine Gustafson, MSN, PNP
Associate Clinical Professor
Pediatric Nurse Practitioner Specialty
School of Nursing
Yale University
New Haven, CT

Shelley Yerger Hawkins, DSN, APRN-BC, FNP, GNP, FAAN
Associate Professor
School of Nursing
Yale University
New Haven, CT

Phoebe M. Heffron, MSN, PNP
School of Nursing
Yale University
New Haven, CT

Joanne DeSanto Iennaco, PhD, PMHCNS-BC, APRN
Assistant Professor
School of Nursing
Yale University
New Haven, CT

Vanessa Jefferson, MSN, BC-ANP, CDE
Lecturer
School of Nursing
Yale University
New Haven, CT

Meredith Wallace Kazer, PhD, APRN, A/GNP-BC
Associate Professor
School of Nursing
Fairfield University
Fairfield, CT

Geraldine F. Marrocco, EdD, APRN, CNS, ANP-BC
Assistant Professor
Adult, Family, Gerontological, and Women's Health
Primary Care Specialty
School of Nursing
Yale University
New Haven, CT

Michelle Wolfe Mayer, MSN, ANP-BC
Assistant Professor
Marymount University
School of Health Professions
Arlington, VA

Mikki Meadows-Oliver, PhD, RN
Assistant Professor
School of Nursing
Yale University
New Haven, CT

Sheila L. Molony, PhD, APRN, GNP-BC
Assistant Professor
School of Nursing
Yale University
New Haven, CT

Julie Murray, MSN, PNP
Pediatric Nurse Practitioner
Southwest Community Health Center
Bridgeport, CT

Jennifer Mygatt, MSN, RN
Family Nurse Practitioner
School of Nursing
Yale University
New Haven, CT

Vanessa Reid, MSN, APRN, CPNP
Pediatric Nurse Practitioner
Child & Family Agency of SE CT, Inc.
New London, CT

Patricia Ryan-Krause, MS, RN, MSN, CPNP
Associate Professor
Pediatric Nurse Practitioner Specialty
Director of Clinical Education
Center for International Nursing Scholarship and Education
School of Nursing
Yale University
New Haven, CT

Mary-Christine Sullivan, MPH, MSN, RN
Family Nurse Practitioner Candidate
School of Nursing
Yale University
New Haven, CT

Katharine Swan, MSN, RN
Family Nurse Practitioner
Yale University
New Haven, CT

Allison A. Vorderstrasse, DSNc, APRN
Assistant Professor
School of Nursing
Duke University
Durham, NC

Kevy Wijaya, MSN, RN, CPNP
Yale University
New Haven, CT

Susannah Young, MSN, RN
Family Nurse Practitioner
School of Nursing
Yale University
New Haven, CT

Preface

This book was written to help clinicians and students in family practice to better understand how to diagnose and manage typical (and some atypical) patient cases. I have often found it difficult to find patient cases that could be assigned to students or used "as is" in the classroom or in practica. I have frequently had to adapt cases I have found in publications or from my own experience. My purpose in writing this book was to make cases available that could be used without the need for adaptation. However, readers and instructors may still find it helpful to change the ages, genders, or locations of the patients in the cases to enable varying perspectives of the diagnoses and treatments of these patients.

The contributing authors in this book are experts in their fields. They have written these cases from real life. These are not textbook situations that do not allow for variations in socioeconomic status or family configuration. Because these cases are adapted from the experiences of the authors, they are realistic and do not result in cookie-cutter resolutions. Critical thinking questions encourage the reader to think carefully about what might happen if there were variations in the case presentation or in the patient's ability to comply with the plan of treatment. It is hoped that these cases will provide a jumping-off place for students and instructors to discuss possible treatment options and to use thoughtful consideration to determine if each case could be handled differently from the way it was presented. Often, in medicine, there is more than one answer to the same question. Therefore, each case should be analyzed carefully to determine the alternatives. Hopefully, this will broaden the scope of the readers' knowledge about family practice.

The sections within this book are presented chronologically from pediatric to adolescent to adult and finally to older adult. Typical cases in family practice within each developmental stage are included with an occasional atypical, but important, case added. Resolutions to the cases are at the end of each case. As tempting as it is to read the resolution before analyzing and discussing the case, it is advised that readers resist that urge in order to optimize the educational experience that this book offers.

Acknowledgments

I would like to thank the many wonderful and expert clinicians who contributed their time and energy to writing this book. It is a great privilege to be among them in this combined effort.

Thanks to all of the patients throughout the years who taught me how to listen, not just hear, and taught me to appreciate that my priorities for their health are not always their priorities and that quality health care requires a partnership between provider and patient that is sacrosanct.

I would also like to thank the editors at Wiley, especially Melissa Wahl, for the opportunity to write and publish this book and Janet Hronek, Editor/Project Manager for Toppan Best-set Premedia Ltd., for her assistance in its publication.

Finally, I'd like to thank Kevin Boylan, my husband, not only for his unending love and support but also for sharing in the writer's lament when things got rough and for giving me sound and helpful advice as a fellow academic author.

Introduction

By Leslie Neal-Boylan, PhD, CRRN, APRN-BC, FNP

Family practice is not simply the practice of caring for individuals across the lifespan. Contrary to the perceptions of many students who enter the world of family practice, it is not simply to care for people "from womb to tomb." Practice that is guided by that philosophy risks missing so much, not only regarding the individual patient's own health but the family dynamics and the tangible and intangible aspects of the family that impact the individual patient. If the "family" aspect of family practice is ignored or neglected, then the clinician is simply caring for individuals as any clinician would and cannot really style themselves as a family practice clinician regardless of title or certification.

To practice as a family practice clinician, it is important to have a basic understanding first about what is meant by "family" and then how the family is integrated into the plan of care and ultimately often becomes the "patient." In previous work about home health clinicians, this author found that home health clinicians care for the "patient entity," which is defined as all those who impact or potentially impact the patient's health. In family practice, the clinician also cares and, at the very least, considers the patient entity when developing and pursuing a plan of care for an individual who seeks health care.

Traditionally, "family" has been considered to be a married heterosexual couple with children. Aunts, uncles, and grandparents have also been traditionally included in documentation of the patient's family history or in genograms. The family history records vital information that can help the clinician assess health risks to the patient by highlighting the health of individual family members, as well as who has died and what caused their death. The age of death can have a significant impact on a sports physical for a patient, for example, by indicating that a family member died at an early age of a cardiac event. This knowledge makes the clinician aware of the need to explore possible cardiac disease in the patient to prevent sudden death brought on by athletic activity. Genograms often go a step further and may indicate who the decision maker in the family is, who the language interpreter is, and who the caregiver is. Clinicians, with the help of technology, have become creative in developing keys or legends for genograms that indicate many different aspects of family members, including physical and psychosocial characteristics that can be helpful in determining the patient's health risks and in planning care that will be realistic and meaningful to the patient.

The meaning of "family" has undergone societal change. Family members may or may not be heterosexual; they may be homosexual. They may not even be couples; single-parent families abound. Family doesn't require the presence of children, nor does anyone necessarily have to be related. Family can mean 2 or more people who have emotional connections to one another and who, in time of illness, will take care of one another. Not infrequently, family members who are related by blood do not have contact with each other and have no desire for contact. The clinician who assumes that blood relations care for one another and decides that he or she will facilitate bringing these people together as if they were all in some sentimental, but unrealistic, movie may find himself or herself ostracized by both the patient and those people who do care for, but may not be related to, the patient.

Consequently, it is important that the clinician not take for granted who is "family" and who is not. It is important to ask the patient who they consider their family. A simple genogram in the patient's chart or electronic medical record (EMR) can help the clinician remember who is considered family and who is important to the patient.

According to theorists, families go through a process of development just as do individuals (Duvall & Miller, 1985). The Family Developmental Theory (Duvall & Miller, 1985) describes 8 developmental stages, with expectations of individuals within the family changing in each stage. Both the family and the individual are engaged in accomplishing tasks. In order to function effectively, the family must promote accomplishment of individual and family tasks. Expectations and tasks required of the individuals and the family as a whole may require role changes and changes in the interactions among family members. If family and individual tasks collide, then there is conflict.

Duvall and Miller (1985) developed their theory based on the traditional family. This author seeks to update the model to make the theory's proposed stages of family development relevant to today's family. Family development begins with the first stage which requires the establishment of a family by joining 2 individuals in a relationship. These individuals leave their originating families to establish a new family. According to Duvall and Miller (1985), the developmental tasks in this first stage are to establish marriage, relate to an expanded network of kin, and plan the family. To update these tasks to conform to modern society, this author suggests that the tasks in this stage consist of establishing a committed relationship, relating to an expanded network of close relationships (that are not necessarily kin or blood relations), and planning a family. The flaw in the original theory by Duvall and Miller (1985) is that the birth of children is required to progress through the stages. What about the couple without children? Aren't they a family, too? Certainly, within the context of family practice, they are. However, for the sake of discussing the developmental tasks of the family with children, let us proceed through the model.

In stage 2, the first child is born and the family must adjust to parenthood and, in so doing, balance the needs of the individuals and of the family. It is not unusual nowadays for new mothers to present in the primary care clinic, lamenting that their partners do not appreciate how much work is involved in caring for a newborn or an infant. Neither partner is getting enough sleep or time to rest. Conflict arises when both partners aren't working together to balance individual and family needs. Stage 3 involves families with preschool-aged children. It then becomes the task of the family to nurture and socialize the children, while the individuals in the family must begin to separate the child from the parents.

In stage 4, the eldest child enters school. The family is expected to promote school achievement, and the individuals must continue to help the child separate from the parents and expand their interactions outside of the family. The couple within the family must work toward maintaining the marriage or committed relationship that they have.

In stage 5, the family copes with teenage children and must work to balance adolescent freedom and independence with the needs of the family. In stage 6, the children prepare to leave the cocoon of the family or the nest. The expectations of the family become coping with the empty nest and discovering new interests as a couple and as individuals.

Stage 7 lasts from the time the last child leaves the home and the retirement of the parents. During this time, the individuals within the couple reestablish and strengthen their own ties while maintaining links with the older and younger generations. In recent times, many adult children have not left the nest or else have returned to it after exploring the outside world. Duvall and Miller's (1985) original theory doesn't speak to this phenomenon, but family practice clinicians encounter this situation on a daily basis.

The adult children who are living in the family home with their parents frequently impact the parent's health status and plan of treatment, whether positively or negatively. They are part of the "patient entity." Just because they live in the home does not mean they will provide care for elderly parents. Often, the parents are financially supporting their adult children and/or are caring for their grandchildren. Caring for grandchildren often puts strains on the psychosocial and physiological status of individuals, as freedom (which has been long awaited) is curtailed and the physical demands of caring for children take their toll. Conversely, older adult parents might move into the home of their adult children. This also puts a strain on the roles and expectations of the individuals and of the family as a whole. Additionally, parents in the earlier stages of family development may need to care for growing children as well as for elder parents.

Stage 8, the final stage, according to this theory, involves the aging family's adjustment to the process of aging; retirement; deaths of partners, spouses, and loved ones; and loneliness. Family practice clinicians often care for older adults suffering from depression due to these losses. Sometimes the partner or loved one is still alive but suffers from dementia and is no longer the person they used to be. The other partner becomes lonely and may or may not seek help for their loneliness. Older adults may be reluctant to admit that they are depressed or that they have the need to seek physical and/or emotional love from someone outside the family. They may worry that this need won't be acceptable to society or, more crucially, to their children or extended family. It is vital that the clinician explore the possibility of depression and present a nonjudgmental attitude toward the patient's needs in this stage. It is also important to recognize that older adults do engage in sexual activity, both within the family and outside of it. Sexually transmitted diseases are a concern and should be discussed.

Individuals have roles within the family unit as well as roles outside of it. Women can be daughters and CEOs. Each of these roles presents its own stressors which may or may not overlap. Men may be brothers and eldest sons who are expected to direct the family if and when the parents are incapable of doing so. That may be a traditional point of view, but it is the family that determines whether roles will be traditional or not. Disease, injury, or illness can drastically change roles both within and outside of the family system. These changes may be temporary or permanent. New roles may be taken up willingly or unwillingly. Take, for example, the 80-year-old husband whose wife has just had a stroke. This man has never done the grocery shopping or the laundry or cleaned the house. Despite his devotion and love for his wife, he may be unwilling to or consider himself unable to assume those domestic responsibilities. Likewise, adult children who live far away from their parents might want to help, but are limited by time and circumstances to intermittent trips to see their parents. They may provide input to the clinician over the phone but are unable to provide care. Sometimes, these children provide monetary support if they cannot be close enough to their parents to care for them in any other way.

Financial circumstances may limit family members from caring for one another when there is illness or infirmity. A family member may not be able to take off time from work to care for a loved one full-time. This can be a source of significant frustration for all involved. Caregivers, regardless of whether or not they are kin of the patient, may suffer from caregiver burden or strain. Regardless of their devotion to the patient, they may become burned out and develop health problems themselves. Clinicians must be alert to this possibility and inquire about the health of the caregiver. Caregiver needs may go unnoticed, because they may not want to draw attention away from the patient. They also may not feel that they can get away to see a health care provider because there is no one else to care for the patient. The clinician can advise about community resources and respite care in these cases.

The patient is also experiencing a change in roles. The patient may no longer be the breadwinner or the household cook or be able to nurture the others in the family. Acute illness can result in temporary role changes, and families and society tend to accept these role changes while the patient is acutely ill or in pain. People with acute illness are often allowed to shirk their usual responsibilities and to take a break, so to speak, from the usual demands and obligations. However, when illness becomes chronic, family members and society are not always so forgiving. Chronic illness may require permanent role changes for the patient and patient entity. Some people might resent this change in expectations and might choose to push the new obligations required of the new roles onto hired caregivers, such as companions, aides, and private duty nurses. Resentment might also manifest itself in depression, anxiety, and difficulties coping.

Continued stressors might cause more serious illness if not identified and treated. For example, some current thought about fibromyalgia suggests that most patients who present with fibromyalgia come from dysfunctional families. This author can think of countless cases of depression, anxiety, and related illnesses that developed because of stressors and conflict within patients' families.

When thinking of family practice, it is also important to recognize that the family is a system. According to Bowen (www.theBowencenter.org), each individual within the family system is expected to interact with other family members in role circumscribed ways. These interactions based on individual roles are determined by each relationship within the family. As behaviors of family members affect the behaviors of other family members, patterns of behavior may develop. If roles change, this can either serve to keep the relationships stable or result in dysfunction and a different level of maintenance.

It is important to recognize that the family is a system that also consists of smaller systems of relationships that work within the family. If something, such as illness or infirmity, occurs and upsets the balance within the smaller systems, then the larger family system may be affected and have disequilibrium among all of the family members.

The cases in this book were chosen in an attempt to illustrate mostly typical (and some atypical) cases that occur in family practice. The reader is encouraged to go beyond simply trying to find the answers regarding the diagnoses and treatment plans for the patients involved in these cases. It will serve to enrich the usefulness of these cases if the reader considers various scenarios for the patient in light of which developmental stage the patient's family might be going through, as well as how the patient's illness or circumstances might affect the family and, consequently, the patient. Remembering that the patient is part of a subsystem within the larger family system can help the reader see that the patient's illness or condition not only impacts the patient but potentially has a ripple effect on many others both within and outside of the family system.

REFERENCES

Bowen Center for the Study of the Family. www.theBowencenter.org
Duvall, E. M. & Miller, B. C. (1985). *Marriage and family development* (6th ed.). New York: Harper and Row.

List of Abbreviations and Acronyms

AAA: Abdominal aortic aneurysm

AAP: American Academy of Pediatrics

ABG: Arterial blood gas

ACL: Anterior cruciate ligament

ADHD: Attention deficit hyperactive disorder

AD LIB: At liberty or whenever the patient wants to do something

AMI: Acute myocardial infarction or heart attack

Apgar: Refers to the score given to newborns at 1 minute and 5 minutes after birth. The newborn is scored on activity (muscle tone), pulse, grimace (reflex irritability), appearance (skin color), and respirations.

AS: Active surveillance

BMI: Body mass index

BMP: Basic metabolic panel

BP: Blood pressure

BS: Bowel sounds

BUN: Blood urea nitrogen

CAD: Coronary artery disease

CAM: Complementary and alternative medicine

CBC: Complete blood count with or without diff (differential)

CBT: Cognitive behavioral therapy

CCRC: Continuing care retirement community

CKD: Chronic kidney disease

CMP: Complete metabolic panel

COC: Combined oral contraceptive pill

COPD: Chronic obstructive pulmonary disease

CT: Computed tomography

CTA: Clear to auscultation

CXR: Chest X-ray

DDVAP: Desmopressin acetate vasopressin

DFA: Direct fluorescent antigen (testing)

DMARD: Disease-modifying antirheumatic drug

DMOA: Depo Provera

DRE: Digital rectal examination

DVT/PE: Deep vein thrombosis/pulmonary embolism

EBV: Epstein Barr Virus

ECG: Electrocardiogram

ED: Emergency department

EEG:	Electroencephalogram
ENT:	Ear, nose, and throat
EOM:	Extraocular movement
ESR:	Erythrocyte sedimentation rate
ETOH:	Alcohol (drinking kind)
FBG:	Fasting blood glucose
FBS:	Fasting blood sugar
FM:	Fibromyalgia
FROM:	Full range of motion
FTT:	Failure to thrive
GABHS:	Group A beta-hemolytic streptococci
GAD:	Glutamic acid decarboxylase
GC/CHL:	Gonorrhea/chlamydia
GCA:	Giant cell arteritis
GCS:	Glascow Coma Scale
GDS:	Geriatric Depression Scale
GERD:	Gastroesophageal reflux disease
GFR:	Glomerular filtration rate
HA1c:	Hemoglobin A1c
HCV:	Hepatitis C virus
HR:	Heart rate
HSDD:	Hypoactive sexual desire disorder
HSM:	Hepatosplenomegaly
HSV:	Herpes simplex virus
IBD:	Inflammatory bowel disease
IBS:	Irritable bowel syndrome
IUC:	Intrauterine contraception
KOH:	Potassium hydroxide
KUB:	Kidneys, ureters, and bladder
LLSB:	Left lower sternal border
LMP:	Last menstrual period
LNMP:	Last normal menstrual period
LR:	Light reflex
LRI:	Lower respiratory infections
LROM:	Limited range of motion
MCI:	Mild cognitive impairment
MCV:	Mean corpuscular volume
MDD:	Major depressive disorder
MDI:	Metered dose inhaler
MGF:	Maternal grandfather
MGM:	Maternal grandmother
MI:	Myocardial infarction
MMSE:	Mini-Mental State Examination
MoCA:	Montreal Cognitive Assessment
MRI:	Magnetic resonance imaging
MSRA:	Methicillin-resistant *Staphylococcus aureus*
MSSA:	Methicillin-susceptible *Staphylococcus aureus*
MVI:	Multiple vitamin
NAD:	No apparent distress
NICU:	Neonatal intensive care unit
NKDA:	No known drug allergies
NKFA:	No known food allergies
NP:	Nurse practitioner
NSAID:	Nonsteroidal antiinflammatory drug

NSVD: Normal sanguineous vaginal delivery
NT/ND: Nontender/nondistended
OA: Osteoarthritis
O2 sat: Oxygen saturation
OCP: Oral contraceptive pill
ODD: Oppositional defiant disorder
OGGT: Oral glucose tolerance test
OSA: Obstructive sleep apnea
OTC: Over-the-counter (medication)
PCOS: Polycystic ovarian syndrome
PCR: Polymerase chain reaction
PDA: Patent ductus arteriosus
PEG: Polyethylene glycol
PERRLA: Pupils equal, round, reactive to light and accommodation
PGF: Paternal grandfather
PGM: Paternal grandmother
PH/G: Pubic hair/gonads
PHN: Postherpetic neuralgia
PID: Pelvic inflammatory disease
PLP: Phantom limb pain
PMDD: Premenstrual dysphoric disorder
PMR: Polymyalgia rheumatica
PMS: Premenstrual syndrome
PNE: Primary nocturnal enuresis
PRN: As needed
QD: Once daily
RAI: Radionucleotide uptake scan with iodine
REM: Rapid eye movement
RICE: Rest, ice, compression, and elevation
ROS: Review of systems
RR: Respiratory rate
RRR: Regular rate and rhythm
RSV: Respiratory syncytial virus
RUQ: Right upper quadrant
SBHC: School-based health center
SEM: Systolic ejection murmur
SJS: Stevens-Johnson Syndrome
SLE: Systemic lupus erythematosus
SNRI: Serotonin norepinephrine reuptake inhibitor
SSRI: Selective serotonin reuptake inhibitor
STI: Sexually transmitted infection
SWS: Slow-wave sleep
TANF: Temporary Assistance for Needy Families
TBSA: Total body surface area
TCA: Tricyclic antidepressant
TEN: Toxic epidermal necrosis
TENS: Transcutaneous electrical nerve stimulation
TM: Tympanic membrane
TPO: Antithydroperoxidase antibody
TRAb: Thyrotropin receptor antibody
TRUS: Transrectal ultrasound
TSH: Thyroid stimulating hormone
TTN: Transient tachypnea of the newborn
TTP: Tenderness to palpation

USPSTF:	U.S. Preventive Services Task Force
UTI:	Urinary tract infection
VCUG:	Voiding cystourethrography
VDRL:	Venereal disease research laboratory
VZV:	Varicella zoster virus
WBC:	White blood cell
WHI:	Women's Health Initiative
WIC:	Women, Infant, and Children's Supplemental Nutrition Program

Clinical Case Studies for the Family Nurse Practitioner

Section 1

The Neonate

Case 1.1 Cardiovascular Screening Exam

By Mikki Meadows-Oliver, PhD, RN

SUBJECTIVE

Joseph, a 10-day-old male, was brought into the primary care office for a weight check. He is accompanied by his parents. His mother is concerned about his feeding habits. She believes that he takes awhile to drink his formula—longer than his siblings did; and she also thinks that he sweats more than they did, even when he doesn't feel warm.

Birth history: Significant for a 36-week gestation. His birth weight was 2600 grams. Because of his premature birth, Joseph was required be hospitalized for the first week of life in the Neonatal Intensive Care Unit (NICU). During his stay in the NICU, he was noted to feed without problems, maintain his temperature without assistance, and gain weight. His weight at discharge from the hospital 3 days ago was 2400 grams. Because of his premature birth status and his decreased weight, the family was told to follow up with the primary care provider in 3 days.

In the office today, his weight is 2490 grams. Further questioning about Joseph's birth history reveals that the mother's pregnancy was normal. She had no infections, falls, or known exposures to environmental hazards. She did not drink alcohol, take prescription medication (other than prenatal vitamins), use tobacco products, or use illicit drugs. During labor, she experienced a failure to progress, which resulted in her having a cesarean birth. The baby's Apgar scores were 8 at 1 minute and 9 at 5 minutes.

Social history: Joseph was born to a single, 29-year-old mother. His father is involved but does not reside in the household. Joseph lives in an apartment with his mother and two other siblings (ages 2 and 4 years). The maternal grandmother (MGM) lives nearby and is able to help Joseph's mother provide care. The family receives several governmental subsidies such as Women, Infants, and Children Supplemental Nutrition Program (WIC), Temporary Assistance for Needy Families (TANF), and Medicaid. Educationally, Joseph's mother has a high school diploma. She works in a local retail store. Joseph's father works in a manufacturing plant. The family has no pets. The MGM smokes but does not smoke in the home.

Diet: Breastfeeding ad lib with supplementation of a milk-based formula.

Elimination: 6–8 wet diapers daily with 3–4 yellow, seedy bowel movements.

Sleep: Sleeps between feedings.

Clinical Case Studies for the Family Nurse Practitioner, First Edition. Edited by Leslie Neal-Boylan.
© 2011 John Wiley & Sons, Inc. Published 2011 by John Wiley & Sons, Inc.

Family medical history: PGF (age 54): diabetes mellitus, heart attack at age 50; PGM (age 53): healthy; MGF: deceased from stroke at age 47; MGM (age 54): asthma; mother (age 29): asthma; father (age 31): healthy; Sibling #1 (age 4): asthma; Sibling #2 (age 2): heart murmur.

Medications: Currently taking no prescription, herbal, or OTC medications.

Allergies: No known allergies to food, medications, or environment.

OBJECTIVE

Vital signs: Weight: 2490 grams; length: 44 centimeters; temperature: 37°C (rectal).

General: Alert, well-nourished, well-hydrated baby.

Skin: Clear with no lesions noted; no cyanosis of lips, nails, or skin; no diaphoresis noted; skin turgor with elastic recoil.

Head: Normocephalic; anterior fontanel open and flat (2 cm × 3 cm); posterior fontanel open and flat (1 cm × 1 cm).

Eyes: Red reflex present bilaterally; pupils equal, round, and reactive to light; no discharge noted.

Ears: Pinnae normal; tympanic membranes gray bilaterally with positive light reflex.

Nose: Both nostrils patent; no discharge.

Oropharynx: Mucous membranes moist; no teeth present; no lesions.

Neck: Supple; no nodes.

Respiratory: RR = 28; clear in all lobes; no adventitious sounds noted; no retractions; no deformities of the thoracic cage noted.

Cardiac/Peripheral vascular: HR = 120; thrill noted in pulmonic area; continuous, systolic, grade 3 heart murmur noted on exam in the pulmonic area of the chest with both the bell and diaphragm; no radiation of the murmur to the back or axilla; brachial and femoral pulses present and *2+* bilaterally.

Abdomen/Gastrointestinal: Soft, nontender, nondistended, no evidence of hepatosplenomegaly. Umbilical cord is in place with no signs and symptoms of infection.

Genitourinary: Normal male; testes descended bilaterally; circumcision healing well.

Back: Spine straight.

Extremities: Full range of motion of all extremities; warm and well perfused; capillary refill <2 seconds. Negative hip click.

Neurologic: Good suck and cry; good tone in all extremities; positive Moro, rooting, plantar, palmar, and Babinski reflexes.

CRITICAL THINKING

Which diagnostic or imaging studies should be considered to assist with or confirm the diagnosis?
___Chest radiograph
___Echocardiogram
___Electrocardiogram

What is the most likely differential diagnosis and why?
___Patent ductus arteriosus
___Venous hum
___Atrioventricular malformation

What is the plan of treatment, and what should be the plan for follow-up care?

Are there any referrals needed?

Does this patient's psychosocial history influence how you might treat the patient?

What if this baby was a baby girl?

What if this baby had been born full term?

What if this baby had been born at a higher altitude?

Are there any standardized guidelines that you should use to assess or treat this case?

RESOLUTION

Diagnostics tests: ECG results are normal. CXR is normal. Echocardiogram reveals a patent ductus arteriosus.

What is the most likely differential diagnosis and why?
Patent ductus arteriosis (PDA):
PDA is the most common congenital heart defect seen in premature infants. Intravenous indomethacin (the drug of choice) often stimulates closure of the ductus arteriosus in premature infants. Nonsteroidal anti-inflammatory drugs (NSAIDs) such as ibuprofen may also be used to stimulate closure of the PDA. Prophylaxis for infective endocarditis is required until the PDA is closed. No long-term sequelae usually occur if the PDA is treated before pulmonary vascular disease develops.

What is the plan of treatment, and what should be the plan for follow-up care?
* Monitor weight and other growth parameters at subsequent visits.
* Provide emotional support. Allow the parents to verbalize their concerns about their baby's health maintenance. Facilitate mother-infant attachment.
* Return to clinic in 4 days for 2-week, well-child check and weight check.
* Discuss signs and symptoms of increased work of breathing (increased respiratory rate; intercostal retractions; nasal flaring) with parents and when to call the office (decreased by-mouth intake; decreased urine output; increased work of breathing; increased temperature ≥100.4°F).

Are there any referrals needed?
* Refer to cardiology for consideration of medication or surgery to aid in the closure of the duct.
* Consider referral for genetic counseling regarding future conception.

Does the patient's psychosocial history influence how you might treat the patient?
Since this mother is a single mother with two other children in the home, it is important for the health care provider to ensure that the family is referred to the appropriate social service agencies. The family should be referred to the Women, Infants, and Children (WIC) program for supplemental food and infant formula services. Mothers with a lower socioeconomic status have been found to be more at risk for postpartum depression, so it will be important for the health care provider to screen this mother for postpartum depression at subsequent visits throughout the baby's first year of life.

What if this baby was a baby girl?
Girls have been noted to be affected by patent ductus arteriosus twice as often as boys.

What if this baby had been born full term?
Functional closure of the ductus occurs within 15 hours of birth in a normal full-term infant, but true closure with the inability to reopen takes about 3 weeks.

What if this baby had been born at a higher altitude?
Babies born at higher altitudes are at increased risk for a patent ductus arteriosus.

Are there any standardized guidelines that you should use to assess or treat this case?
There are no standardized guidelines located in the literature for the assessment and/or treatment of patent ductus arteriosus.

REFERENCES AND RESOURCES

Giliberti, P., De Leonibus, C., Giordano, L., & Giliberti, P. (2009). The physiopathology of the patent ductus arteriosus. *The Journal of Maternal-Fetal & Neonatal Medicine, 22*(Suppl. 3), 6–9.

Katakam, L., Cotton, C., Goldberg, R., Dang, C., & Smith, P. (2010). Safety and effectiveness of indomethacin versus ibuprofen for treatment of patent ductus arteriosus. *American Journal of Perinatology, 27,* 425–429.

Lin, Y., Huang, H., Lien, R., Yang, P., Su, W., Chung, H., . . . Liu, W. (2010). Management of patent ductus arteriosus in term or near-term neonates with respiratory distress. *Pediatrics & Neonatology, 51,* 160–165.

Taggart, N., Cetta, F., O'Leary, P., Seward, J., & Eidem, B. (2010). Left atrial volume in children without heart disease and in those with ventricular septal defect or patent ductus arteriosus or hypertrophic cardiomyopathy. *The American Journal of Cardiology, 106,* 1500–1504.

Tavera, M., Bassareo, P., Biddau, R., Montis, S., Neroni, P., & Tumbarello, R. (2009). Role of echocardiography on the evaluation of patent ductus arteriosus in newborns. *The Journal of Maternal-Fetal & Neonatal Medicine, 22*(Suppl. 3), 10–13.

Case 1.2 Pulmonary Screening Exam

By Mikki Meadows-Oliver, PhD, RN

SUBJECTIVE

Caitlin, a 12-hour-old female, was born at home via planned home birth. She was brought into the office for an initial health maintenance visit. On initial examination, she was found to have rapid breathing when the office nurse weighed her. Caitlin is accompanied by both parents. There are no parental concerns.

Birth history: Caitlin is the product of a 40-week gestation. She was delivered vaginally at home by a certified nurse midwife. During the pregnancy, Caitlin's mother had no falls, infections, or known exposures to environmental hazards. She did not drink alcohol, take prescription medication (other than prenatal vitamins), use tobacco products, or use illicit drugs. The total labor duration was 2 hours. Caitlin's birth weight was 3380 g and her Apgars were 9 at 1 minute and 9 at 5 minutes.

Social history: Caitlin was born to a 37-year-old mother. Caitlin is the second child and has a 3-year-old sibling. She lives at home with both parents and her older sibling. The family employs an au pair who also resides in the home. Both parents are college educated. The mother works as a research assistant, and the father works as an accountant. There are no pets or smokers in the home.

Diet: Breastfeeding ad lib, but mother feels that Caitlin is having problems latching on. Colostrum is present. Milk has not come in yet.

Elimination: Urinated at birth, and has had 3 wet diapers since that time. Passed meconium at 10 hours of age.

Sleep: Sleeps between feedings.

Family medical history: PGF (age 67): sarcoidosis; PGM (age 63): healthy; MGF (age 64): Type 2 diabetes; MGM (age 64): history of MI at age 63; mother (age 37): healthy; father (age 42): healthy; Sibling #1 (age 3): healthy; history of bronchiolitis.

Medications: Currently taking no prescription, herbal, or over-the-counter medications.

Allergies: No known allergies to food, medications, or environment.

Clinical Case Studies for the Family Nurse Practitioner, First Edition. Edited by Leslie Neal-Boylan.
© 2011 John Wiley & Sons, Inc. Published 2011 by John Wiley & Sons, Inc.

OBJECTIVE

Vital signs: Weight in the office today is 3360 g; length: 48 cm; temperature: 37.2°C (rectal); pulse oximeter reading: 95% on room air.

General: Alert, active baby.

Skin: Clear with no lesions noted; no cyanosis of skin, lips, or nails; no diaphoresis noted; skin turgor intact.

Head: Molding present; anterior fontanel open and flat (2 cm × 2 cm); posterior fontanel open and flat (1 cm × 1 cm).

Eyes: Red reflex present bilaterally; pupils equal, round, and reactive to light; no discharge noted.

Ears: Pinnae normal; Tympanic membranes gray bilaterally with positive light reflex.

Nose: Both nostrils patent; no discharge; mild nasal flaring.

Oropharynx: Mucous membranes moist; no teeth present; no lesions.

Neck: Supple; no nodes.

Respiratory: RR = 68; crackles present in lower lung fields bilaterally; mild intercostal retractions; no grunting. No deformities of the thoracic cage noted.

Cardiac/Peripheral vascular: HR = 120; regular rhythm; no murmur noted; brachial and femoral pulses present and 2+ bilaterally.

Abdomen/Gastrointestinal: Soft, nontender, nondistended, no evidence of hepatosplenomegaly. Umbilical is cord in place with no signs and symptoms of infection.

Genitourinary: Normal female genitalia.

Back: Spine straight.

Extremities: Full range of motion of all extremities; warm and well-perfused; capillary refill <2 seconds; negative hip click.

Neurologic: Good suck and cry; good tone in all extremities; positive Moro, rooting, gag, plantar, palmar, and Babinski reflexes.

CRITICAL THINKING

Which diagnostic or imaging studies should be considered to assist with or confirm the diagnosis?
___Chest radiograph
___Arterial blood gas (ABG)
___Pulmonary function tests

What is the most likely differential diagnosis and why?
___Transient tachypnea of the newborn
___Pneumonia
___Neonatal sepsis

What is your plan of treatment, referral, and follow-up care?

Are there any demographic characteristics that would affect this case?

What if the patient lived in a rural, isolated setting?

Are there any standardized guidelines that you should use to assess or treat this case?

RESOLUTION

Diagnostic tests: It is important to obtain an arterial blood gas (ABG) to determine the level of gas exchange and acid-base balance. The ABG results reveal mild respiratory and metabolic acidosis.

Chest radiography is the diagnostic standard for transient tachypnea of the newborn. The chest radiograph shows generalized overexpansion of the lung (hypoaeration of alveoli) and flattened contours of the diaphragm which are consistent with transient tachypnea of the newborn.

What is the most likely differential diagnosis and why?
Transient tachypnea of the newborn (TTN):
Transient tachypnea of the newborn (TTN) is a self-limited disease. Approximately 1% of neonates have some form of respiratory distress that is not associated with infection such as transient tachypnea of the newborn. TTN results from a delay in clearance of fetal liquid from the lungs. Infants with TTN usually present with tachypnea within the first few hours of life. It has been associated with precipitous deliveries and births by cesarean section. The use of medications in TTN is minimal, although empiric antibiotics are often used for 48 hours after birth until sepsis has been ruled out. Medical care of TTN is supportive. As the retained lung fluid is absorbed by the infant's lymphatic system, the pulmonary status of the infant typically improves. TTN resolves over a 24-hour to 72-hour period.

What is your plan of treatment, referral, and follow-up care?

- Begin oxygen therapy in the office.
- Refer the patient and family to the local emergency department for support of the respiratory system, a workup for possible sepsis (complete blood count, blood cultures, lumbar puncture for culture of cerebrospinal fluid, and urine culture), and consultation with a neonatologist. An ambulance should be called to transport the baby from the office to the emergency department so that the baby's airway and respiratory status may be maintained.
- Provide emotional support to the parents. Allow the parents to verbalize their concerns about their baby's health status. Facilitate mother-infant attachment.

Are there any demographic characteristics that would affect this case?
The risk for TTN is equal in males and females. There has been no association with race or ethnicity reported. TTN presents as respiratory distress in full-term or near-term infants.

What if the patient lived in a rural, isolated setting?
Health care providers practicing in rural, isolated settings should have emergency office plans in place for patients experiencing respiratory distress.

Are there any standardized guidelines that you should use to assess or treat this case?
There were no standardized guidelines located in the literature for the assessment and/or treatment of transient tachypnea of the newborn.

REFERENCES AND RESOURCES

Kasap, B., Duman, N., Ozer, E., Tatli, M., Kumral, A., & Ozkan, H. (2008). Transient tachypnea of the newborn: Predictive factor for prolonged tachypnea. *Pediatrics International, 50*, 81–84.

Liem, J., Huq, S., Ekuma, O., Becker, A., & Kozyrskyj, A. (2007). Transient tachypnea of the newborn may be an early clinical manifestation of wheezing symptoms. *The Journal of Pediatrics, 151*, 29–33.

Takaya, A., Igarashi, M., Nakajima, M., Miyake, H., Shima, Y., & Suzuki, S. (2008). Risk factors for transient tachypnea of the newborn in infants delivered vaginally at 37 weeks or later. *Journal of Nippon Medical School, 75*, 269–273.

Case 1.3 Skin Screening Exam

By Mikki Meadows-Oliver, PhD, RN

SUBJECTIVE

Sarah is a 4-day-old infant in the office with her mother for an initial visit and weight check. Her mother states that Sarah has a rash on her chest and arms that has been intermittent for the past 2 days. There do not seem to be any triggers for the rash. Sarah's mother has washed all of the baby's clothes in a hypoallergenic cleanser only and has not used any moisturizers on the skin since the baby was discharged from the hospital. The rash also appears when Sarah is clad in only a diaper. The rash does not appear to cause discomfort for Sarah. Sarah's mother has not found anything that makes the rash better or worse.

Birth history: Sarah is the product of a 40-week gestation. Her birth weight was 3600 g. Further questioning about Sarah's birth history reveals that the mother's pregnancy was normal. She had no infections, falls, nor known exposures to environmental hazards. She did not use alcohol, take prescription medication (other than prenatal vitamins), use tobacco products, or use illicit drugs. During labor, Sarah's mother received a narcotic analgesic 1 hour prior to birth. Sarah was delivered via spontaneous vaginal delivery and her A scores were 7 at 1 minute and 9 at 5 minutes.

Social history: Sarah was born to a single, 18-year-old mother. Sarah's father is involved but does not reside in the household. Sarah lives in a 2-bedroom apartment with her mother and maternal grandmother (MGM). The MGM is able to help Sarah's mother provide care. Sarah's mother receives several governmental subsidies such as Women, Infants, and Children (WIC) Supplemental Nutrition Program, Temporary Assistance for Needy Families (TANF), and Medicaid. Educationally, Sarah's mother is completing coursework for her high school diploma. Sarah's father is also a high school student. There are no smokers in the home. The family has a dog.

Diet: Sarah is being fed a milk-based formula—2 oz every 3–4 hours.

Elimination: 6–8 wet diapers daily with 3–4 yellow, seedy bowel movements.

Sleep: Sleeps between feedings

Family medical history: PGF (age 40): asthma; PGM (age 38): obesity, high cholesterol, hypertension; MGF (age 36): sickle cell trait; MGM (age 34): bipolar disorder; mother (age 18): sickle cell trait; father (age 17): eczema.

Medications: Currently taking no prescription, herbal, or over-the-counter medications.

Allergies: No known allergies to food, medications, or environment.

OBJECTIVE

Vital signs: Weight: 3690 g; length: 44 cm; temperature: 36.8°C (rectal).

General: Alert; well-nourished; well-hydrated baby.

Skin: Scattered 1-cm, yellow-white papules on an erythematous base on the trunk, upper arms, and thighs; lesions are nontender to touch; lanugo over shoulders; no cyanosis of lips, nails, or skin; no diaphoresis noted; good skin turgor.

Head: Normocephalic; anterior fontanel open and flat (0.3 cm × 3 cm); posterior fontanel open and flat (0.5 cm × 0.5 cm).

Eyes: Red reflex present bilaterally; pupils equal, round, and reactive to light; no discharge noted.

Ears: Pinnae normal; tympanic membranes gray bilaterally with positive light reflex.

Nose: Both nostrils patent; no discharge.

Oropharynx: Mucous membranes moist; no teeth present; no lesions.

Neck: Supple; no nodes.

Respiratory: RR = 28; clear in all lobes; no adventitious sounds noted; no retractions; no deformities of the thoracic cage noted.

Cardiac/Peripheral vascular: HR = 120; regular rhythm; no murmur noted; brachial and femoral pulses present and 2+ bilaterally.

Abdomen/Gastrointestinal: Soft, nontender, nondistended, no evidence of hepatosplenomegaly. Umbilical cord is in place without signs and symptoms of infection.

Genitourinary: Normal male; testes descended bilaterally; circumcision healing well.

Back: Spine straight.

Extremities: Full range of motion of all extremities; warm and well-perfused; capillary refill <2 seconds; negative hip click.

Neurologic: Good suck and cry; good tone in all extremities; positive Moro, rooting, plantar, palmar, and Babinski reflexes.

CRITICAL THINKING

Which diagnostic or imaging studies should be considered to assist with or confirm the diagnosis?
___Skin biopsy
___Peripheral blood smear
___Bacterial/viral culture from the lesion

What is the most likely differential diagnosis and why?
___Milia
___Erythema toxicum
___Herpes simplex virus

What is your plan of treatment?

Does the patient's psychosocial history impact how you might treat this patient?

Are any referrals needed?

Does the patient's psychosocial history impact how you might treat this patient?

Are there any demographic characteristics that would affect this case?

Are there any standardized guidelines that you should use to assess or treat this case?

RESOLUTION

Diagnostic tests: Eosinophils will be noted on microscopic examination using a Wright stain. Eosinophilia may also be noted on peripheral blood studies. However, the diagnosis of erythema toxicum is usually made on the basis of clinical findings from the history and physical examination. No diagnostic testing is usually needed.

What is the most likely differential diagnosis and why?
Erythema toxicum:
Erythema toxicum, also called erythema toxicum neonatorum or toxic erythema of the newborn, is a common skin condition seen in newborns. It is self-limited and only occurs in the neonatal period. Herpes usually has more of a clustered and vesicular appearance whereas the lesions of erythema toxicum are scattered. Milia are whitish, pearly bumps in the skin of newborns. The lesions are not on erythematous bases. Milia lesions typically occur on the cheeks, nose, and chin—and not on the trunk.

The etiology of erythema toxicum is unknown. It may appear in up to 70% of newborns between 3 days and 2 weeks of life. Although the condition is harmless, it can be of great concern to the new parent.

What is your plan of treatment?
Erythema toxicum is not contagious and does not require any medical treatment. It usually resolves within 2 weeks after birth. Follow-up care is not needed unless the condition persists or does not resolve by 2 weeks of life.

Are any referrals needed?
Erythema toxicum neonatorum is often diagnosed easily by pediatricians and family physicians. If the features are atypical, if the newborn appears ill, or if the newborn has risk factors for sepsis, consultation with a pediatric dermatologist may be advisable.

Does the patient's psychosocial history impact how you might treat this patient?
The family has a pet dog. The lesions from erythema toxicum may sometimes resemble flea bites. Flea bites also should be considered among the differential diagnoses.

Are there any demographic characteristics that would affect this case?
There have been significant differences noted in the incidence of erythema toxicum based on race or gender. This condition is limited to the neonatal period. If an infant older than 28 days of age has a similar rash, then other diagnoses should be strongly considered.

Are there any standardized guidelines that you should use to assess or treat this case?
There are currently no standardized guidelines for the assessment and/or treatment of erythema toxicum.

REFERENCES AND RESOURCES

Liu, C., Feng, J., Qu, R., Zhou, H., Ma, H., Niu, X., & Tian, Z. (2005). Epidemiologic study of the predisposing factors in erythema toxicum neonatorum. _Dermatology, 210_, 269–272.

Marchini, G., Nelson, A., Edner, J., Lonne-Rahm, S., Stavreus-Evers, A., & Hultenby, K. (2005). Erythema toxicum neonatorum is an innate immune response to commensal microbes penetrated into the skin of the newborn infant. _Pediatric Research, 58_, 613–616.

Morgan, A., Steen, C., Schwartz, R., & Janniger, C. (2009). Erythema toxicum neonatorum revisited. _Cutis, 83_, 13–16.

Case 1.4 Oxygenation

By Mikki Meadows-Oliver, PhD, RN

SUBJECTIVE

Michael, a 27-day-old infant, arrives at the office with complaints of "breathing fast" and congestion since yesterday. He is accompanied by both parents. He has had no fever. At home, his rectal temperature was 37.2 degrees this morning. The parents tried using a humidifier to alleviate the symptoms, but they do not feel that this helped. They also used a bulb syringe with nasal saline to help relieve nasal congestion. Michael has had several visitors at his home during the first few weeks of his life, including small children who attend day-care centers. His mother thinks that some of those visitors may have had cold symptoms, although she tried to keep anyone who seemed sick away from Michael.

Diet: Normally breast-feeding every 2–3 hours; occasionally supplementing with a milk-based formula. Since yesterday, intake has decreased.

Elimination: 4–6 wet diapers since yesterday, which is decreased from his normal urine output. 2–3 bowel movements.

Sleep: Normally sleeps approximately 5 hours at night with several naps throughout the day. However, since yesterday, Michael's sleep has been interrupted.

Medications: Currently taking no prescription, herbal, or over-the-counter medications.

Allergies: No known allergies to food, medications, or environment.

Birth history: Michael was the product of a 39-week gestation. He was delivered via planned cesarean section. Michael's mother had no falls or known exposures to environmental hazards. She has a history of chlamydia during the pregnancy at 36-weeks' gestation. She was treated with antibiotics. The only other prescription medications taken during the pregnancy were prenatal vitamins. She did not use tobacco products or use illicit drugs. She stated that she drank an occasional glass of wine during the third trimester. Michael's birth weight was 3250 g, and his Apgar scores were 9 at 1 minute and 9 at 5 minutes.

Clinical Case Studies for the Family Nurse Practitioner, First Edition. Edited by Leslie Neal-Boylan.
© 2011 John Wiley & Sons, Inc. Published 2011 by John Wiley & Sons, Inc.

Social history: Michael was born to a 32-year-old mother. He lives at home with both parents. Neither parent has any other children. The mother works as a secretary, and the father works in construction. Michael's father is a smoker. The family has 2 cats.

Family medical history: PGF (age 65): Type 2 diabetes mellitus; PGM (age 64): breast cancer at age 55; MGF (age 60): asthma; MGM (age 64): healthy; mother (age 32): asthma; father (age 32): seasonal allergies.

OBJECTIVE

Vital signs: Weight: 4050 grams; length: 48 cm; temperature: 37.2°C (rectal); pulse oximeter reading: 93% on room air.

General: Alert baby; well-hydrated; well-nourished; in mild respiratory distress.

Skin: Clear with no lesions noted; no cyanosis of skin, lips, or nails; no diaphoresis noted; good skin turgor.

Head: Normocephalic; anterior fontanelle open and flat (2 cm × 2 cm); posterior fontanelle open and flat (0.5 cm × 0.5 cm).

Eyes: Red reflex present bilaterally; pupils equal, round, and reactive to light; no discharge noted.

Ears: Pinnae normal; tympanic membranes gray bilaterally with positive light reflex.

Nose: Both nostrils congested; cloudy discharge present in nares; mild nasal flaring.

Oropharynx: Mucous membranes moist; no teeth present; no lesions.

Neck: Supple; no nodes.

Respiratory: RR = 42; expiratory wheezing present in all lobes; intercostal retractions present; no grunting; no deformities of the thoracic cage noted.

Cardiac/Peripheral vascular: HR = 120; regular rhythm; no murmur noted; brachial and femoral pulses present and 2+ bilaterally.

Abdomen/Gastrointestinal: Soft, nontender, nondistended, no evidence of hepatosplenomegaly.

Genitourinary: Normal male genitalia; testes descended bilaterally.

Back: Spine straight.

Extremities: Full range of motion of all extremities; warm and well-perfused; capillary refill <2 seconds; negative hip click.

Neurologic: Good suck and cry; good tone in all extremities; positive Moro, rooting, plantar, palmar, and Babinski reflexes.

CRITICAL THINKING

Which diagnostic or imaging studies should be considered to assist with or confirm the diagnosis?
___Chest radiograph (anterior-posterior [AP] and lateral views)
___Direct fluorescent antibody (DFA) test to detect respiratory syncytial virus (RSV)
___Complete blood count

What is the most likely differential diagnosis and why?
___Bronchiolitis
___Upper respiratory infection (URI)
___Chlamydial pneumonia

What is your plan of treatment, referral, and follow-up care?

What are demographic characteristics that might affect this case?

Does the patient's psychosocial history impact how you might treat this patient?

What if the patient lived in a rural, isolated setting?

RESOLUTION

Diagnostic tests: The DFA test was positive for RSV. A complete blood count (CBC) is seldom useful since the white blood cell (WBC) count is usually within normal limits. Chest radiographs are not routinely necessary. The nonspecific findings of hyperinflation and patchy infiltrates may be seen on the chest radiograph.

What is the most likely differential diagnosis and why?
Bronchiolitis:
The most likely differential diagnosis is bronchiolitis related to an infection with RSV. Michael's history and physical examination form the primary basis for the diagnosis of bronchiolitis. Bronchiolitis is usually due to a viral infection of the small lower airways (bronchioles). Infection is spread by direct contact with respiratory secretions. Previous infection does not confer immunity. Reinfection can be common. Early symptoms are those of a viral URI, including mild rhinorrhea, cough, and sometimes low-grade fever. It is unlikely to be chlamydial pneumonia since the mother was successfully treated during the pregnancy. Scattered crackles with good breath sounds are characteristic of chlamydial pneumonia, and wheezing is usually absent. Conjunctivitis and middle-ear abnormality may be present in half the infants with chlamydial pneumonia. Chest radiographs will show bilateral interstitial infiltrates with hyperinflation.

What is your plan of treatment, referral, and follow-up care?

- Begin oxygen therapy in the office, and monitor Michael's cardiac and respiratory status.
- Place Michael in an upright position to facilitate respirations.
- Consider a trial of a bronchodilator. (The use of bronchodilators is controversial. These agents relieve reversible bronchospasm by relaxing smooth muscles of the bronchi. Metaanalyses of clinical studies show little or no benefit from treatment with inhaled beta-adrenergic agents [with or without ipratropium bromide]. Empiric treatment with beta-agonists seems to be the standard of care. Clinical trials demonstrate that corticosteroids have no benefit in the treatment of bronchiolitis, and thus they should not be used routinely. Antibiotics are not routinely used unless a bacterial infection is present. Ribavarin, an antiviral drug specifically available for RSV treatment is reserved for cases of severe disease such as infants with complicated CHD or who are immunocompromised. Prophylaxis with Synagis is used for some infants at risk for RSV.)
- Refer patient and family to the local emergency department for support of the respiratory system, a workup for possible sepsis (complete blood count, blood cultures, lumbar puncture for culture of cerebrospinal fluid, and urine culture), and consultation with a neonatologist. An ambulance should be called to transport the baby from the office to the emergency department so that the baby's airway and respiratory status may be maintained.
- Provide emotional support to the parents. Allow the parents to verbalize their concerns about their baby's health status. Facilitate mother-infant attachment.

What are demographic characteristics that might affect this case?
Race and socioeconomic status may affect the frequency of contracting bronchiolitis. Lower socioeconomic status may increase the likelihood of hospitalization. Bronchiolitis occurs as much as 1.25 times more frequently in males than in females. Although infection with etiologic agents may occur at any age, the clinical entity of bronchiolitis includes only infants and young children. In cases of bronchiolitis, 75% of the cases occur in children younger than 1 year, and 95% occur in children younger than 2 years. Incidence peaks in those aged 2–8 months.

Does the patient's psychosocial history impact how you might treat this patient?
Michael's father is a smoker; and the family has 2 cats. Both of these things may be lung irritants.

What if the patient lived in a rural, isolated setting?
Health care providers practicing in rural, isolated settings should have emergency office plans in place for patients experiencing respiratory distress.

REFERENCES AND RESOURCES

Al-Ansari, K., Sakran, M., Davidson, B., El Sayyed, R., Mahjoub, H., & Ibrahim, K. (2010). Nebulized 5% or 3% hypertonic or 0.9% saline for treating acute bronchiolitis in infants. *Journal of Pediatrics, 157*, 630–634.

Fernandes, R., Bialy, L., Vandermeer, B., Tjosvold, L., Plint, A., Patel, H., & Hartling, L. (2010). Glucocorticoids for acute viral bronchiolitis in infants and young children. *Cochrane Database of Systematic Reviews*, (10), CD004878.

Petruzella, F. & Gorelick, M. (2010). Current therapies in bronchiolitis. *Pediatric Emergency Care, 26*, 302–307.

Sumner, A., Coyle, D., Mitton, C., Johnson, D., Patel, H., Klassen, T. & Pediatric Emergency Research Canada (2010). Cost-effectiveness of epinephrine and dexamethasone in children with bronchiolitis. *Pediatrics, 126*, 623–631.

Case 1.5 Nutrition and Weight

By Mikki Meadows-Oliver, PhD, RN

SUBJECTIVE

Alicia is a 2-week-old Hispanic female in for her well-child check. She is accompanied by her 15-year-old mother. The family speaks only Spanish. A Spanish-speaking interpreter is used for the visit. Alicia's mother is concerned that Alicia spits up a lot after eating. The mother states that the vomit is not projectile. The mother is worried that, since the baby is vomiting so much, she is not getting enough food. Therefore, the mother has been feeding Alicia even more formula. Also, Alicia's mother is worried that she will run out of formula since the baby takes so much.

Diet: Formula feeding: 5 oz every 2–3 hours.

Elimination: 6 wet diapers and 3 bowel movements since yesterday.

Sleep: Sleeps approximately 4 hours at night with several naps throughout the day.

Medications: Currently taking no prescription, herbal, or over-the-counter medications.

Allergies: No known allergies to food, medications, environment.

Birth history: Alicia was the product of a 38-week gestation. She was delivered via spontaneous vaginal delivery. Alicia's mother had no falls, infections, or known exposures to environmental hazards. The only prescription medications taken during the pregnancy were prenatal vitamins. She did not use alcohol, tobacco products, or illicit drugs during the pregnancy. Alicia's birth weight was 3250 g and her APGAR scores were 8 at 1 minute and 9 at 5 minutes. Her discharge weight was 3180 g.

Social history: Alicia lives at home with her teenage mother and her maternal grandmother who immigrated from Mexico. The father of the baby is involved. Neither parent has any other children. Both parents are students at a local high school. The family has a dog.

Family medical history: PGF (age 37): high blood pressure; PGM (age 33): thyroid problems; MGF (age 35): health history unknown; MGM (age 30): healthy; mother (age 15): healthy; father (age 15): healthy.

Clinical Case Studies for the Family Nurse Practitioner, First Edition. Edited by Leslie Neal-Boylan.
© 2011 John Wiley & Sons, Inc. Published 2011 by John Wiley & Sons, Inc.

OBJECTIVE

Vital signs: Weight: 4050 g; length: 48 cm; temperature: 37.3°C (rectal).

General: Alert baby; well-developed.

Skin: Clear with no lesions noted; no cyanosis of skin, lips, or nails; no diaphoresis noted; good skin turgor.

Head: Normocephalic; anterior fontanel is open and flat (3 cm × 2 cm); posterior fontanel is open and flat (1.0 cm × 0.5 cm).

Eyes: Red reflex present bilaterally; pupils equal, round, and reactive to light; no discharge noted.

Ears: Pinnae normal; tympanic membranes gray bilaterally with positive light reflex.

Nose: Both nostrils congested; cloudy discharge present in nares; mild nasal flaring.

Oropharynx: Mucous membranes moist; no teeth present; no lesions.

Neck: Supple; no nodes.

Respiratory: RR = 24; lungs with clear breath sounds in all lobes; no retractions present; no grunting; no deformities of the thoracic cage noted.

Cardiac/Peripheral vascular: HR = 120; regular rhythm; no murmur noted; brachial and femoral pulses present and 2+ bilaterally.

Abdomen/Gastrointestinal: Soft, nontender, nondistended, no evidence of hepatosplenomegaly.

Genitourinary: Normal female genitalia.

Back: Spine straight.

Extremities: Full range of motion of all extremities; warm and well-perfused; capillary refill <2 seconds; negative hip click.

Neurologic: Good suck and cry; good tone in all extremities; positive Moro, rooting, plantar, palmar, and Babinski reflexes.

CRITICAL THINKING

Which diagnostic or imaging studies should be considered to assist with or confirm the diagnosis?
___Upper gastrointestinal (GI) imaging series
___Manometry to assess esophageal motility and lower esophageal sphincter function
___Complete blood count

What is the most likely differential diagnosis and why?
___Overfeeding
___Gastroesophageal reflux disease
___Gastroenteritis

What is your plan of treatment and follow-up care?

Does the patient's psychosocial history impact how you might treat this patient?

What demographic characteristics might affect this case?

Are there any standardized guidelines that you should use to assess or treat this case?

RESOLUTION

Diagnostic test results: No tests are needed based on the history and physical examination.

What is the most likely differential diagnosis and why?
Overfeeding:
Based on the history of the baby taking 5 oz of formula every 2 hours, the significant weight gain in the first 2 weeks of life, and the unremarkable physical examination, the most likely differential is overfeeding. Gastroesophageal reflux disease (GERD) is often associated with failure to thrive. Neonates with GERD may also present with respiratory symptoms. Neonates with gastroenteritis may present with diarrhea and fever—which this baby does not have.

What is your plan of treatment and follow-up care?

*   Via a Spanish-speaking medical interpreter, provide education about feeding, proper mixing of formula, and signs of satiety in neonates.
*   Discuss ways to comfort the baby that do not involve feeding.
*   Refer the family to the Women, Infants, and Children (WIC) for a consultation with a nutritionist and assistance with obtaining formula.

Does the patient's psychosocial history impact how you might treat this patient?
Having a teenage mother who has limited English proficiency is an aspect of the patient's psychosocial history that may affect his treatment. Working with the mother and her family will require extra time during visits to ensure that the patient education and anticipatory guidance are properly understood.

What demographic characteristics might affect this case?
There are no particular race or socioeconomic characteristics that would affect overfeeding.

Are there any standardized guidelines that you should use to assess or treat this case?
There are no known guidelines that focus on overfeeding in the neonate. The American Academy of Pediatrics has guidelines about the introduction of solids.

REFERENCES AND RESOURCES

Gawron, A., & Hirano, I. (2010). Advances in diagnostic testing for gastroesophageal reflux disease. *World Journal of Gastroenterology*, *16*, 3750–3756.

Herbella, F., & Patti, M. (2010). Gastroesophageal reflux disease: From pathophysiology to treatment. *World Journal of Gastroenterology*, *16*, 3745–3749.

Lacy, B., Weiser, K., Chertoff, J., Fass, R., Pandolfino, J., Richter, J., & Vaezi, M. (2010). The diagnosis of gastroesophageal reflux disease. *The American Journal of Medicine*, *123*, 583–592.

Section 2

The Infant

Case 2.1 Nutrition and Weight

By Mikki Meadows-Oliver, PhD, RN

SUBJECTIVE

Nelson, a 12-month-old infant, presents to the office for a well-baby visit. He is accompanied by his mother, Kylie. Kylie states that Nelson has been healthy since his last well-baby visit at 9 months of age. He has had no visits to the urgent care clinic or to the emergency room in the interim. Kylie is concerned that Nelson's appetite has diminished. She states that he is not eating as much lately as he had been.

Diet: Nelson's nutrition history reveals that he has successfully transitioned to a diet with whole milk. He drinks five 8-oz bottles of whole milk daily. Nelson is a "picky eater." He rarely eats foods that are offered to him and, instead, prefers to drink from the bottle. He is not currently taking any multivitamins.

Elimination: Kylie states that Nelson has 4–6 wet diapers daily. He does not have any diarrhea but does have occasional constipation that is relieved with prune juice.

Sleep: Nelson sleeps 13 hours nightly but does not take any naps during the day. He does not have any problems falling asleep or staying asleep. His nighttime bedtime routine includes a bath and bedtime story read to him by Kylie.

Developmental: Nelson is able to walk while holding onto furniture. He can also stand unassisted for about 5 seconds. Nelson says "dada" and "mama" and has words for bottle and milk.

Birth history: Nelson was the product of a 37-week gestation. He was delivered vaginally with the assistance of a vacuum. During the pregnancy, Kylie had no falls or infections. She did not drink alcohol, take over-the-counter or prescription medications (other than prenatal vitamins), use tobacco products, or use illicit drugs. Nelson's birth weight was 3000 g, and his Apgar scores were 8 at 1 minute and 9 at 5 minutes. Past medical history reveals that Nelson has had 3 episodes of acute otitis media since birth. He has had no injuries or illnesses requiring visits to the emergency department.

Social history: Nelson was born to a 20-year-old mother. He has a 2-month-old younger sibling. He lives at home with his mother and his paternal grandmother. Nelson's father is currently incarcerated. Nelson's mother does not currently work outside the home. The family receives rent subsidy from Section 8 and food subsidy from the Women, Infants, and Children (WIC) program and food stamps.

Clinical Case Studies for the Family Nurse Practitioner, First Edition. Edited by Leslie Neal-Boylan.
© 2011 John Wiley & Sons, Inc. Published 2011 by John Wiley & Sons, Inc.

The family also receives monthly cash assistance from the Temporary Aid to Needy Families (TANF) program. The family has no pets and there are no smokers in the home.

Family medical history: Nelson's mother has no health problems. His father is 32 years old and has no history of chronic medical conditions. His maternal grandmother has a history of breast cancer. His maternal grandfather has high blood pressure. His paternal grandmother (48 years of age) is healthy with no health problems. The health history of his paternal grandfather is unknown.

Nelson is not currently taking any over-the-counter, prescription, or herbal medications. He has no known allergies to food, medications, or the environment. He is up to date on required immunizations.

OBJECTIVE

Nelson's vital signs were taken in the office. His weight is 6.4 kg, and his length is 66 cm. His temperature is within the normal range at 36.8°C (temporal). When observing Nelson's general appearance, he is alert, active, and playful. He appears well hydrated and well nourished.

Skin: Clear of lesions; no cyanosis of his skin, lips, or nails; no diaphoresis noted. Nelson has good skin turgor on examination.

HEENT: Nelson's head is normocephalic. His anterior fontanel is open and flat (0.5 cm × 0.5 cm). Red reflex is present bilaterally; and his pupils are equal, round, and reactive to light. There is no discharge noted. Pinnae are normal, and the tympanic membranes are gray bilaterally with positive light reflexes. Bony landmarks are visible, and there is no fluid noted behind the tympanic membrane. Both nostrils are patent. There is no nasal discharge; and there is no nasal flaring. Nelson's mucous membranes are noted to be moist when examining his oropharynx. He has 8 teeth present with white spots present on both upper central incisors. There are no lesions present in the oral cavity.

Neck: Supple and able to move in all directions without resistance; shotty nodes present in the posterior cervical region.

Respiratory: Respiratory rate is 20 breaths per minute, and his lungs are clear to auscultation in all lobes. There is good air entry, and no retractions or grunting are noted on examination. No deformities of the thoracic cage noted.

Cardiovascular: Heart rate is 106 beats per minute with a regular rhythm. There is no murmur noted upon auscultation; brachial and femoral pulses are present and 2+ bilaterally.

Abdomen: Normoactive bowel sounds are present throughout; soft and nontender. There is no evidence of hepatosplenomegaly.

Genitourinary: Normal male genitalia. Nelson is circumcised and his testes are descended bilaterally.

Neuromusculoskeletal: Good tone in all extremities; full range of motion in all extremities. His extremities are warm and well perfused. Capillary refill is less than 2 seconds, and his spine is straight.

CRITICAL THINKING

Which laboratory tests should be ordered as part of a 12-month, well-child visit?

Other than "well child," what additional diagnoses should be considered for Nelson?

What is your plan of treatment, referral, and follow-up care?

Does this patient's psychosocial history affect how you might treat this case?

What if the patient lived in a rural setting?

Are there any demographic characteristics that might affect this case?

Are there any standardized guidelines that you should use to assess or treat this case?

RESOLUTION

Diagnostic tests: According to the American Academy of Pediatrics (AAP) *Recommendations for Preventive Pediatric Health Care* guidelines, there are several tests that are recommended for the 12-month well-child visit. A hemoglobin or hematocrit is recommended at the well-child visit to screen for iron deficiency anemia. A blood lead test is also recommended to screen for an elevated blood lead level. A tuberculin test is recommended if the child has risk factors for contracting tuberculosis, such as travel to an endemic area, residing in a homeless shelter, or visiting someone in jail. Nelson's father is incarcerated. If he visits in father in jail, he should receive a screening for tuberculosis.

Other than "well child," what additional diagnoses should be considered for Nelson?
Based on the information gathered during his history and on his physical examination, there are several additional diagnoses that may be considered. Related to Nelson's nutrition, there are 2 potential diagnoses: at risk for constipation and at risk for iron deficiency anemia. Nelson is drinking nearly 40 oz of cow's milk daily. This amount of milk is excessive for his age (recommended amount is 20–24 oz daily). Excessive milk intake is associated with iron-deficiency anemia, as well as constipation. Regarding his weight, Nelson is currently in the age range to develop physiologic anorexia of the toddler. Because the rate of growth decreases during the second year of life (between 1–2 years of age), this diagnosis signifies that the child needs fewer calories and therefore may be more likely to eat less. Another consideration is that Nelson is becoming full from his excessive milk intake and may be less likely to be hungry for solid foods.

What is your plan of treatment, referral, and follow-up care?
The plan of treatment for this visit would be to discuss the excessive milk intake, discuss iron rich foods, and discuss the decreased caloric needs of the young toddler compared to the young infant. Kylie should be advised to feed Nelson solid foods before offering him milk. She would also be advised to wean Nelson off the bottle and to feed him liquids from a cup only, limiting juice to 4 oz and cow's milk to 24 oz per day. A daily pediatric multivitamin may also be prescribed for Nelson.

Since Kylie already receives TANF and WIC services, she can be referred to the SNAP Food Stamp Assistance Program for additional help in acquiring nutritious foods for Nelson. If further nutritional concerns arise, the family can be referred to a nutritionist. Nelson should return to the office for a well-child visit in 3 months for his 15-month checkup. He should return sooner if there are signs and symptoms of illness.

Does this patient's psychosocial history affect how you might treat this case?
Nelson's family is likely to be of a lower socioeconomic status (SES) based on their eligibility for governmental subsidies such as WIC, TANF, and Section 8. Because of their SES, the family may be less likely to be able to afford nutritious foods. This could affect Nelson's weight and growth patterns.

What if the patient lived in a rural setting?
Living in a rural setting might further limit access to nutritious foods since there may be fewer local facilities where nutritious foods can be readily purchased.

Are there any demographic characteristics that might affect this case?
The family's low income status is the demographic factor in this case. Other demographic characteristics such as gender and ethnicity are not likely to affect this case.

Are there any standardized guidelines that you should use to assess or treat this case?
Refer to the American Dietetic Association (2007) and American Heart Association (2005) resources in the References and Resources below for standardized guidelines on nutrition and weight that might be used to assess or treat this case.

REFERENCES AND RESOURCES

American Dietetic Association. (2007). *Pediatric weight management evidence-based nutrition practice guideline.* American Dietetic Association.

American Heart Association. (2005). *Dietary recommendations for children and adolescents: A guideline for practitioners: Consensus statement from the American Heart Association.* American Heart Association.

Daher, S., Tahan, S., Sole, D., Naspitz, C., Da Silva-Patricio, R., Neto, U., & De Morais, M. (2001). Cow's milk protein intolerance and chronic constipation in children. *Pediatric Allergy and Immunology, 12,* 339–342.

Food Stamp Assistance. http://foodstamp-assistance.com

Oliveira, M., & Osorio, M. (2005). Cow's milk consumption and iron deficiency anemia in children. (Portuguese—English Abstract). *Jornal de Pediatria, 81,* 361–367.

Supplemental Nutrition Assistance Program (2010). Food stamp assistance.

Case 2.2 Health Maintenance

By Mikki Meadows-Oliver, PhD, RN

SUBJECTIVE

Juancarlos, a 9-month-old male, presents to the office for a well-baby visit. He is accompanied by his mother, Lupe. Lupe is Spanish speaking, so a medical interpreter is used for the visit. Lupe has no concerns and states that Juancarlos has been healthy since his last well-child visit at 6 months of age. He has had no visits to the urgent care clinic or to the emergency room in the interim.

Diet: Juancarlos' nutrition history reveals that he is still being breastfed but that he is also being supplemented with a low-iron, milk-based formula. Lupe states that she gives Juancarlos low-iron formula because formula that is not low-iron makes him constipated. He eats a diet of regular food that the family eats. He eats fruits and vegetables daily. Lupe introduced finely chopped meats into Juancarlos' diet last week, and he has tolerated the addition well. Juancarlos also enjoys Cheerios® which he is able to grasp and bring to his mouth without assistance. He is not currently taking any multivitamins.

Elimination: Lupe states that Juancarlos has 4–6 wet diapers daily and voids easily with a straight urine stream. He does not have any diarrhea or constipation since beginning the low-iron formula.

Sleep: Juancarlos is sleeping 10 hours at night and takes one 2-hour nap daily. He does not have any problems falling asleep or staying asleep. At night, he has a bedtime routine that includes a bath and bedtime story read to him by an older sibling.

Development: Juancarlos is crawling and pulling up to stand. He makes lots of vocalizations and is saying "da-da," although Lupe is not sure if he is just making sounds or referring to his father when he says "da-da." Juancarlos has a beginning pincer grasp that allows him to eat small items such as Cheerios®.

Birth history: Juancarlos is the product of a 40-week gestation. He was delivered vaginally without complications. During the pregnancy, his mother had no falls or infections. Lupe did not drink alcohol, take over-the-counter or prescription medications (other than prenatal vitamins), use tobacco products, or use illicit drugs. Juancarlos's birth weight was 3500 g, and his Apgar scores were 9 at 1 minute and 9 at 5 minutes. Past medical history reveals that he was hospitalized at 4 months of age for bronchiolitis. He has had no episodes of wheezing since that time.

Social history: Juancarlos was born to a 31-year-old mother. He has 2 older siblings (7 and 9 years old). He lives at home with both parents and his maternal grandfather. The family is from Ecuador.

Clinical Case Studies for the Family Nurse Practitioner, First Edition. Edited by Leslie Neal-Boylan.
© 2011 John Wiley & Sons, Inc. Published 2011 by John Wiley & Sons, Inc.

His mother works as a housekeeper, and his father works in construction. The family has a pet bird. There are no smokers in the home.

Family medical history: Juancarlos's mother has asthma and seasonal allergies. His 33-year-old father is healthy and has no history of chronic medical conditions. Juancarlos's maternal grandmother died at age 55 years from a myocardial infarction. His maternal grandfather has a history of Type 2 diabetes mellitus and obesity. His paternal grandparents are both deceased; both died in a motor vehicle accident several years ago.

Juancarlos is not currently taking any over-the-counter, prescription, or herbal medications. He has no known allergies to food, medications, or the environment. He is up to date on required immunizations.

OBJECTIVE

Juancarlos's vital signs were taken in the office today. His weight is 6.0 kg, and his length is 64 cm. Juancarlos's temperature is within the normal range at 37°C (temporal). When observing his general appearance, he is alert, active, and playful. He appears well hydrated and well nourished.

Skin: His skin is clear of lesions. There is no cyanosis of his skin, lips, or nails. There was no diaphoresis noted. Juancarlos has good skin turgor on examination.

HEENT: Juancarlos's head is normocephalic. His anterior fontanel is open and flat (0.5 cm × 0.5 cm). Red reflexes are present bilaterally and pupils are equal, round, and reactive to light. There is no discharge noted. Pinnae are normal; tympanic membranes are gray bilaterally with positive light reflexes. Bony landmarks are visible, and there is no fluid noted behind the tympanic membrane. Both nostrils are patent. There is no nasal discharge; and there is no nasal flaring. Juancarlos' mucous membranes are noted to be moist when examining his oropharynx. He has 2 teeth present without evidence of caries. There are no lesions present in the oral cavity.

Neck: Supple and able to move in all directions without resistance. There is no cervical lymphadenopathy.

Respiratory: Respiratory rate is 22 breaths per minute and his lungs are clear to auscultation in all lobes. There is good air entry, and no retractions or grunting are noted on examination. No deformities of the thoracic cage are noted.

Cardiovascular: Heart rate is 102 beats per minute with a regular rhythm. There is no murmur noted upon auscultation; brachial and femoral pulses are present and 2+ bilaterally.

Abdomen: Normoactive bowel sounds are present throughout; soft and nontender. There is no evidence of hepatosplenomegaly.

Genitourinary: Genitourinary examination reveals normal male genitalia. Juancarlos is uncircumcised, and his testes are descended bilaterally.

Neuromusculoskeletal: Good tone in all extremities; full range of motion of all extremities. His extremities are warm and well perfused. Capillary refill is less than 2 seconds, and his spine is straight.

CRITICAL THINKING

Which laboratory or diagnostic imaging tests should be ordered as part of a 9-month, well-child visit?
___CBC
___Lead screening test

___Liver function tests
___Cholesterol level
___Baseline chest radiograph

What is the most likely differential diagnosis and why?
___Iron deficiency anemia
___Constipation
___Other

What is your plan of treatment, referral, and follow-up care?

Does this patient's psychosocial history affect how you might treat this case?

What if the patient lived in a rural setting?

Are there any demographic characteristics that might affect this case?

Are there any standardized guidelines that you should use to assess or treat this case?

RESOLUTION

Diagnostic tests: According to the American Academy of Pediatrics (AAP) *Recommendations for Preventive Pediatric Health Care* guidelines, there are no recommended laboratory tests or diagnostic imaging tests for the 9-month, well-child visit. However, based on Juancarlos' history of receiving a low-iron formula, the health care provider may consider obtaining a hemoglobin test to screen for iron-deficiency anemia. If the hemoglobin is abnormally low, then the health care provider can obtain a full complete blood count to confirm the diagnosis of iron deficiency anemia. The AAP guidelines recommend that children at risk for lead poisoning (those children living at or below the poverty line who live in older housing) receive a risk-assessment screening for lead poisoning at 9 months of age.

What is the most likely differential diagnosis and why?
__Iron deficiency anemia and constipation:__
Based on the history provided by Juancarlos' mother, diagnoses to consider would be iron deficiency anemia and constipation.

What is your plan of treatment, referral, and follow-up care?
The plan of treatment would be to discuss nutrition, anticipatory guidance and safety. For the 9-month visit, the health care provider should discuss safety issues such as car safety (having the child in a rear-facing car seat) and water safety (water temperature < 120 degrees; never leaving the baby in the bathtub alone; keeping the toilet lid and the bathroom door closed; empty mop buckets after each use). In addition, the health care provider should discuss firearm safety, the prevention of burns, and the need for working smoke and carbon monoxide detectors.

The health care provider should discuss anticipatory guidance topics such as introducing the cup and beginning to wean Juancarlos off the bottle; reading to him each night; and discouraging television watching and encouraging more interactive activities that promote proper brain development, such as talking, playing, singing, and reading together.

Nutrition topics such as the need for iron-fortified formula, not low-iron formula, to prevent iron deficiency anemia should be discussed. Nutritional suggestions should be given to prevent constipation associated with iron intake such as pureed prunes or prune juice.

The family may be referred to the WIC (Women, Infants, and Children) program for assistance with obtaining formula and iron-fortified infant cereals. The WIC program has nutritionists on staff that will be able to provide Juancarlos's family with nutritional education.

Juancarlos should follow up for a well-child visit at 1 year of age or sooner as needed for signs and symptoms of illness.

Does this patient's psychosocial history affect how you might treat this case?

The language difference between the health care provider and the patient's family may be a potential barrier to receiving effective health care—even with the use of a certified medical interpreter. Because of this barrier, the health care provider may need to spend extra time when working with this family.

What if the patient lived in a rural setting?

It may be difficult to obtain appropriate medical translator services for families living in rural settings. This may prompt health care providers to use family members for interpretation, which could compromise patient confidentiality. Telephone translator services are available for use for practices without in-person translators. Also, obtaining supplemental nutrition services such as WIC may be difficult because of lack of access to nearby WIC distribution centers.

Are there any demographic characteristics that might affect this case?

Besides being of Hispanic ethnicity and not speaking English, age is a demographic factor that might affect this case. At 9 months of age, Juancarlos likely has no maternal iron stores; and since he is consuming low-iron formula and not taking multivitamins, he is at risk for iron deficiency anemia.

Are there any standardized guidelines that you should use to assess or treat this case?

The American Academy of Pediatrics has issued several clinical practice guidelines that may assist health care providers during well-child visits. For more information, refer to the resources below and their web links.

REFERENCES AND RESOURCES

American Academy of Pediatrics. (2010). Recommendations for preventive pediatric health care. http://practice.aap.org/content.aspx?aid=1599

American Academy of Pediatrics. (2010).Recommended childhood and adolescent immunization schedules—United States. http://aappolicy.aappublications.org/cgi/content/full/pediatrics;125/1/195

Baker, R. D., Greer, F. R., & Committee on Nutrition American Academy of Pediatrics (2010). Diagnosis and prevention of iron deficiency and iron-deficiency anemia in infants and young children (0–3 years of age). *Pediatrics, 126,* 1040–1050.

Centers for Disease Control and Prevention. (2009). Lead prevention tips. http://www.cdc.gov/nceh/lead/tips.htm

Constipation Guideline Committee of the North American Society for Pediatric Gastroenterology, Hepatology and Nutrition (2006). Evaluation and treatment of constipation in infants and children: Recommendations of the North American Society for Pediatric Gastroenterology, Hepatology and Nutrition. *Journal of Pediatric Gastroenterology and Nutrition, 43,* e1–e13.

Food and Nutrition Program. (2010). Women, Infants, and Children. http://www.fns.usda.gov/wic/

Magar, N. A., Dabova-Missova, S., & Gjerdingen, D. K. (2006). Effectiveness of targeted anticipatory guidance during well-child visits: A pilot trial. *Journal of the American Board of Family Medicine: JABFM, 19,* 450–458.

Schempf, A. H., Minkovitz, C. S., Strobino, D. M., & Guyer, B. (2007). Parental satisfaction with early pediatric care and immunization of young children: The mediating role of age-appropriate well-child care utilization. *Archives of Pediatrics & Adolescent Medicine, 161,* 50–56.

Case 2.3 Growth and Development

By Mikki Meadows-Oliver, PhD, RN

SUBJECTIVE

Kierra, a 9-month-old infant, presents to the office for a well-baby visit. She is accompanied by her foster mother, Ann. Ann states that Kierra has been in her care for the past 7 months. Kierra is the first infant that Ann has cared for. According to Ann, Kierra has been healthy since her last well-child visit at 6 months of age. She has had no visits to the urgent care clinic or to the emergency room in the interim. Ann is concerned that Kierra appears thin.

Diet: Kierra's nutrition history reveals that she drinks three 8-oz bottles of milk-based formula daily. Kierra also eats 1 jar of stage 1 baby food twice daily. She is not currently taking any multivitamins.

Elimination: Ann states that Kierra has 4–6 wet diapers daily. She does not have any diarrhea or constipation.

Sleeps: Kierra sleeps 10 hours nightly and takes 2 naps daily. Ann states that Kierra does not have any problems falling asleep or staying asleep. The family does not currently have a bedtime routine for Kierra.

Birth history: Ann does not know any of the details of Kierra's birth history or family history.

Past medical history: Kierra has been healthy since being placed in Ann's care. Since placement, Kierra has had no injuries or illnesses requiring visits to the emergency department. Developmentally, Kierra is able to crawl. She is able to pick up small objects such as Cheerios® using only her thumb and forefinger. Kierra makes many sounds and is beginning to say "dada."

Social history: Kierra lives at home with her foster mother Ann. Ann does not currently work outside the home. The family receives rent subsidy from Section 8, food subsidies from the Women, Infants, and Children (WIC) program, and food stamps. The family also receives monthly cash assistance from the Temporary Aid to Needy Families (TANF) program. The family has no pets, and there are no smokers in the home.

Medications: Kierra is not currently taking any over-the-counter, prescription, or herbal medications.

Allergies: No known allergies to food, medications, or the environment. She is up to date on required immunizations.

Clinical Case Studies for the Family Nurse Practitioner, First Edition. Edited by Leslie Neal-Boylan.
© 2011 John Wiley & Sons, Inc. Published 2011 by John Wiley & Sons, Inc.

OBJECTIVE

General: Appears thin but alert, active, and playful.

Vital signs: Weight in the office today is 6.4 kg and his length is 66 centimeters. Kierra's temperature is within the normal range at 36.8°C (temporal). Kierra's weight has not changed since her last well child visit.

Skin: She appears well hydrated, and her skin was clear of lesions. There is no cyanosis of her skin, lips, or nails. There was no diaphoresis noted. Kierra has good skin turgor on examination.

HEENT: Kierra's head is normocephalic. Her anterior fontanel is open and flat (0.5 cm × 0.5 cm). Red reflexes are present bilaterally; and pupils are equal, round, and reactive to light. There is no discharge noted. Pinnae are normal; the tympanic membranes were gray bilaterally with positive light reflexes. Bony landmarks are visible and there was no fluid noted behind the tympanic membrane. Both nostrils are patent. There is no nasal discharge, and there is no nasal flaring. Kierra's mucous membranes are noted to be moist when examining her oropharynx. She has 2 teeth present—lower central incisors. There are no lesions present on the teeth or in the oral cavity.

Neck: Supple and able to move in all directions without resistance. There are no lymph nodes present in the neck area.

Respiratory: Rate is 22 breaths per minute, and her lungs are clear to auscultation in all lobes. There is good air entry, and no retractions or grunting are noted on examination. No deformities of the thoracic cage noted.

Cardiovascular: Heart rate is 110 beats per minute with a regular rhythm. There is no murmur noted upon auscultation; brachial and femoral pulses are present and 2+ bilaterally.

Abdomen: Normoactive bowel sounds are present throughout; soft and nontender. There is no evidence of hepatosplenomegaly.

Genitourinary: Genitourinary examination reveals normal female genitalia.

Neuromusculoskeletal: Good tone in all extremities. She has full range of motion in all extremities and her extremities are warm and well perfused. Capillary refill is less than 2 seconds, and his spine is straight.

CRITICAL THINKING

Which diagnostic or imaging studies should be considered to assist with or confirm the diagnosis?
___CBC count
___Urinalysis
___Urine culture
___Electrolytes, including creatinine and BUN
___Liver function tests, including total protein and albumin
___Barium swallow
___Chest radiograph

What is the most likely differential diagnosis and why?
___Organic failure to thrive (FTT)
___Nonorganic FTT (FTT)
___Constitutional growth delay
___Fetal alcohol spectrum disorder

What is your plan of treatment, referral, and follow-up care?

Does this patient's psychosocial history affect how you might treat this case?

What if the patient lived in a rural setting?

Are there any demographic characteristics that might affect this case?

Are there any standardized guidelines that you should use to assess or treat this case?

RESOLUTION

Diagnostic tests: Many cases of children not gaining weight are nonorganic, so a history and physical examination are normally all that are needed. Certain laboratory tests may help to screen for an underlying pathologic condition. A complete blood count (CBC) can be ordered as well as a urinalysis and urine culture. If an electrolyte imbalance is suspected, electrolytes including blood urea nitrogen (BUN) and creatinine can be ordered. Liver function tests may also be ordered to rule out an underlying liver condition.

If it is suspected that the infant is having a physical problem such as difficulty swallowing, a modified barium swallow may be ordered. This test would be done under the directions of a feeding therapist and a radiologist. During the test, the infant would be given liquids and solids differing in consistency. The infant's swallows would be filmed to determine if there are swallowing difficulties that are contributing to the lack of weight gain. A chest radiograph would be helpful in assessing whether a cardiopulmonary disease is a contributing factor.

What is the most likely differential diagnosis and why?
Nonorganic failure to thrive:
With an infant who is not gaining weight, there are several differential diagnoses to consider including organic failure to thrive, nonorganic failure to thrive (FTT), constitutional growth delay, and fetal alcohol spectrum disorder. We do not know much about Kierra's birth and past history—only that she was removed from her mother's care and placed in foster care. Because it is unknown whether or not she was exposed to substances, including alcohol in utero, it would be wise to initially consider a diagnosis of fetal alcohol spectrum disorder as a contributing factor to the failure to gain weight. Children with true fetal alcohol syndrome display a failure to gain weight, as well as distinct facial anomalies; and they typically have cognitive/developmental impairment. Those with fetal alcohol spectrum disorder may display growth and cognitive delays but may or may not have the distinct facial features that are associated with fetal alcohol syndrome. Given Kierra's history, there was nothing on the physical examination or in the history to indicate that she has distinct facial anomalies or any delays in development. Based on these findings, it is likely that both fetal alcohol spectrum disorder and fetal alcohol can be ruled out as causes for Kierra's growth impairment.

Constitutional growth delay may also be considered in the differential diagnoses for a failure to gain weight. Children with constitutional growth delay may have linear growth velocity and weight gain that slows beginning as early as age 3–6 months. We do not have information on this child's linear growth velocity. We have only one length measurement, which would not tell us whether or not the linear growth velocity is stable, increasing, or decreasing. However, most children who have constitutional growth delay do not seek medical attention until puberty, when a lack of sexual development becomes apparent and a discrepancy in height from peers is noted because of the delay in pubertal growth spurt. This makes it likely that Kierra does not have constitutional growth delay and that her care provider should consider other diagnoses.

Organic FTT usually results from problems such as neuromuscular abnormalities, craniofacial abnormalities, or lack of appetite. Other conditions that may result in organic FTT include breathing difficulties, significant developmental delay, and primary gastrointestinal disease or dysfunction. The information obtained in Kierra's history and on her physical examination does not indicate that she suffers from any of the aforementioned problems, making organic FTT an unlikely diagnosis.

Nonorganic FTT usually results from adverse environmental and psychosocial factors. It may be associated with abnormal interactions between the caregiver and the infant. This may result in an inadequate provision of food and/or inadequate intake of food. Nonorganic FTT is most common in the setting of poverty. It may include a combination of poverty and lack of preparation for parenting. An important part of the evaluation of all children is observation of the infant while feeding. Observing infants while they are feeding sheds light on maternal-infant interactions. Given Kierra's history and physical examination and the elimination of the previous diagnoses, nonorganic FTT is the most likely diagnosis at this time. Kierra's caregiver has not cared for an infant in the past, so it may be possible that she is unaware of the caloric needs of a 9-month-old. A 9-month-old infant needs an approximate caloric intake of 140 kilocalories (kcal)/kilogram (kg) per day. Calculating Kierra's daily caloric needs (6.4 kg × 140 kcal) means that she would need 896 kcal per day. Calculating her caloric intake based on her reported history, Kierra's daily caloric intake is less than her calculated caloric needs. Calories in regular infant formula are 20 kcal/oz. Kierra's stated intake is 24 oz of formula daily, which provides her with 480 kcal/day. She also eats 2 jars of stage 1 baby food daily. Stage 1 baby foods typically have 25–50 kcal/jar, providing Kierra with an additional 50–100 kcal per day. Kierra's approximate caloric intake per day is 530–580 kcal, far below her daily caloric need of 896 kcal. Also, Kierra's foster mother does not work outside the home and receives several government housing and food subsidies. Her eligibility for these subsidies makes it likely that she lives at or near the poverty line, a risk factor for nonorganic FTT.

What is your plan of treatment, referral, and follow-up care?

The goal for Kierra would to provide her with adequate caloric intake for growth. In this case, it would appear that Kierra can be treated for her nonorganic FTT on an outpatient basis. However, frequent follow-up visits are necessary (initially at 2–4 weeks, then at least monthly thereafter). Kierra's weight gain, linear growth velocity, head circumference, and daily caloric intake should be recorded at each follow-up visit. Her weight, length, and head circumference should be plotted on the same age-appropriate growth chart over time. Ann should be instructed on proper caloric intake for Kierra and on ways to increase calories in Kierra's diet. Home visits, from the health care provider or an outreach worker may assist in determining the underlying reason for the nonorganic FTT.

If outpatient treatment does not lead to documented weight gain, hospitalization may be necessary for diagnostic and therapeutic reasons. When treating an infant with FTT, a multidisciplinary team approach should be used. A pediatric health care provider, nutritionist, and social worker should be a part of the team. A mental health care professional may also be included. This team should complete a thorough evaluation of the family's psychosocial situation and determine if future support is required. A home visit can help to support the caregiver. The family may also be referred to a local food bank if food affordability is a problem.

Does this patient's psychosocial history affect how you might treat this case?

Kierra's psychosocial history does affect how this case would be treated. Kierra is in foster care. It is essential that her foster care worker be informed of diagnosis. Through the state's child protective services, Kierra's foster care worker may be able to provide additional support (social and financial) for Ann. They may also need to determine if Kierra would be better cared for in a foster home where the foster mother is knowledgeable about infant nutrition and care.

What if the patient lived in a rural setting?

If this patient and her foster family lived in a rural setting, having frequent follow-up appointments in the office might not feasible. In that case, the health care provider could consider employing the services of a visiting nurse service to visit the home monthly to monitor Kierra's weight and nutritional status. The family's ability to obtain additional food through a source such a food bank may be limited as there may not be one in the area.

Are there any demographic characteristics that might affect this case?

While failure to thrive can occur in any socioeconomic strata, nonorganic FTT is more likely to occur in families living in poverty. There is an increased incidence of nonorganic FTT in children receiving Medicaid, children living in rural areas, and those who are homeless. While the exact reason is unknown, nonorganic FTT is more likely to occur in females than in males. In regard to age in the pediatric population, the most likely age groups to have nonorganic FTT are infants and toddlers.

Are there any standardized guidelines that you should use to assess or treat this case?
For two guidelines for the detection and treatment of failure to thrive, see Cincinnati Children's Hospital Medical Center (2009) and Block & Krebs (2005) in References and Resources below.

REFERENCES AND RESOURCES

Block, R., & Krebs, N. (2005). Failure to thrive as a manifestation of child neglect. *Pediatrics, 116*, 1234–1237.

Cincinnati Children's Hospital Medical Center. (2009). Best evidence statement (BESt) failure to thrive treatment protocol. Cincinnati, OH: Cincinnati Children's Hospital Medical Center. http://www.guidelines.gov/content.aspx?id=14794&search=failure+to+thrive

Daniel, M., Kleis, L., & Cemeroglu, A. (2008). Etiology of failure to thrive in infants and toddlers referred to a pediatric endocrinology outpatient clinic. *Clinical Pediatrics, 47*, 762–765.

Ficicioglu, C., & An Haack, K. (2009). Failure to thrive: When to suspect inborn errors of metabolism. *Pediatrics, 124*, 972–979.

Panetta, F., Magazzu, D., Sferlazzas, C., Lombardo, M., Magazzu, G., & Lucanto, M. (2008). Diagnosis on a positive fashion of nonorganic failure to thrive. *Acta Paediatrica, 97*, 1281–1284.

Case 2.4 Heart Murmur

By Mikki Meadows-Oliver, PhD, RN

SUBJECTIVE

Jacob, a 12-month-old infant, presents to the primary care office for a well-child visit. He is accompanied by his parents. His mother is concerned that Jacob is eating less than usual but says that he is drinking his normal amount. His activity level has not changed.

Birth history: Jacob was born at 39 weeks' gestation. His birth weight was 3200 g. There were no complications during the labor or delivery. The mother had no infections, falls, or known exposures to environmental hazards. She did not drink alcohol, take prescription medication (other than prenatal vitamins), use tobacco products, or use illicit drugs. The immediate neonatal period was unremarkable. Jacob was discharged at 2 days of age to home with his mother.

The social history reveals that Jacob was born to a single, 23-year-old mother. His father is involved but does not reside in the household. Jacob lives in an apartment with his mother and 19-year-old cousin. The maternal grandmother (MGM) lives in the neighborhood and is able to help Jacob's mother with child care. The family receives assistance from governmental subsidies such as Women, Infants, and Children supplemental nutrition program (WIC), Temporary Assistance for Needy Families (TANF), and Medicaid. Educationally, both Jacob's mother and father have high school diplomas. She works at a fast-food restaurant. Joseph's father works as a construction worker. The family has no pets. There are no smokers in the home.

Diet: Jacob eats a balanced diet of table foods. Still breast-feeds but is transitioning to whole milk. Takes a daily multivitamin.

Elimination: 4–6 wet diapers daily with 1 bowel movement.

Sleep: Takes one 2-hour nap daily and sleeps 12 hours at night.

Family medical history: PGF (age 54): healthy; PGM (age 53): diabetes mellitus; MGF (age 46) high blood pressure; MGM (age 44): asthma; mother (age 23): asthma; father (age 32): healthy.

Medications: Currently taking no prescription, herbal, or over-the-counter medications.

Immunizations: Up to date.

Allergies: No known allergies to food, medications, or environment.

Clinical Case Studies for the Family Nurse Practitioner, First Edition. Edited by Leslie Neal-Boylan.
© 2011 John Wiley & Sons, Inc. Published 2011 by John Wiley & Sons, Inc.

OBJECTIVE

Vital signs: Weight: 10 kg; length: 84 cm; temperature: 37°C (axillary).

General: Alert; well nourished; well hydrated; interactive.

Skin: Clear with no lesions noted; no cyanosis of lips, nails, or skin; no diaphoresis noted; good skin turgor.

Head: Normocephalic; anterior fontanel is open and flat (1 cm × 1 cm).

Eyes: Red reflexes present bilaterally; pupils equal, round, and reactive to light; no discharge noted.

Ears: Pinnae normal; tympanic membranes gray bilaterally with positive light reflex.

Nose: Both nostrils are patent; no discharge.

Oropharynx: Mucous membranes are moist; no teeth are present; no lesions.

Neck: Supple; no nodes.

Respiratory: RR = 24; clear in all lobes; no adventitious sounds noted; no retractions; no deformities of the thoracic cage noted.

Cardiac/Peripheral vascular: HR = 120; vibratory, systolic, grade 2 heart murmur noted on exam at the lower left sternal border area of the chest with both the bell and diaphragm; heard best in the supine position; no heaves or thrills noted; no radiation of the murmur to the back or axilla; brachial and femoral pulses present and 2+ bilaterally.

Abdomen/Gastrointestinal: Soft, nontender, nondistended, no evidence of hepatosplenomegaly.

Genitourinary: Normal circumcised male genitalia; testes descended bilaterally.

Back: Spine straight.

Ext: Full range of motion of all extremities; warm and well perfused; capillary refill < 2 seconds.

Neurologic: Good strength and tone.

CRITICAL THINKING

Which diagnostic or imaging studies should be considered to assist with or confirm the diagnosis?
___Chest radiograph
___Echocardiogram
___Electrocardiogram

What is the most likely differential diagnosis and why?
___Patent ductus arteriosus (PDA)
___Ventricular septal defect (VSD)
___Still murmur

What is your plan of treatment, referral, and follow-up care?

Are there any referrals needed?

Does the patient's psychosocial history impact how you might treat this patient?

What if this baby were a girl?

What if this baby was 6 months old?

Are there any standardized guidelines that you should use to assess or treat this case?

RESOLUTION

Diagnostic tests: Based on the history and physical examination, no imaging studies are needed. However, if any of the above studies were ordered, no abnormalities would be noted on the test.

What is the most likely differential diagnosis and why?
Still murmur:
Still murmur is a murmur that is classified as "functional," "innocent," or "physiologic." It is not a structural defect of the heart and may be a result of noise flowing through a normal heart. There is no known cause. Neither a PDA nor a VSD are position-dependent (heard louder in the supine position). Also, the vibratory quality of the murmur is consistent with a Still murmur. PDA is more common in infants born prematurely.

What is your plan of treatment, referral, and follow-up care?

- Discuss physiologic murmurs with the parents and explain that no limitation on activity is required.
- Monitor weight and other growth parameters at subsequent visits.
- Allow the parents to verbalize their concerns about their baby's health maintenance.
- Discuss signs and symptoms of increased work of breathing (increased respiratory rate; intercostal retractions; nasal flaring) with parents and when to call the office (decreased by mouth intake; decreased urine output; increased work of breathing; increased temperature).
- Return to clinic in 3 months for well-child check or sooner as needed.

Are there any referrals needed?
Consider a referral to cardiology. However, a referral for a Still murmur in a child one year old or greater is not required.

Does the patient's psychosocial history impact how you might treat this patient?
There are no known psychosocial factors that would affect the treatment of this patient.

What if this baby were a girl?
There are no known gender differences in the occurrences of Still murmur.

What if this baby was 6 months old?
Infants less than one year of age should be referred to a cardiologist for evaluation of all murmurs.

Are there any standardized guidelines that you should use to assess or treat this case?
There were no standardized guidelines located in the literature for the assessment and/or treatment of Still murmur.

REFERENCES AND RESOURCES

Frommelt, M. (2004). Differential diagnosis and approach to a heart murmur in term infants. *Pediatric Clinics of North America, 51,* 1023–1032.

Geggel, R., Horowitz, L., Brown, E., Parsons, M., Wang, P., & Fulton, D. (2002). Parental anxiety associated with referral of a child to a pediatric cardiologist for evaluation of a Still's murmur. *The Journal of Pediatrics, 140,* 747–752.

Lessard, E., Glick, M., Ahmed, S., & Saric, M. (2005). The patient with a heart murmur: Evaluation, assessment and dental considerations. *The Journal of the American Dental Association, 136,* 347–356.

Poddar, B., & Basu, S. (2004). Approach to a child with a heart murmur. *Indian Journal of Pediatrics, 71,* 63–66.

Case 2.5 Cough

By Mikki Meadows-Oliver, PhD, RN

Katherine, a 7-month-old infant, presents to the office with complaints of cough for 2 days and "breathing heavy" since this morning. Katherine is accompanied by both parents. She has had a fever for 2 days. Her maximum temperature at home was 101°F (rectal). She also has a runny nose. Her mother has tried an over-the-counter cough medicine without much relief. Katherine's mother has not found much that helps the symptoms; but she notices that, when Katherine cries, the breathing sounds get worse. Katherine attends day care and her mother states that many of the kids there have coughs and runny noses. Katherine's mother also has had cold symptoms for nearly 5 days.

Birth history: Katherine was the product of a 40-week gestation. She was delivered vaginally without complications. During the pregnancy, Katherine's mother had no falls, infections, or known exposures to environmental hazards. She did not drink alcohol, take over-the-counter or prescription medication (other than prenatal vitamins), use tobacco products, or use illicit drugs. Katherine's birth weight was 3300 g and her Apgar scores were 9 at 1 minute and 9 at 5 minutes.

Social history: Katherine was born to a 31-year-old mother. Katherine has a 2-year-old sibling. She lives at home with both parents and her older sibling. Both parents have high school diplomas. The mother works as an administrative assistant, and the father works as a maintenance worker. There are no pets or smokers in the home.

Diet: Decreased solid and liquid intake since yesterday.

Elimination: Decreased urine output; no diarrhea or constipation.

Sleep: Sleep is interrupted by coughing.

Family medical history: Paternal grandfather (PGF) (age 60): history of prostate cancer; paternal grandmother (PGM) (age 59): healthy; maternal grandfather (MGF)(age 61): Type 2 diabetes mellitus, high cholesterol, high blood pressure; maternal grandmother (MGM) (age 61): asthma; mother (age 31): asthma; father (age 30): healthy; sibling (age 2): healthy; history of bronchiolitis.

Medications: Currently taking no prescription or herbal medications. Taking a children's over-the-counter cough suppressant.

Clinical Case Studies for the Family Nurse Practitioner, First Edition. Edited by Leslie Neal-Boylan.
© 2011 John Wiley & Sons, Inc. Published 2011 by John Wiley & Sons, Inc.

Immunizations: Up to date.

Allergies: No known allergies to food, medications, or environment.

OBJECTIVE

Vital signs: Weight: 7.1 kg; length: 65 c; temperature: 37.9° Celsius (rectal); pulse oximeter reading: 95% on room air.

General: Alert, active, well-hydrated, interactive baby.

Skin: Clear with no lesions noted; no cyanosis of skin, lips, or nails; no diaphoresis noted; good skin turgor.

Head: Normocephalic; anterior fontanel is open and flat (1.5 cm × 1.5 cm).

Eyes: Red reflexes present bilaterally; pupils equal, round, and reactive to light; no discharge noted.

Ears: Pinnae normal; tympanic membranes gray bilaterally with positive light reflex.

Nose: Both nostrils patent; no discharge; mild nasal flaring.

Oropharynx: Mucous membranes moist; no teeth present; no lesions.

Neck: Supple; no nodes.

Respiratory: RR = 32; barking cough noted; inspiratory stridor with activity; no intercostal, suprasternal, or subcostal retractions; no grunting; no deformities of the thoracic cage noted.

Cardiac/Peripheral vascular: HR = 120; regular rhythm; no murmur noted; brachial and femoral pulses present and 2+ bilaterally.

Abdomen/Gastrointestinal: Soft, nontender, nondistended, no evidence of hepatosplenomegaly.

Genitourinary: Normal female genitalia.

Back: Spine straight.

Extremities: Full range of motion of all extremities; warm and well perfused; capillary refill < 2 seconds.

Neurologic: Good tone in all extremities.

CRITICAL THINKING

Which diagnostic or imaging studies should be considered to assist with or confirm the diagnosis?
___Chest radiograph (CXR)
___Arterial blood gas (ABG)
___Complete blood count (CBC)

What is the most likely differential diagnosis and why?
___Croup (laryngotracheobronchitis)
___Bronchiolitis
___Epiglottitis

What is your plan of treatment, referral, and follow-up care?

Are there any demographic characteristics that would affect this case?

What if the patient lived in a rural, isolated setting?

RESOLUTION

Diagnostic tests: Based on the history and physical findings, there are no laboratory or imaging studies needed other than a CXR. However, if a CBC were obtained, the results would show nonspecific findings such as an elevated white blood count. An ABG examination is not necessary since the child does not appear to be in respiratory distress. The CXR reveals a steeple sign; it signifies subglottic narrowing during inspiration.

What is the most likely differential diagnosis and why?
Croup:
Croup is the most likely differential diagnosis based on the history, physical examination findings, and the chest radiograph findings of steeple sign. The presence of inspiratory stridor, low grade fever, and barking cough support the diagnosis of croup. With epiglottitis, the child usually appears toxic, and the fever is usually 40°C or higher. With epiglottitis, marked restlessness and extreme anxiety may be present. Infants with bronchiolitis are more likely to have expiratory wheezing and rales, as opposed to inspiratory stridor.

What is your plan of treatment, referral, and follow-up care?
Begin oxygen therapy in the office. The child should be kept as comfortable as possible. She should be allowed to remain in her parent's arms. Unnecessary painful interventions that may cause agitation and increased oxygen requirements by the child should be avoided. Monitor heart rate, respiratory rate/effort, and pulse oximetry.

A single dose of dexamethasone (0.15 mg/kg) should be administered in the office, and the child should be monitored for improvement. If no improvement is seen, refer the patient and family to the local emergency department for support of the respiratory system. An ambulance should be called to transport the baby from the office to the emergency department so that the baby's airway and respiratory status may be maintained. Antibiotics are not indicated. Provide emotional support to the parents. Allow the parents to verbalize their concerns about their baby's health status.

Are there any demographic characteristics that would affect this case?
Male-to-female ratio for croup is approximately 1.4:1. Croup occurs most frequently between the ages of 7 months and 36 months. While croup is rare after 6 years of age, it may present as late as 15 years.

What if the patient lived in a rural, isolated setting?
Health care providers practicing in rural, isolated setting should have emergency office plans in place for patients experiencing respiratory distress.

REFERENCES AND RESOURCES

Eboriadou, M., Chryssanthopoulou, D., Stamoulis, P., Damianidou, L., & Haidopoulou, K. (2010). The effectiveness of local corticosteroids therapy in the management of mild to moderate viral croup. *Minerva Pediatrica*, *62*, 23–28.

Mazza, D., Wilkinson, F., Turner, T., Harris, C., & Health for Kids Guideline Development Group (2008). Evidence based guideline for the management of croup. *Australian Family Physician*, *37*, 14–20.

Rajapaksa, S., & Starr, M. (2010). Croup—Assessment and management. *Australian Family Physician*, *39*, 280–282.

Wall, S., Wat, D., Spiller, O., Gelder, C., Kotecha, S., & Doull, I. (2009). The viral aetiology of croup and recurrent croup. *Archives of Disease in Childhood*, *94*, 359–360.

Case 2.6 Diarrhea

By Mikki Meadows-Oliver, PhD, RN

SUBJECTIVE

Daniel, an 11-month-old infant, presents to the office with complaints of watery diarrhea for 1 day. Daniel is accompanied by his mother. In addition to the diarrhea, he has had vomiting for 1 day and a fever for 2 days. His maximum temperature at home was 102°F (rectal). Daniel has not vomited today although the fever continues and the diarrhea seems to be getting worse. He has had at least 10 diapers with diarrhea since yesterday. Daniel's mother is unsure of his urine output because each diaper is so full of stool. No blood or mucus has been noted in the stool. His mother believes that a rash is starting on his buttocks due to the diarrhea. She knows that another child in the day care center had diarrhea a few days ago. No one at home has any similar symptoms.

Yesterday, Daniel completed a course of amoxicillin for otitis media. Daniel's mother states that earlier in the week she began to introduce whole milk into his diet and that she also gave him Indian take-out food with a strong curry flavor. She is concerned that one of these factors may have caused or contributed to Daniel's diarrhea. Further review of systems reveals that Daniel has had decreased solid food and soy formula intake since yesterday and that he has been sleeping more than usual.

Birth history: Daniel is the product of a 41-week gestation. He was delivered vaginally without complications. During the pregnancy, his mother had no falls or infections. She was in a car accident when she was 6 months pregnant and had to receive an X-ray of her right wrist. There was no break in the wrist, and she was told to take Tylenol for pain. Daniel's mother did not drink alcohol, take prescription medication (other than prenatal vitamins), use tobacco products, or use illicit drugs. His birth weight was 3480 g, and his Apgar scores were 7 at 1 minute and 8 at 5 minutes.

Social history: Daniel was born to a 39-year-old mother. He is an only child. He lives at home with his mother. She works as a psychologist with her own private practice. Daniel's father is not involved. There are no pets or smokers in the home.

Family medical history: The health history of Daniel's father and the paternal grandparents is unknown. Daniel's mother is positive for Crohn disease. His maternal grandmother has a history of Type 2 diabetes, and the maternal grandfather has a history of prostate cancer.

Clinical Case Studies for the Family Nurse Practitioner, First Edition. Edited by Leslie Neal-Boylan.
© 2011 John Wiley & Sons, Inc. Published 2011 by John Wiley & Sons, Inc.

Daniel is currently taking no prescription or herbal medications. His mother gave him an over-the-counter antiemetic, Emetrol ®, to help reduce nausea and vomiting. She has not given him any antidiarrheal agents. Daniel has no known allergies to food, medications, or the environment. He is up to date for required vaccinations, but he did not receive a rotavirus vaccination due to a recall of the vaccination.

OBJECTIVE

Daniel's vital signs were taken in the office today. His weight is 6.8 kg, and his length is 69 cm. Daniel's temperature is elevated at 38°C (rectal). When observing Daniel's general appearance, he is alert and consolable by his mother when crying.

Skin: The skin on Daniel's buttocks is mildly erythematous. There is no cyanosis of his skin, lips, or nails. There is no diaphoresis noted. Daniel has good skin turgor on examination.

HEENT: Daniel's head is normocephalic. His anterior fontanel is open and flat (0.5 cm × 0.5 cm). Upon examination of Daniel's eyes, his red reflexes are present bilaterally and his pupils are equal, round, and reactive to light. There is no discharge noted, and tears are present when crying. Daniel's external ear reveals that the pinnae are normal. On otoscopic examination, the tympanic membranes are pink bilaterally with positive light reflex. Bony landmarks are visible, and there is no fluid noted behind the tympanic membrane. Both nostrils are patent. There is no nasal discharge, and there is no nasal flaring. Daniel's mucous membranes are noted to be moist when examining his oropharynx. He has 4 teeth present without evidence of caries. There are no lesions present in the oral cavity.

Neck: Daniel's neck is supple and able to move in all directions without resistance. There is no cervical lymphadenopathy.

Respirations: Respiratory rate is 28 breaths per minute, and lungs are clear to auscultation in all lobes. There is good air entry, and no retractions or grunting are noted on examination. No deformities of the thoracic cage are noted.

Cardiovascular: Heart rate is 110 beats per minute with a regular rhythm. There is no murmur noted upon auscultation. Brachial and femoral pulses are present and 2+ bilaterally.

Abdomen: Hyperactive bowel sounds are present throughout. Daniel has diffuse tenderness on abdominal palpation. His abdomen is mildly distended; there is no evidence of hepatosplenomegaly.

Genitourinary: Genitourinary examination revealed normal male genitalia. Daniel is circumcised, and his testes are descended bilaterally.

Neuromusculoskeletal: Daniel was noted to have good tone in all extremities. He has full range of motion of all extremities. His extremities are warm and well perfused. Capillary refill is less than 2 seconds. Daniel's spine is straight.

CRITICAL THINKING

Which laboratory or imaging studies should be considered to assist with or confirm the diagnosis?
___Complete blood count (CBC)
___Stool culture
___Electrolyte levels
___Hydrogen breath test
___Lactose tolerance test

What is the most likely differential diagnosis and why?

What is your plan of treatment, referral, and follow-up care?

Are there any demographic factors that should be considered?

Are there any standardized guidelines that you should use to assess or treat this case?

RESOLUTION

Diagnostic tests: A CBC would not provide any clinically useful information in this case. The white blood count (WBC) may be elevated but that is a nonspecific finding as the WBC is likely to be elevated with most infectious processes. A stool culture may provide identification of an infectious organism that is causing the diarrhea. They are not done routinely for acute cases of pediatric diarrhea that is being treated in the outpatient setting. Electrolyte levels can be obtained if there is a concern of dehydration. A hydrogen breath test may be helpful in diagnosing older children with lactose intolerance, but this test is not usually done on babies and very young children because it can cause severe diarrhea. Similarly, a lactose tolerance test can aid in the diagnosis of lactose intolerance, but it is usually not performed on babies and very young children.

What is the most likely differential diagnosis and why?
Viral gastroenteritis:
The complaint of diarrhea can lead to several differential diagnoses. The most common differentials for someone with Daniel's history are viral gastroenteritis, antibiotic-associated diarrhea, and lactose intolerance. Differentiating between these conditions requires a thorough history and review of systems. Viral gastroenteritis should be considered as Daniel has had diarrhea, vomiting, and fever. He also recently started a new day care, which is a risk factor for viral gastroenteritis. Daniel recently finished a course of antibiotics which could be a possible source of diarrhea. Whole milk was introduced into the diet which may lead the health care provider to consider lactose intolerance.

Based on the history and physical exam, viral gastroenteritis due to rotavirus is the most likely of the differential diagnoses. The presence of fever likely rules out noninfectious causes of diarrhea. Rotavirus is one of several viruses known to cause gastroenteritis. It commonly affects children in the winter months in the United States but may occur year-round in developing countries. Many children under the age of 5 years have come into contact with this virus at some point in their lives.

What is your plan of treatment, referral, and follow-up care?
In the majority of cases of viral gastroenteritis infection related to rotavirus, no medications are necessary. Antidiarrheal agents should typically be avoided in young children. Antibiotics are not indicated and may include diarrhea as a side effect—worsening the diarrhea. Hyperosmolar beverages such as sports drinks should be avoided because they may cause infants to develop hypernatremia. Excessive plain water intake may cause infants to develop hyponatremia. Beverages such as Pedialyte® have the correct balance of glucose, sodium, and potassium and should be encouraged in small, frequent feedings for the child with viral gastroenteritis secondary to rotavirus. Because rotavirus is contagious, family members should be encouraged to practice good hand washing after changing diapers and before preparing meals. Daniel's mother should be instructed that the diarrhea may last 1 full week. She should also be instructed about the signs and symptoms of dehydration and told to seek care immediately if any of these signs and symptoms develops. Based on the history and physical findings, no referrals are needed at this time.

Daniel's mother should be allowed to express her concerns regarding his illness status, especially since he is just recovering from acute otitis media and also since she believed that she may have contributed to the diarrhea with the introduction of food with curry or the introduction of whole milk.

Are there any demographic factors that should be considered?
There have been no racial/ethnic factors that contribute to the development of rotavirus, but it has been shown that it is more prevalent among those of lower socioeconomic status.

Are there any standardized guidelines that you should use to assess or treat this case?
The Advisory Committee on Immunization Practices (ACIP) has developed guidelines for the prevention of rotavirus in infants and small children (Cortese & Parashar, 2009).

REFERENCES AND RESOURCES

Cortese, M. M., & Parashar, U.D. (2009 Feb). Centers for Disease Control and Prevention (CDC). Prevention of rotavirus gastroenteritis among infants and children: Recommendations of the Advisory Committee on Immunization Practices (ACIP). MMWR Recomm Report, 58(RR-2):1–25.

Henker, J., Laass, M. W., Blokhin, B. M., Maydannik, V. G., Bolbot, Y. K., Elze, M., & De Morais, M. (2008). Probiotic *Escherichia coli* Nissle 1917 versus placebo for treating diarrhea of greater than 4 days duration in infants and toddlers. *The Pediatric Infectious Disease Journal, 27*, 494–499.

Misra, S., Sabui, T. K., & Pal, N. K. (2009). A randomized controlled trial to evaluate the efficacy of lactobacillus GG in infantile diarrhea. *The Journal of Pediatrics, 155*, 129–132.

Vernacchio, L., Vezina, R. M., Mitchell, A. A., Lesko, S. M., Plaut, A. G., & Acheson, D. W. (2006). Diarrhea in American infants and young children in the community setting: Incidence, clinical presentation and microbiology. *The Pediatric Infectious Disease Journal, 25*, 2–7.

Case 2.7 Fall off Changing Table

By Mikki Meadows-Oliver, PhD, RN

SUBJECTIVE

Vance, a 2-month-old infant, presents in the office for an examination after he fell off the changing table. He is accompanied by his mother, Amy. Amy states that she was preparing to change Vance's diaper, and she placed him on the changing table. She then realized that she had forgotten to bring the diaper wipes to the changing table. When she turned around to retrieve the wipes, Vance rolled off the table and onto the floor. Amy states that Vance cried immediately after falling. She did not notice any bleeding after the fall but she did notice bruising on the left side of Vance's head, which prompted her to bring him in to the office. The injury occurred approximately 1 hour ago. Since that time, Vance has not had anything to eat or drink. He has not had any wet diapers. Amy stated that she did not let Vance sleep after his head injury.

Diet: Normally, Vance takes six 4-oz bottles of soy-based formula daily. He has not yet started any solids.

Elimination: Amy states that Vance normally has 6–8 wet diapers daily. He has 2 bowel movements daily. Amy denies that Vance has diarrhea or constipation.

Sleep: Vance normally sleeps 2–3 hours at a time between feedings. He has one 5-hour stretch of sleep during the night.

Birth history: Vance is the product of a 40-week gestation. He was born via spontaneous vaginal delivery. During the pregnancy, Amy had no falls or infections. She did not drink alcohol, take over-the-counter or prescription medications (other than prenatal vitamins), use tobacco products, or use illicit drugs. His birth weight was 3280 g, and his Apgar scores were 9 at 1 minute and 9 at 5 minutes. Since birth, he has had no other injuries or illnesses.

Social history: Vance was born to an 18-year-old mother. He lives at home with his mother and his maternal grandmother. Vance's father is not involved in his care. His mother does not currently work outside the home but plans to return to work at a local fast-food restaurant soon. She is looking for child care. The family receives rent subsidy from Section 8, food subsidies from the Women, Infants, and Children (WIC) program, and food stamps. The family also receives monthly cash assistance from the Temporary Aid to Needy Families (TANF) program. The family has no pets, and there are no smokers in the home.

Clinical Case Studies for the Family Nurse Practitioner, First Edition. Edited by Leslie Neal-Boylan.
© 2011 John Wiley & Sons, Inc. Published 2011 by John Wiley & Sons, Inc.

Family medical history: Vance's mother has no health problems. His father is 17-years-old and has no history of chronic medical conditions. His maternal grandmother (38 years of age) has a history of high blood pressure. His maternal grandfather (39 years of age) also has high blood pressure. His paternal grandmother (48 years of age) is healthy with no health problems, and his paternal grandfather's health history is unknown.

Medications: Vance is not currently taking any over-the-counter, prescription, or herbal medications. He has no known allergies to food, medications, or the environment. He has not yet received any recommended immunizations other than the hepatitis B vaccination received at 1 day of age.

OBJECTIVE

Vance's vital signs are taken, and his weight in the office today is 5.24 kg. His temperature is within the normal range at 37.1°C (rectal). He is alert, active, and playful. He appears well hydrated and well nourished.

Skin: His skin shows a 1.5 × 1.0 cm area of ecchymosis over the left forehead. The area appears mildly tender to touch. There is no cyanosis of his skin, lips, or nails. There is no diaphoresis noted, and he has good skin turgor on examination.

HEENT: Normocephalic with no swelling of the scalp. His anterior fontanel is open and flat (2 cm × 2 cm). Vance's red reflexes are present bilaterally; and his pupils are equal, round, and reactive to light. He is able to fix and follow the examination past midline. There is no ocular discharge noted. The external ear reveals that the pinnae are normal. On otoscopic examination, the tympanic membranes are gray bilaterally with positive light reflexes. Bony landmarks are visible, and there is no fluid noted behind the tympanic membrane. Both nostrils are patent. There are no nasal discharge and no nasal flaring. Vance's mucous membranes are noted to be moist when examining his oropharynx. He has no teeth, and there are no lesions present in the oral cavity.

Neck: Vance's neck is supple and able to move in all directions without resistance. He has no cervical lymphadenopathy.

Respiratory: Respiratory rate is 24 breaths per minute, and lungs are clear to auscultation in all lobes. There is good air entry, and no retractions or grunting are noted on examination. No deformities of the thoracic cage noted.

Cardiovascular: Heart rate is 116 beats per minute with a regular rhythm. There is no murmur noted upon auscultation. When palpating, brachial and femoral pulses are present and 2+ bilaterally.

Abdomen: Normoactive bowel sounds are present throughout; soft and nontender. There is no evidence of hepatosplenomegaly.

Genitourinary: Normal male genitalia. Vance is uncircumcised and his testes are descended bilaterally.

Neuromusculoskeletal: Good tone in all extremities; full range of motion in all extremities. His extremities are warm and well perfused. Capillary refill is less than 2 seconds, and his spine is straight.

CRITICAL THINKING

Which laboratory tests should be ordered as part of a workup after a fall from a height?

What is the most likely differential diagnosis and why?

What is your plan of treatment, referral, and follow-up care?

Does this patient's psychosocial history affect how you might treat this case?

What if the patient lived in a rural setting?

Are there any demographic characteristics that might affect this case?

Are there any standardized guidelines that you should use to assess or treat this case?

RESOLUTION

Diagnostic tests: Since Vance hit his head, any laboratory tests or imaging studies would be geared toward diagnosing an intracranial bleed. There is no clear consensus regarding whether all patients with mild head injuries should have neuroimaging. Patients who have lost consciousness should, in general, receive a computed tomography (CT) scan. While magnetic resonance imaging (MRI) has been demonstrated to be more sensitive than CT scans, it has usually been reserved for patients who have mental status abnormalities that are unexplained by CT scan findings. Electroencephalogram (EEG) testing has been shown to be of limited usefulness in patients with head injuries. Skull radiographs are rarely used in patients with a closed head injury. Cerebral angiography is rarely used in the evaluation of acute head injury.

If imaging is determined to be necessary, a CT scan is the diagnostic study of choice in the evaluation of a head injury because it has a rapid acquisition time, is nearly universally available, is easily interpretable, and is reliable. Health care providers should consider a CT scan for children with a head injury if they are less than 1 year of age or have a Glascow Coma Scale score (GCS) of less than 14/15. An additional indication for a CT in an infant would be the presence of bruising, swelling, or laceration that is more than 5 cm. MRIs have a limited role in the initial evaluation of a head injury because of their long acquisition times and the difficulty in obtaining them for persons who are critically ill.

What is the most likely differential diagnosis and why?

There are several diagnoses that should be considered for a child with a head injury including minor closed head injury, subdural hematoma, subarachnoid hemorrhage, and epidural hematoma. There are several factors from this case which lead to the diagnosis of minor head injury. Vance's Glascow Coma Scale (GCS) was 15/15, there were no focal neurological deficits, and there was no seizure activity. These factors support a diagnosis of mild closed injury. Additional factors that support this diagnosis are that there was no vomiting, there was no loss of consciousness, the fall was less than 1 meter, and there was no fluid or drainage from Vance's nose or ears. Patients with a subarachnoid hemorrhage typically have vomiting and loss of consciousness. There were no focal neurologic findings, and there was a GCS of 15/15. Patients with a subdural hematoma generally lose consciousness (this is not an absolute) and typically experience moderate to severe blunt head trauma. Epidural hematoma may present with loss of consciousness, vomiting, and seizures.

What is your plan of treatment, referral, and follow-up care?

Based on Vance's history, physical examination, and likely diagnosis of a mild closed head injury, he should be observed in the office and would likely not need radiographic evaluation or neuroimaging. There will be no limitations on his activity or diet. His mother can be told to apply ice for 20 minutes at a time (every 2–4 hours as needed) to his head wound for 24 hours. This will help to reduce or prevent swelling of the injured area. Vance can be discharged to home if it is determined that he has a reliable caregiver at home who can monitor him for signs of complications related to his head injury. Vance's caregivers should be given an instruction sheet for head injury care that explains that he should be awakened every 2 hours and assessed neurologically. Vance's caregivers should be instructed to seek medical attention if he develops persistent nausea and vomiting, seizures, unusual behavior, or watery discharge from either the nose or the ears. There are no referrals necessary based on Vance's history and physical examination findings.

Does this patient's psychosocial history affect how you might treat this case?

An aspect of Vance's psychosocial history that might affect the handling of his case is that both of his parents are teenagers. Research has shown that children of adolescent mothers (when compared to children of adult mothers) have an increased rate of unintentional injuries during the first 5 years of life (Koniak-Griffin et al., 2003).

What if the patient lived in a rural setting?
A patient living in a rural setting may not be able to access a health care center in a timely fashion for assessment and diagnostic testing of a head injury after a fall.

Are there any demographic characteristics that might affect this case?
There are no specific demographics that affect this case. There are no known associations of unintentional head injury with ethnicity or gender in the pediatric population.

Are there any standardized guidelines that you should use to assess or treat this case?
National Institute for Health and Clinical Excellence & National Collaborating Centre for Acute Care offer guidelines in the reference below.

REFERENCES AND RESOURCES

Koniak-Griffin, D., Verzemnieks, I., Anderson, N., Brecht, M., Lesser, J., Kim, S., & Turner-Pluta, C. (2003). Nurse visitation for adolescent mothers: Two-year infant health and maternal outcomes. *Nursing Research, 52,* 127–136.

National Institute for Health and Clinical Excellence & National Collaborating Centre for Acute Care. (2007). Head injury. Triage, assessment, investigation and early management of head injury in infants, children and adults. Clinical guideline; no. 56. London (U.K.): National Institute for Health and Clinical Excellence.

Section 3

The Toddler/Preschool Child

Case 3.1 Earache

By Mikki Meadows-Oliver, PhD, RN and Susannah Young, MSN, RN

SUBJECTIVE

Julie, a 3-year-old preschool child, presents to the office with a complaint of left ear pain for 2 days. She is accompanied by her mother, Mary. She has had an intermittent fever and her maximum temperature at home was 101°F (axillary). The pain is worse sometimes when she is lying down. The pain is occasionally relieved with the use of over-the-counter pain relievers. Julia has had no vomiting or diarrhea. She has had a slight runny nose, but no cough.

Diet: Julia's nutrition history reveals that she has a balanced diet with enough dairy, protein, fruits, and vegetables. Her appetite has decreased over the past 2 days since the ear pain began.

Elimination: She is voiding well with no complaints of dysuria.

Sleep: Julia sleeps approximately 10 hours at night and takes one 1-hour nap at her preschool. She usually has no problems falling or staying asleep but since the ear pain has started, her sleep has been interrupted.

Past medical history: Julia was born via vaginal delivery at 40 weeks' gestation. Since being discharged at 2 days of age, she has had no emergency department (ED) visits or hospitalizations. Julia has had 2 episodes of otitis media that were cleared with antibiotics. She has had no injuries or illnesses since that time. Julia passed her developmental screening at her last well-child visit. She currently attends preschool and is doing well according to Mary. She has no chronic illnesses and is currently taking no medications.

Social history: Julia lives at home with both parents. Her mother works as a teacher, and her father is a commercial fisherman. The family has a pet cat. Julia's father smokes, but not in the home.

Family medical history: Julia's mother (31 years old) and father (30 years old) are healthy and have no history of chronic medical conditions. Her maternal grandmother (age 52 years) has a history of lupus. Her maternal grandfather (54 years of age) has a history of prostate cancer (in remission). Julia's paternal grandfather (age 59 years) has a history of hypertension. Her paternal grandmother (53 years of age) has a history of asthma.

Clinical Case Studies for the Family Nurse Practitioner, First Edition. Edited by Leslie Neal-Boylan.
© 2011 John Wiley & Sons, Inc. Published 2011 by John Wiley & Sons, Inc.

Medications: Julia is currently taking no prescription or herbal medications. She has been taking over-the-counter pain relievers/antipyretics to relieve symptoms associated with ear pain. Julia has an allergy to penicillin. She gets hives when she takes penicillin. Julia has no known allergies to food or the environment. She is up to date on required immunizations.

OBJECTIVE

Julia's vital signs are taken, and her weight in the office today is 14 kg. Her temperature is slightly elevated at 38°C (temporal). Julia is alert and quiet, sitting in her mother's lap. She appears well hydrated and well nourished.

Skin: Her skin is clear of lesions and warm to touch. There is no cyanosis of her skin, lips, or nails. There is no diaphoresis noted. Julia has good skin turgor on examination.

HEENT: Julia's head is normocephalic. Her red reflexes are present bilaterally; and her pupils are equal, round, and reactive to light. There is no ocular discharge noted. Julia's external ear reveals that the pinnae are normal, and there is no tenderness to touch on the external ear. On otoscopic examination, the right tympanic membrane (TM) is gray, in normal position, with positive light reflexes. Bony landmarks are visible, and there is no fluid noted behind the TM. The left TM is erythematous and bulging with purulent fluid visible behind the TM. The TM is opaque with no light reflex or bony landmarks present. Both nostrils are patent. There is no nasal discharge, and there is no nasal flaring. Julia's mucous membranes are noted to be moist. She has 20 teeth present without evidence of caries. There are no lesions present in the oral cavity.

Neck: Julia's neck is supple and able to move in all directions without resistance. There are shotty anterior cervical nodes present on the left side of the neck. There is no erythema or tenderness of the nodes.

Respiratory: Julia's respiratory rate is 26 breaths per minute and her lungs are clear to auscultation in all lobes. There is good air entry, and no retractions or grunting are noted on examination. No deformities of the thoracic cage are noted.

Cardiovascular: Julia's heart rate is 102 beats per minute with a regular rhythm. There is no murmur noted upon auscultation.

Abdomen: Normoactive bowel sounds are present throughout. Julia's abdomen is soft and non-tender. There is no evidence of hepatosplenomegaly.

Genitourinary: Genitourinary examination reveals normal female genitalia.

Neuromusculoskeletal: Julia is noted to have good tone in all extremities. She has full range of motion of all extremities. Her extremities are warm and well perfused. Capillary refill is less than 2 seconds, and her spine is straight.

CRITICAL THINKING

Are there laboratory tests or diagnostic imaging studies that should be ordered as part of a workup for ear pain?

What is the most likely differential diagnosis and why?

What is the plan of treatment, referral, and follow-up care?

Does this patient's psychosocial history affect how you might treat this case?

What if the patient lived in a rural setting?

Are there any demographic characteristics that might affect this case?

Are there any standardized guidelines that you should use to assess or treat this case?

RESOLUTION

Diagnostic tests: Middle ear effusion may be confirmed with the observation of decreased or absent tympanic membrane mobility with pneumatic otoscopy. Unfortunately, when performing pneumatic otoscopy in infants and young children, it can be very difficult to maintain a tight fitting seal for the exam. Tympanometry may be performed to determine the presence of fluid (infected or uninfected) in the middle ear. Tympanometry is useful if cerumen makes visualization of the tympanic membrane difficult on otoscopic exam. Tympanocentesis, though not often done, may be performed to acquire a sample of the fluid behind the tympanic membrane for culture and sensitivity if the child is immunocompromised or has failed previous courses of antibiotic therapy.

What is the most likely differential diagnosis and why?
Otitis media:
The complaint of ear pain can lead to several differential diagnoses. Acute otitis media, otitis externa, cholesteatoma, foreign body, and hemotympanum (blood behind the tympanic membrane) are some of the more common causes of ear pain in a child. A thorough history and careful physical exam will help to differentiate among these diagnoses.

Otitis media is the most likely diagnosis for Julia based on the history and physical examination findings. Julia had a fever, sleep and eating disturbances, and a previous history of otitis media. On examination, the left TM was erythematous and bulging. It is unlikely to be otitis externa as there is no ear pain elicited by palpation of the external ear, a characteristic sign of otitis externa. Cholesteatoma should be considered in the differential because of Julia's past diagnosis of otitis media. However, there was no pocket of retraction, keratinous debris, or mass on the tympanic membrane, ruling out a diagnosis of cholesteatoma.

What is the plan of treatment, referral, and follow-up care?
The first line treatment for uncomplicated otitis media in a child with a temperature less than 39°C (102.2°F) is amoxicillin, 80–90 mg/kg per day for 10 days. For children 6 years and older, a 5–7 day course of amoxicillin is appropriate. For children with a temperature over 39°C (102.2°F) or if *H. Influenza* or *M. Catarrhalis* are suspected, therapy should start with amoxicillin-clavulanate, (90 mg/kg per day of amoxicillin and 6.4 mg/kg per day of clavulanate) in 2 divided doses per day.

In patients with non–Type 1 allergic reactions to amoxicillin, a cephalosporin may be used (cefdinir 14 mg/kg per day in 1 or 2 doses, cefpodoxime 10 mg/kg per day once daily or cefuroxime 30 mg/kg per day in 2 divided doses). If the child has experienced a Type 1 reaction in the past (anaphylaxis or urticaria), azithromycin (10 mg/kg per day on the first day, then 5 mg/kg for 4 days) or clarithromycin (15 mg/kg per day in 2 divided doses) may be used. Because Julia has had hives in the past when using penicillin, azithromycin is the best choice for her. At 14 kg, her dose on day 1 would be 140 mg and on days 2 through 5, her dose would be 70 mg. Using the 100 mg/5 mL oral suspension, she would be instructed to take 7 mL on day 1, then 3.5 mL for days 2 through 5.

Based on the history and physical exam findings, no referrals are needed at this time.

Julia's mother, Mary, should be instructed to follow up with a call to the office or to seek medical attention if no improvement is seen in 48–72 hours after the first dose of medication. Julia's fever should be lowered, and her sleeping and eating should also improve in 48–72 hours.

Does this patient's psychosocial history affect how you might treat this case?
Julia's psychosocial history contains elements that may increase her risk for developing otitis media. Her enrollment in a child care center places her at an increased risk for developing otitis media. Julia's father is a smoker. Exposure to passive cigarette smoke has been found to be a risk factor for the development of otitis media in preschool children. This information can be discussed with Julia's parents. Julia's father can be given information on smoking cessation resources.

What if the patient lived in a rural setting?

If Julia lived in a rural setting, her parents should be given clear instructions about when and how to follow up if there is no improvement in the 48–72 hour window or if symptoms worsen. If an emergency department is not easily accessible, Julia should be followed closely by her primary care provider to ensure that worsening symptoms are not left unnoticed.

Are there any demographic characteristics that might affect this case?

Otitis media has been found to be more frequent in certain racial groups, such as the Inuit and American Indians. The difference in the frequency of occurrence compared to other racial groups is likely due to anatomic differences in the eustachian tube. Regarding gender, boys have been found to be affected more commonly than girls. No specific causative factors for this have been found in the literature. Age is a demographic characteristic that affects otitis media. Otitis media occurs more commonly in infants, toddlers, and preschool children between the ages of 6 months and 3 years of age. This age distribution may be due to a combination of several factors. These factors can be immunologic, such as lack of pneumococcal antibodies, and/or anatomic. Younger children have a low angle of the eustachian tube with relation to the nasopharynx.

Are there any standardized guidelines that you should use to assess or treat this case?

The American Academy of Pediatrics and American Academy of Family Physicians have developed clinical practice guidelines for the management of otitis media (Liberthal, Ganiats, et al., 2004).

REFERENCES AND RESOURCES

Bellussi, L., & Mandala, M. (2005). Quality of life and psycho-social development in children with otitis media with effusion. *Acta Otorhinolaryngologica Italica, 25*(6), 359–364.

Greenberg, D., Hoffman, S., Leibovitz, E., & Dagan, R. (2008). Acute otitis media in children: Association with day care centers—Antibacterial resistance, treatment, and prevention. *Paediatric Drugs, 10,* 75–83.

Hughes, E., & Lee, J. (2001). Otitis externa. *Pediatrics in Review, 22,* 191–197.

Liberthal, A., Ganiats, T., et al. (2004). Diagnosis and management of acute otitis media: Clinical practice guideline. *Pediatrics, 113*(5), 1451–1465.

Nguyen, C., & Parikh, S. (2008). Cholesteatoma: In brief. *Pediatrics in Review, 29*(9), 330–331.

Sophia, A., Isaac, R., Rebekah, G., Brahmadathan, K., & Rupa, V. (2010). Risk factors for otitis media among preschool, rural Indian children. *International Journal of Pediatric Otorhinolaryngology, 74,* 677–683.

Case 3.2 Bedwetting

By Mikki Meadows-Oliver, PhD, RN and Mary-Christine Sullivan, MPH, MSN, RN

SUBJECTIVE

Four-year-old J'Quan presents to the office with his mother, Regina, with a complaint of bedwetting. Regina states that J'Quan consistently wets the bed each night although he remains dry throughout the day. According to his mother, J'Quan has never been dry at night but has been toilet trained during the daytime for 2 years. Regina is frustrated with this behavior because she is frequently washing bedsheets and having to buy new mattresses. She has a 5-year-old daughter who achieved daytime and nighttime dryness by the age of 3 years old. Regina said that J'Quan's father is also frustrated with the bedwetting and will sometime spank J'Quan when he wets the bed. Regina says that her 5-year-old daughter teases J'Quan and calls him names such as "pee-pee boy." She says that she has already tried strategies such as limiting his liquid intake 2 hours before bed and waking him to urinate before she goes to bed. Regina states that often, when she goes to wake J'Quan before going to bed herself, he has already wet the bed. She does not know what to do now and has come to the office today because she would like assistance in resolving this issue. J'Quan has no other symptoms of illness.

Diet: J'Quan's nutrition history reveals that he has a balanced diet with enough dairy, protein, fruits, and vegetables. He does not appear to eat or drink large amounts.

Elimination: He is voiding well (normal amounts) with no complaints of dysuria. J'Quan does have occasional constipation that is relieved with an over-the-counter laxative.

Sleep: J'Quan sleeps 11 hours at night and has no trouble falling or staying asleep.

Past medical history: Born via cesarean section at 38 weeks' gestation. This was a repeat C-section for Regina. Since being discharged at 4 days of age, he has had no hospitalizations. J'Quan had 4 teeth removed at 2 years of age, under general anesthesia, due to early childhood caries. He had an emergency department (ED) visit at 3 years of age for a broken arm after he fell from the jungle gym at day care. J'Quan passed his developmental screening at his last well-child visit. He currently attends preschool and is doing well. He has no chronic illnesses and is taking no medications.

Social history: J'Quan lives at home with both parents and a 5-year-old sibling. His mother works as a store clerk, and his father is a school custodian. The family has a no pets. There are no smokers in the home.

Clinical Case Studies for the Family Nurse Practitioner, First Edition. Edited by Leslie Neal-Boylan.
© 2011 John Wiley & Sons, Inc. Published 2011 by John Wiley & Sons, Inc.

Family medical history: J'Quan's mother (26 years old) and father (26 years old) are healthy and have no history of chronic medical conditions. His mother has sickle cell trait. His maternal grandmother (age 48 years old) has a history of heart disease. His maternal grandfather (50 years old) has a history of liver disease. J'Quan's paternal grandfather (51 years old) has a history of vertigo. His paternal grandmother (50 years old) has a history of high cholesterol.

Medications: J'Quan is currently taking no over-the-counter, prescription, or herbal medications. He has no known allergies to medication, food, or the environment. He is up to date for required immunizations.

OBJECTIVE

J'Quan's vital signs are taken, and his weight in the office is 20 kg. His temperature is within the normal range at 36.7° C (temporal). When observing J'Quan's general appearance, he is alert, pleasant, and interactive. He appears well hydrated and well nourished.

Skin: His skin is clear of lesions. There is no cyanosis of his skin, lips, or nails. There is no diaphoresis noted, and J'Quan has good skin turgor on examination.

HEENT: J'Quan's head is normocephalic. His red reflexes are present bilaterally; and his pupils are equal, round, and reactive to light. There is no ocular discharge noted. J'Quan's external ear reveals that the pinnae are normal and that there is no tenderness to touch on the external ear. On otoscopic examination, the tympanic membranes are gray bilaterally, in normal position with positive light reflexes. Bony landmarks are visible, and there is no fluid noted behind the tympanic membranes. Both nostrils are patent. There is no nasal discharge, and there is no nasal flaring. J'Quan's mucous membranes are noted to be moist. He has 16 teeth present. There are no lesions present in the oral cavity.

Neck: J'Quan's neck is supple and able to move in all directions without resistance. There is no cervical lymphadenopathy present.

Respiratory: J'Quan's respiratory rate is 20 breaths per minute, and his lungs are clear to auscultation in all lobes. There is good air entry, and no retractions or grunting are noted on examination. No deformities of the thoracic cage are noted.

Cardiovascular: J'Quan's heart rate is 96 beats per minute with a regular rhythm. There is no murmur noted upon auscultation.

Abdomen: Normoactive bowel sounds are present throughout, and J'Quan's abdomen is soft and nontender. J'Quan has shotty nodes present in his inguinal area bilaterally. These nodes are mobile, nontender, and nonerythematous. There is no evidence of hepatosplenomegaly.

Genitourinary: Normal circumcised male genitalia without erythema or lesions. His testes are descended bilaterally.

Neuromusculoskeletal: Good tone and full range of motion in all extremities; extremities are warm and well perfused. Capillary refill is less than 2 seconds, and his spine is straight.

CRITICAL THINKING

What laboratory tests or diagnostic imaging studies should be ordered as part of a workup for bedwetting?

What is the most likely differential diagnosis and why?

What is the plan of treatment, referral, and follow-up care?

Does this patient's psychosocial history affect how you might treat this case?

What if the patient lived in a rural setting?

Are there any demographic characteristics that might affect this case?

Are there any standardized guidelines that you should use to assess or treat this case?

RESOLUTION

Diagnostic testing: A urine dipstick will provide information on hydration, infection, diabetes insipidus, or diabetes mellitus by measuring the urine specific gravity, nitrites, glucose, and ketones. A urine culture can be done if infection is suspected to identify the organism. In preschool-aged children with enuresis and a urinary tract infection (UTI), consider a renal and bladder ultrasound. If abnormalities are found on the ultrasound, a voiding cystourethrography (VCUG) to identify structural abnormalities and measure bladder filling can be obtained. An X-ray of the kidney, ureters, and bladder can be done if constipation or abnormalities of the spine are suspected. Urodynamic studies measure the flow of urine qualitatively and quantitatively and may be used if a neurological disorder is suspected or in children with daytime wetting who do not respond to traditional therapies.

What is the most likely differential diagnosis and why?
Enuresis:
Bedwetting, or enuresis, has many etiologies. Enuresis refers to involuntary urinary incontinence beyond the expected age of 4 years for daytime dryness and 5 years for night dryness. It may involve genetic factors, changes in vasopressin secretion, sleep factors, structural abnormalities, infection, or pyschological factors. Primary nocturnal enuresis (PNE) is defined as a child > 5 years who is incontinent at night with no previous history of dryness at night for an extended period of time. Secondary enuresis refers to episodes of bedwetting after a period of dryness > 6 months and can be precipitated by a stressful event in the child's life.

The most common differentials for enuresis are urinary tract infection, diabetes mellitus, diabetes insipidus, structural abnormalities of the genitourinary tract, constipation, excessive caffeine, spinal cord injury, or psychological stress. A UTI may be the source when there is dysuria, urinary frequency, and a positive urine culture. High glucose or ketones in the urine dip would indicate diabetes mellitus, and a low specific gravity would indicate diabetes insipidus. Abdominal palpation of stool or stool visible on a KUB (kidneys, ureters, and bladders) x-ray would indicate constipation. Abnormal physical exams of the spine or reflexes can indicate an underlying neurologic disorder or spinal cord injury. Structural abnormalities are identified with a renal and bladder ultrasound, VCUG, or urodynamic studies. In the absence of clinical evidence for enuresis, a thorough history should review psychological stressors, abuse, or dietary patterns that include caffeine or liquids before bed.

J'Quan's mother states he has "never been dry at night but has been toilet trained during the daytime for 2 years." Because enuresis refers to involuntary urinary incontinence beyond the expected age of 4 years for daytime dryness and 5 years for night dryness, J'Quan is within the normal age range for his bedwetting to be considered nonpathologic.

What is the plan of treatment, referral, and follow-up care?
The plan of treatment would be to provide counseling and reassurance for the family after ruling out any other physiologic, psychologic, or organic causes of bedwetting. You can reassure the family that J'Quan is developmentally appropriate for his age. Bedwetting is more frequent in boys than girls, and 5%–10% of children have primary nocturnal enuresis (PNE) at age 5. It is important to emphasize that J'Quan might be experiencing stress and embarrassment related to his bedwetting and that this is exacerbated by teasing from his sister, being spanked for wetting the bed by his father, and seeing his mother's frustration. Parents should avoid punishment and criticism of a child's bedwetting and provide positive reinforcement when the child has a night without wetting the bed.

The health care provider may recommend children's books on bedwetting or making a sticker chart to keep track of dry nights. J'Quan's mother should be reminded to limit nighttime fluids to 2 hours before bed. She can also ensure that J'Quan has easy access to the toilet. The family can be helped to set a goal for J'Quan to use the toilet when he has to go to the bathroom at night, rather than staying dry all night. Based on history and physical exam, J'Quan does not need a referral at this time. Telephone followup can be conducted with J'Quan's family to monitor progress over the course of the next year until his 5-year-old, well-child visit. His family should be encouraged to come to the office sooner as needed for signs and symptoms of illness.

For children with true enuresis, there are several options that can be used in the treatment of this condition, such as bedwetting alarms or medications. Bedwetting alarms work best with children 7 years or older and can be very effective. The alarm conditions the child to get up to use the toilet in order to avoid the alarm going off. They must be used every night for 3–4 months, the family must be counseled on proper use, and the family must wake the child if the child does not awaken to the noise of the alarm.

Medications can also help to manage enuresis. First-line treatment is desmopressin acetate vasopressin (DDVAP) in children ages 6 years and older to reduce the volume of urine produced at night. In patients with nocturnal enuresis and daytime incontinence or those who fail with DDVAP alone, adding anticholinergic agents such as oxybutynin chloride or imipramine, a tricyclic antidepressant, in children age 5 years and older can be helpful in reducing uninhibited bladder contractions. Children older than 5 years may also benefit from complementary medicine including acupuncture/acupressure, hypnosis, and biofeedback although there is limited evidence for the success of these interventions.

Daytime wetting can also be a stressful issue for children. Its origin can be neurologic, anatomic, muscular, or functional which results in problems with storage or emptying of the bladder. Similar to nocturnal enuresis, a full workup should be done to determine the cause. Daytime enuresis is treated with the same medications and behavioral strategies as nighttime enuresis.

Does this patient's psychosocial history affect how you might treat this case?
In J'Quan's situation, the health care provider should reinforce with the parents and sibling that J'Quan should not be teased or punished for bedwetting.

What if the patient lived in a rural setting?
If this patient lived in a rural setting, it might not be convenient for them to return to clinic for a follow-up visit. Telephone followup with the family to discuss J'Quan's bedwetting and to evaluate any strategies the family has tried may be more feasible for families living in a rural setting.

Are there any demographic characteristics that might affect this case?
There is no racial or ethnic predisposition regarding the development of enuresis. In relation to gender, males are affected more than females. The incidence of enuresis decreases as children age. J'Quan's mother reports frustration with having to wash sheets frequently and buy new mattresses because of bedwetting. Considering the socioeconomic status of the parents, it is possible that this is causing additional financial strain for the family. As the provider, you can suggest plastic coverings for the mattress or plastic reusable underpads to protect the mattress from getting wet, as well as absorbent briefs for J'Quan to wear at night.

Are there any standardized guidelines that you should use to assess or treat this case?
Guidelines for the treatment of enuresis are available from the International Children's Continence Society (Neveus, et al., 2010).

REFERENCES AND RESOURCES

Gim, C., Lillystone, D., & Caldwell, P. (2009). Efficacy of the bell and pad alarm therapy for nocturnal enuresis. *Journal of Paediatrics and Child Health, 45*, 405–408.

Glazener, C., Evans, J., & Cheuk, D. (2005). Complementary and miscellaneous interventions for nocturnal enuresis in children. *Cochrane Database of Systematic Reviews*, (2), CD005230.

Neveus, T., Eggert, P., Evans, J., Macedo, A., Rittig, S., Tekgul, S. International Children's Continence Society. (2010). Evaluation of and treatment for monosymptomatic enuresis: A standardization document from the International Children's Continence Society. Journal of *Urology, 183*, 441–447.

Case 3.3 Burn

By Mikki Meadows-Oliver, PhD, RN

SUBJECTIVE

Two-year-old Fatima presents to the office with her mother, Khalila, with a complaint of a burn to the right hand. Khalila states that she was curling her hair in the bathroom when her telephone rang. She left the bathroom to retrieve the telephone. While she was answering the telephone, Fatima entered the bathroom and pulled on the curling iron cord that was hanging down below. The incident was unwitnessed, but Khalila heard Fatima scream. She ran to the bathroom to find both Fatima and the curling iron on the floor. She then noticed that Fatima's right hand was red and swollen. She immediately brought her in to the office. Fatima has no symptoms of illness.

Diet: Fatima's nutrition history reveals that she has a balanced diet with enough dairy, protein, fruits, and vegetables. She has not eaten since she burned her hand.

Elimination: She is voiding well with no complaints of dysuria. She is not yet toilet trained.

Sleep: Fatima sleeps 10 hours at night and has no trouble falling or staying asleep. She takes one 2-hour nap during the day.

Past medical history: Born via vaginal delivery at 37 weeks' gestation. Since being discharged at 2 days of age, she has had no hospitalizations. She had an emergency department (ED) visit 3 months ago for ingestion of cigarette butts. Fatima passed her developmental screening at her last well-child visit. She currently attends an in-home day care while her mother is working. Fatima has no chronic illnesses and is currently taking no medications.

Social history: Fatima lives at home with her 18-year-old mother, 6-month-old sibling, and maternal grandmother. Her father is not involved. Fatima's mother works as a nurse's aide in a long-term care facility. The family has 2 cats. There are no smokers in the home.

Family medical history: Fatima's mother (18 years old) and father (19 years old) are healthy and have no history of chronic medical conditions. Khalila did have high blood pressure with both pregnancies but the condition resolved after she delivered her children. Her maternal grandmother (age 34 years) has thalassemia trait. Her maternal grandfather (35 years old) is healthy with no chronic illnesses. The health history of Fatima's paternal grandfather is unknown. Her paternal grandmother (40 years old) has a history of obesity and high blood pressure.

Clinical Case Studies for the Family Nurse Practitioner, First Edition. Edited by Leslie Neal-Boylan.
© 2011 John Wiley & Sons, Inc. Published 2011 by John Wiley & Sons, Inc.

Medications: Fatima is not currently taking any over-the-counter, prescription, or herbal medications. She has no known allergies to medication, food, or the environment. She is up to date on required immunizations, although her mother declines the flu vaccine yearly.

OBJECTIVE

Fatima's vital signs are taken, and her weight in the office is 14 kg. Her temperature is within the normal range at 37.2°C (temporal). She is alert, crying at times, but consolable. She appears well hydrated and well nourished.

Skin: The skin on the palm of her right hand is erythematous and beginning to blister. The affected area is painful to touch. The rest of her skin is without lesions. There is no cyanosis of her skin, lips, or nails. There is no diaphoresis noted, and Fatima has good skin turgor on examination.

HEENT: Fatima's head is normocephalic. Her red reflexes are present bilaterally; and her pupils are equal, round, and reactive to light. There is no ocular discharge noted. Fatima's external ear reveals that the pinnae are normal, and there is no tenderness to touch on the external ear. On otoscopic examination, the tympanic membranes are gray bilaterally and in normal position with positive light reflexes. Bony landmarks are visible, and there is no fluid noted behind the tympanic membranes. Both nostrils are patent. There is no nasal discharge and no nasal flaring. Fatima's mucous membranes are noted to be moist. She has 20 teeth present. There are no lesions present in the oral cavity.

Neck: Fatima's neck is supple and able to move in all directions without resistance. There is no cervical lymphadenopathy present.

Respiratory: Her respiratory rate is 28 breaths per minute, and her lungs are clear to auscultation in all lobes. There is good air entry, and no retractions or grunting are noted on examination. No deformities of the thoracic cage are noted.

Cardiovascular: Fatima's heart rate is 106 beats per minute with a regular rhythm. There is no murmur noted upon auscultation.

Abdomen: Normoactive bowel sounds are present throughout and Fatima's abdomen is soft and nontender. There is no evidence of hepatosplenomegaly.

Genitourinary: Normal female genitalia without erythema or lesions.

Neuromusculoskeletal: Good tone and full range of motion in all extremities. Her extremities are warm and well perfused. Capillary refill is less than 2 seconds, and her spine is straight.

CRITICAL THINKING

Are there any laboratory tests or diagnostic imaging studies that should be ordered as part of a workup for a burn?

What additional diagnoses should be considered for a pediatric patient with a burn?

What is your plan of treatment, referral, and follow-up care?

Does this patient's psychosocial history affect how you might treat this case?

What if the patient lived in a rural setting?

Are there any demographic characteristics that might affect this case?

Are there any standardized guidelines that you should use to assess or treat this case?

RESOLUTION

Diagnostic tests: There are no recommended laboratory or imaging studies for a burn such as the one described in the physical examination.

What is the most likely differential diagnosis?
Partial thickness burn:
When examining a pediatric patient with a burn, it is important to determine the thickness of the burn. Older descriptions of burns were first, second, or third degree. Now burns are classified as superficial, superficial partial thickness, deep partial thickness, and full thickness injuries. Superficial burns (first degree) affect only the surface of the skin (epidermis). The skin will be erythematous and painful but will not develop blisters. Superficial burns usually tend to heal within 1 week without scarring. A partial-thickness (second-degree) burn damages not only the epidermis but extends down into the dermis. These burns will typically be painful. Partial-thickness burns are subdivided into two categories: superficial partial-thickness burns and deep partial-thickness burns. Superficial partial-thickness burns develop blisters within approximately 2 to 3 weeks. Superficial partial-thickness burns usually heal without significant scarring. Deep partial-thickness burns are at risk for significant scarring due to the depth of the injury. Healing time for deep partial-thickness burns is weeks to months. Full-thickness burns (third degree) require an extensive healing time if not excised and grafted. Full thickness burns may not be painful because the nerves are damaged. These burns have a poor cosmetic outcome.

Based on the history and physical examination, it appears that Fatima has a partial-thickness burn to her right hand.

What is your plan of treatment, referral, and follow-up care?
Immediate treatment of the injury in the home environment should be documented. It is preferable to cool a partial-thickness burn for approximately 20 minutes to diminish the burning of the skin. Evaluation of a burn includes an investigation as to the type of heat source, estimation of temperature, and duration of contact. Ascertaining this information may give insight into the depth of burn.

The initial management of a burn involves determining the burn depth and total body surface area (TBSA) affected. Only partial- and full-thickness burns are included in the calculation. The TBSA may be calculated using either the rule of nines burn chart (Table 3.3.1) or the Lund and Browder burn chart (Tables 3.3.2 and 3.3.3). For the pediatric patient, the Lund and Browder burn chart is preferred. Calculating the percentage of TBSA affected is important when deciding the need for hospitalization versus outpatient management. Criteria for determining whether or not a burn can be treated at home vary based on the experience and resources of the treating health care center. Burns that *may* be treated on an outpatient basis include those that affect less than 15% TBSA and those that have no airway involvement. The ability of the child to drink and tolerate oral fluids and having a dependable family able to transport the patient for clinic appointments are also key factors. If the burn is the result of suspected abuse, the patient may not be treated on an outpatient basis.

For small burns, a rough estimate of the affected BSA can be made by comparing the burn with the size of child's palm (which represents approximately 1% of the BSA). Since Fatima's burn is only

TABLE 3.3.1. Rule of Nines Burn Chart.

Body Part	Percent of Body Surface Area		
	Infant	Child	Adolescent/Adult
Head	18%	13%	9%
Anterior trunk	18%	18%	18%
Posterior trunk	18%	18%	18%
Upper extremity (each one)	9%	9%	9%
Lower extremity (each one)	14%	16%	18%
Genitalia	1%	1%	1%

TABLE 3.3.2. Lund and Browder Burn Chart (Part 1).

Body Part	Percent of Body Surface Area
Head	See chart below (Part 2) as this measurement changes with age
Neck	1%
Anterior trunk	13%
Posterior trunk	13%
Upper extremity (each one)	5%
Buttocks	5%
Lower extremity (each one)	See chart below (Part 2) as this measurement changes with age
Genitalia	1%

TABLE 3.3.3. Lund and Browder Burn Chart (Part 2).

Age (years)	0	1	5	10	15	Adult
1/2 of head	9 ½%	8 ½%	6 ½%	5 ½%	4 ½%	3 ½%
1/2 of one thigh	2 ¾%	3 ¼%	4%	4 ¼%	4 ½%	4 ¾%
1/2 of one leg	2 ½%	2 ½%	2 ¾%	3%	3 ¼%	3%

on her right palm, it is estimated that her burn represents only 1% of her TBSA. Although the burn represents only a minute portion of Fatima's TBSA, all burns of the hands, mouth, or genitals require immediate medical attention. Hand burns are susceptible to functional limitations, as a consequence of scar formation and contractures. The treatment of hand burns in the pediatric patient should involve careful followup to gauge not only the healing and restoration of function to the hand but also to assess for psychological and emotional trauma. Current American Burn Association (2006) guidelines recommend burn unit referral for burns involving the hands. However, many hand burns are treated in primary care settings, such as the emergency room, primary care office, or an urgent care center.

Goals of treatment for Fatima's partial-thickness (second-degree) burn are to reduce pain and prevent infection. Pain relievers such as acetaminophen or ibuprofen can help with inflammation and pain and should be used according to directions. Children under the age of 18 years should not be given aspirin for the relief of pain or inflammation because of the risk of developing Reye syndrome. Topical antimicrobials of choice include bacitracin and neomycin for partial-thickness burns. Since this is a hand burn at risk for contractures, the primary care health care provider in this case should refer Fatima to the local emergency department or to a burn specialist if one is accessible.

Fatima's mother should be educated regarding the signs and symptoms of infection and when to call or return to the primary care office. She should also be educated about the prevention of burns.

Does this patient's psychosocial history affect how you might treat this case?
An aspect of Fatima's psychosocial history that might affect the handling of her case is that her mother is a teenager. Research has shown that when compared to children of adult mothers, children of adolescent mothers have an increased rate of unintentional injuries during the first 5 years of life (Koniak-Griffin et al., 2003). It would be important to provide extensive education regarding safety to prevent future unintentional injuries. It would also be important to have close followup to ensure that the family follows up as necessary.

What if the patient lived in a rural setting?
If Fatima and her family lived in a rural setting, gaining rapid access to a health care provider skilled in treating hand burns in pediatric patients might be delayed. Also, the family may experience barriers in attending follow-up appointments to monitor the healing. For this reason, if Fatima's family lived in a rural setting, she might have to be hospitalized for the initial treatment of her burn.

Are there any demographic characteristics that might affect this case?
Both age and ethnicity are demographic factors that may affect the incidence of burns in the pediatric patient. Children less than 6 years of age are more likely to suffer from burns than children under

the age of 6 years of age. This may be due to a natural curiosity on the part of the younger child, coupled with their slower reaction time when contacting a hot object. African-American children are most commonly affected by burns, followed by Caucasians, Hispanics, and Asians (Goodis, 2010).

Are there any standardized guidelines that you should use to assess or treat this case?

The American Burn Association has listed guidelines for the management of burns and burn centers. See the reference listed below.

REFERENCES AND RESOURCES

American Burn Association. (2006). Guidelines for the operation of burn centers. http://www.ameriburn.org/Chapter14.pdf?PHPSESSID=bee7bcc69446242993f78c00abb01ead

Choi, M., Armstrong, M., & Panthaki, Z. (2009). Pediatric hand burns: Thermal, electrical, chemical. *Journal of Craniofacial Surgery, 20*, 1045–1048.

Cuttle, L., Kravchuk, O., Wallis, B., & Kimble, R. (2009). An audit of first-aid treatment of pediatric burns patients and their clinical outcome. *Journal of Burn Care & Research, 30*, 1028–1034.

Goodis, J. (2010). Thermal burns in emergency medicine. Retrieved on May 12, 2011, from http://emedicine.medscape.com/article/769193-overview#a0199

Kassira, W., & Namias, N. (2008). Outpatient management of pediatric burns. *Journal of Craniofacial Surgery, 19*, 1007–1009.

Koniak-Griffin, D., Verzemnieks, I., Anderson, N., Brecht, M., Lesser, J., Kim, S., & Turner-Pluta, C. (2003). Nurse visitation for adolescent mothers: Two-year infant health and maternal outcomes. *Nursing Research, 52*, 127–136.

Palmieri, T. (2009). Initial management of acute pediatric hand burns. *Hand Clinics, 25*, 461–467.

Reis, E., Yasti, A., Kerimoglu, R., Dolapci, M., Doganay, M., & Kama, N. (2009). The effects of habitual negligence among families with respect to pediatric burns. *Turkish Journal of Trauma & Emergency Surgery: TJTES, 15*, 607–610.

Scott, J. R., Costa, B. A., Gibran, N. S., Engrav, L. H., Heimbach, D. H., & Klein, M. B. (2008). Pediatric palm contact burns: A ten-year review. *Journal of Burn Care & Research, 29*, 614–618.

The Royal Children's Hospital Melbourne (2010). Clinical practice guidelines: Burns. Retrieved from http://www.rch.org.au/clinicalguide/cpg.cfm?doc_id=5158

University of Wisconsin Hospitals and Clinic Authority (2008). Assessing burns and planning resuscitation: The rule of nines. Retrieved from http://www.uwhealth.org/emergency-room/assessing-burns-and-planning-resuscitation-the-rule-of-nines/12698

Case 3.4 Toothache

By Mikki Meadows-Oliver, PhD, RN

Five-year-old Lamin presents to the office with his father, Alieu, with a complaint of a toothache. Alieu states that Lamin woke in the middle of the night, crying, stating that his tooth (on the back, left side of his mouth) hurt. Alieu gave Lamin an over-the-counter pain reliever to help with the pain. The pain reliever helped, and Lamin went back to sleep. However, when Lamin awakened this morning, he was again complaining of a toothache; and Alieu decided to bring him in for a visit. Alieu states that he thinks that Lamin had a fever. The family does not have a thermometer, but Lamin's forehead felt hot. Lamin has no cough, runny nose, vomiting, or diarrhea.

Diet: Lamin's nutrition history reveals that he has a balanced diet with enough dairy, protein, fruits, and vegetables. He also ingests quite a bit of junk food, including chips and cookies. Alieu admits that Lamin sometimes drinks juice and soda from a baby bottle.

Elimination: Lamin is voiding well with no complaints of dysuria. He has 1 bowel movement daily and denies constipation or diarrhea.

Sleep: Lamin sleeps approximately 10 hours at night and has no trouble falling asleep or staying asleep.

Past medical history: Born via vaginal birth in Senegal. His birth was a home birth attended by a local midwife. The exact number of weeks' gestation is unknown, but Lamin's parents state that his was a full-term birth. Lamin has had no injuries or illnesses requiring visits to the emergency department. He passed his developmental screening at his last well-child visit. He currently attends kindergarten and is doing well.

He has no chronic illnesses and is currently taking no medications.

Social history: Lamin lives at home with both parents and his 1-year-old sibling. The family has been in the United States for 2 years. They are in the United States so that Lamin's father can study biology at a local university. His mother is currently not working because her visa does not allow her to work. The family has a no pets. There are no smokers in the home.

Family medical history: Lamin's mother (26 years old) and father (30 years old) both have sickle cell trait, but neither has a history of chronic medical conditions. Lamin's 1-year-old sister also has sickle

Clinical Case Studies for the Family Nurse Practitioner, First Edition. Edited by Leslie Neal-Boylan.
© 2011 John Wiley & Sons, Inc. Published 2011 by John Wiley & Sons, Inc.

cell trait. His maternal grandmother (46 years old) has a history of hepatitis. His maternal grandfather (50 years old) has a history of tuberculosis (successfully treated before Lamin was born). Lamin's paternal grandfather (51 years old) has no known history of health problems. His paternal grandmother (50 years old) has a history of malaria.

Medications: Lamin is not currently taking any over-the-counter, prescription, or herbal medications. He has no known allergies to medication, food, or the environment. He is up to date on required immunizations.

OBJECTIVE

Lamin's vital signs are taken, and his weight in the office was 24 kg. His temperature is 37.5°C (temporal). He is alert, cooperative, and interactive. He appears well hydrated and well nourished.

Skin: His skin is clear of lesions. There is no cyanosis of his skin, lips, or nails. There was no diaphoresis noted, and Lamin had good skin turgor on examination.

HEENT: Lamin is normocephalic. Red reflexes are present bilaterally; and his pupils are equal, round, and reactive to light. There is no ocular discharge noted. Lamin's external ear reveals that the pinnae are normal and that there is no tenderness to touch on the external ear. On otoscopic examination, the tympanic membranes are gray bilaterally, in normal position with positive light reflexes. Bony landmarks are visible, and there is no fluid noted behind the tympanic membranes. Both nostrils are patent. There is no nasal discharge, and there is no nasal flaring. Lamin's mucous membranes are noted to be moist when examining his oropharynx. He has 20 teeth present. Both premolars on the lower, left side are noted to have visible caries. The gingival area surrounding those 2 teeth is erythematous and edematous. The area is tender to touch. There are no other lesions present in the oral cavity.

Neck: Supple and able to move in all directions without resistance. There is a 1-cm diameter left, anterior cervical node present. The node is nonerythematous, mobile, and mildly tender to touch.

Respiratory: Respiratory rate is 20 breaths per minute, and lungs are clear to auscultation in all lobes. There is good air entry, and no retractions or grunting are noted on examination. No deformities of the thoracic cage are noted.

Cardiovascular: Heart rate is 92 beats per minute with a regular rhythm. There is no murmur noted upon auscultation.

Abdomen: Normoactive bowel sounds throughout; soft and nontender. No evidence of hepatosplenomegaly.

Genitourinary: Normal uncircumcised male genitalia without erythema or lesions. His testes are descended bilaterally.

Neuromusculoskeletal: Good tone and full range of motion in all extremities, warm, and well-perfused. Capillary refill is less than 2 seconds, and his spine is straight.

CRITICAL THINKING

Which diagnostic or imaging studies should be considered to assist with or confirm the diagnosis?
___Complete blood count
___Erythrocyte sedimentation test
___Dental X-ray

What are the most likely differential diagnoses and why?
___Gingivitis
___Dental caries
___Periodontitis

What is your plan of treatment, referral, and follow-up care?

Does this patient's psychosocial history affect how you might treat this case?

What if the patient lived in a rural setting?

Are there any demographic characteristics that might affect this case?

Are there any standardized guidelines that you should use to assess or treat this case?

RESOLUTION

Diagnostic tests: Unless a systemic infection is suspected, there are no laboratory tests needed for a diagnosis associated with tooth pain. Imaging studies such as a dental X-ray will be able to detect caries not visible to the naked eye.

What are the most likely differential diagnoses and why?
Gingivitis and dental caries:
When considering the symptom of tooth pain, there are several differential diagnoses to consider, including gingivitis, dental caries, and periodontitis. Gingivitis is an inflammatory process of the gum tissues surrounding the teeth. With gingivitis, the gingiva (gums) may appear to be erythematous and swollen. This is prevalent in people with inadequate oral hygiene, inadequate plaque removal, poor nutrition, and lack of periodic dental examinations. Caries (cavities) are decayed areas of the teeth that develop into openings or holes. Caries are caused by a combination of factors, including not cleaning the teeth well, eating frequent sugary snacks, and drinking sugary drinks. Periodontitis is a serious gum infection that damages the soft tissues and bones that support the teeth. Like gingivitis and caries, periodontitis is usually the result of poor oral hygiene. People who have periodontitis will likely have receding gums. They may also display pus between their teeth and gums. Based on the history of erythematous and edematous gums and holes in his teeth, it would appear that Lamin has both gingivitis and dental caries. He was not reported to have any receding of his gums, so it is unlikely that he has developed periodontitis.

What is your plan of treatment, referral, and follow-up care?
Treatment for Lamin's tooth pain related to his gingivitis and caries will encompass several aspects. Proper oral hygiene (including brushing and flossing) should be stressed. Because of a probable lack of hand dexterity in a 5-year-old, Lamin's parents should assist him in brushing his teeth at least once daily and flossing the teeth that are in contact with other teeth. Using a power toothbrush with an oscillating motion has been shown to be better at removing plaque than a manual toothbrush. These actions will help to reduce plaque associated with gingivitis and caries. Lamin should use a warm saline rinse several times per day to help resolve his gingival inflammation. An oral rinse with a hydrogen peroxide 3% solution may also help. Nonsteroidal anti-inflammatory drugs (NSAIDs) have been shown to assist with the resolution of pain and inflammation associated with gingivitis and caries. Prevention of dental disease (good oral hygiene and regular dental checkups) should be discussed with Lamin's parents. Proper nutrition, including foods that do not contain simple sugars, should be stressed. Research has shown that foods containing milk or milk components (e.g., yogurt) may have cariostatic properties. These foods should be encouraged as part of a balanced diet for Lamin. Drinking from the bottle should be discontinued. Lamin should be referred to a dentist for a professional cleaning of his teeth and for the management of his caries. He should follow up in the primary care office if his tooth pain worsens or if he develops a fever before his dental appointment.

Does this patient's psychosocial history affect how you might treat this case?

Children who immigrate to the United States tend to have a higher rate of dental disease and lower rates of dental health care utilization than do children born in the United States (Maserejian, Trachtenberg, & Hayes (2008). Lamin's family may not have had access to preventive dental care and teaching about good dental hygiene in their home country. In addition, Lamin has a cariogenic diet. His history revealed that he eats quite a bit of junk food. Lamin also still drinks sugary drinks from a bottle.

What if the patient lived in a rural setting?

Children in rural locations may have decreased access to dental care based on the lack of availability to a nearby dentist. However, research reveals that children in rural settings have fewer cavities than children in urban areas.

Are there any demographic characteristics that might affect this case?

Preschool age is a common time for the development of dental problems because the responsibility of oral hygiene (such as tooth brushing) shifts to the child. The preschool-age child does not always have the manual dexterity to brush and floss correctly. Therefore, they are at risk for developing dental problems such as gingivitis and dental decay. It is estimated that 9%–17% of children aged 3–11 years have gingivitis; and 70%–90% adolescents have gingivitis. In adults, gingivitis is slightly more common in males than in females, because females are more likely to have better oral hygiene.

Are there any standardized guidelines that you should use to assess or treat this case?

The American Academy of Pediatric Dentistry has developed guidelines for pediatric dental health. See their reference below.

REFERENCES AND RESOURCES

American Academy of Pediatric Dentistry (AAPD). (2009). Guideline on Periodicity of Examination, Preventive Dental Services, Anticipatory Guidance/Counseling, and Oral Treatment for Infants, Children, and Adolescents. AAPD Reference Manual, 32 (6), 93–100. Retrieved from: http://www.aapd.org/media/Policies_Guidelines/G_Periodicity.pdf

Horton, S., & Barker, J. (2009). Rural Mexican immigrant parents' interpretation of children's dental symptoms and decisions to seek treatment. *Community Dental Health*, 26, 216–221.

Mariath, A., Haas, A., Fischer, C., de Araujo, F., & Rösing, C. (2009). Professional toothbrushing as a method for diagnosing gingivitis in 3- to 6-year-old preschool children. *Oral Health & Preventive Dentistry*, 7, 315–321.

Maserejian, N., Trachtenberg, F., Hayes, C., & Tavares, M. (2008). Oral health disparities in children of immigrants: Dental caries experience at enrollment and during follow-up in the New England Children's Amalgam Trial. *Journal of Public Health Dentistry*, 68(1), 14–21.

Maserejian, N., Tavares, M., Hayes, C., Soncini, J., & Trachtenberg, F. (2008). Rural and urban disparities in caries prevalence in children with unmet dental needs: The New England Children's Amalgam Trial. *Journal of Public Health Dentistry*, 68, 7–13.

Tanaka, K., Miyake, Y., & Sasaki, S. (2010). Intake of dairy products and the prevalence of dental caries in young children. *Journal of Dentistry*, 38, 579–583.

Walsh, T., Worthington, H., Glenny, A., Appelbe, P., Marinho, V., & Shi, X. (2010). Fluoride toothpastes of different concentrations for preventing dental caries in children and adolescents. *Cochrane Database of Systematic Reviews*, (1), CD007868.

Case 3.5 Abdominal Pain

By Mikki Meadows-Oliver, PhD, RN and Anna Faria, MSN, PNP-BC

SUBJECTIVE

Four-year-old Jasmine presents to the office with a complaint of abdominal pain for 2 days. She is accompanied by her mother, Anna. Anna states that Jasmine's pain is intermittent and is mainly on the left side of her abdomen. She states that the pain is sometimes worse after eating and that the pain is sometimes relieved by passing gas. Jasmine is unable to describe the quality of the pain, but Anna states that Jasmine will sometimes "double over" in pain. Jasmine has had no vomiting or diarrhea. She has had no cough or runny nose.

Diet: Jasmine's nutrition history reveals that she eats bananas and rice almost daily. She drinks 4–5 cups of whole milk daily.

Elimination: She is voiding well with no complaints of dysuria. Jasmine has 2–3 bowel movements per week. Anna is unsure of the amount or consistency, since she rarely accompanies Jasmine into the bathroom.

Sleep: Jasmine sleeps approximately 10 hours at night. She has no problems falling asleep or staying asleep. Her sleep has not been interrupted by her abdominal pain.

Past medical history: Born via Cesarean section at 37 weeks' gestation. Since being discharged at 4 days of age, she has had no emergency department visits or hospitalizations. Jasmine had bronchiolitis at 6 months of age but has had no injuries or illnesses since that time. Jasmine passed her developmental screening at her last well-child visit. She currently attends prekindergarten and is doing well, according to Anna. She has no chronic illnesses and is not currently taking any medications.

Social history: Jasmine lives at home with both parents and a 2-year-old sibling. Her mother works as a nurse, and her father is a firefighter. The family has a pet chihuahua. There are no smokers in the home.

Family medical history: Jasmine's mother (29 years old) and father (29 years old) are healthy and have no history of chronic medical conditions. Her 2-year-old sibling is healthy as well. Her maternal grandmother (52 years old) has a history of Crohn disease. Her maternal grandfather (54 years old) has a history of asthma. Jasmine's paternal grandfather passed away at age 47 years of age from stomach cancer. Her paternal grandmother (53 years old) has a history of obesity and Type 2 diabetes.

Clinical Case Studies for the Family Nurse Practitioner, First Edition. Edited by Leslie Neal-Boylan.
© 2011 John Wiley & Sons, Inc. Published 2011 by John Wiley & Sons, Inc.

Medications: Jasmine is currently taking no over-the-counter, prescription, or herbal medications. She has no known allergies to medications, food, or the environment. She is up to date on required immunizations.

OBJECTIVE

Jasmine's vital signs are taken, and her weight in the office today is 27 kg. Her temperature is 37°C (temporal). She is alert, cooperative, and interactive. She appears well hydrated and well nourished.

Skin: Her skin is clear of lesions. There is no cyanosis of her skin, lips, or nails. There is no diaphoresis noted. Jasmine has good skin turgor on examination.

HEENT: Jasmine's head is normocephalic. Red reflexes are present bilaterally; and pupils are equal, round, and reactive to light. There is no ocular discharge noted. Julia's external ear reveals that the pinnae are normal and that there is no tenderness to touch on the external ear. On otoscopic examination, the tympanic membranes are gray bilaterally and in normal position with positive light reflexes. Bony landmarks are visible, and there is no fluid noted behind the tympanic membranes. Both nostrils are patent. There is scant nasal discharge, and there is no nasal flaring. Jasmine's mucous membranes are noted to be moist when examining her oropharynx. She has 20 teeth present without evidence of caries. There are no lesions present in the oral cavity.

Neck: Supple and able to move in all directions without resistance; no cervical lymphadenopathy.

Respiratory: Respiratory rate is 24 breaths per minute, and lungs are clear to auscultation in all lobes. There is good air entry, and no retractions or grunting are noted on examination. No deformities of the thoracic cage are noted.

Cardiovascular: Heart rate is 104 beats per minute with a regular rhythm. There is no murmur noted upon auscultation.

Abdomen: Normoactive bowel sounds are present throughout; abdomen is soft and mildly tender in the lower left quadrant. There is no evidence of hepatosplenomegaly.

Genitourinary: Normal female genitalia.

Neuromusculoskeletal: Good tone in all extremities; full range of motion of all extremities. Extremities are warm and well perfused. Capillary refill is <2 seconds, and spine is straight.

CRITICAL THINKING

Are there laboratory tests or diagnostic imaging studies that should be ordered as part of a workup for abdominal pain?
___Stool test for occult blood
___Anorectal manometry
___Digital rectal exam
___Abdominal radiograph
___Blood test for celiac disease
___Erythrocyte sedimentation rate (ESR)
___Barium enema
___Total colonic motility studies
___Thyroid function test
___Stool culture
___Endoscopy/Colonoscopy

What is the most likely differential diagnosis and why?
___Functional dyspepsia
___Functional constipation
___Irritable bowel syndrome
___Cyclic vomiting syndrome
___Abdominal migraine
___Functional abdominal pain syndrome
___Gastrointestinal infection
___Hirschsprung disease
___Intussusception
___Celiac disease
___Crohn disease
___Dietary intolerances

What is your plan of treatment, referral, and follow-up care?

Does this patient's psychosocial history affect how you might treat this case?

What if the patient lived in a rural setting?

Are there any demographic characteristics that might affect this case?

Are there any standardized guidelines that you should use to assess or treat this case?

RESOLUTION

Diagnostic tests: An abdominal radiograph may be helpful if constipation is suspected. It may reveal a full rectal vault and fecal loading. There would be no signs of obstruction. A stool test for occult blood would reveal the presence of blood in the stool and may suggest rectal or anal tearing during stooling. Anorectal manometry evaluates internal sphincter relaxation with rectal distention. This test would be used if Hirschsprung disease is suspected. A digital rectal exam should reveal a full rectal vault in functional constipation, while Hirschsprung disease is more likely to present with an empty rectum on physical exam. Patients with constipation and failure to thrive should be evaluated with a celiac panel for celiac disease and a thyroid function test for hypothyroidism. While Jasmine's history and physical are not consistent with Crohn disease, it would be important to consider this diagnosis if her abdominal pain were persistent and unrelieved by treatment, given the family history for this disease. In a patient with Crohn disease, ESR may be elevated. An endoscopy and colonoscopy would be warranted if this diagnosis was suspected.

What is the most likely differential diagnosis and why?
Constipation:
While the differential for abdominal pain is extensive, it is important to bear in mind that the majority of abdominal pain in children is functional and not the result of an underlying pathological process. Included in the differential for functional abdominal pain are functional dyspepsia, functional constipation, irritable bowel syndrome, cyclic vomiting syndrome, abdominal migraine, and functional abdominal pain syndrome.

Organic etiologies of abdominal pain include gastrointestinal infection, anatomic abnormalities such as Hirschsprung or intussusception, inflammatory diseases such as celiac disease, Crohn disease, and dietary intolerances. Red flags for organic etiologies of abdominal pain include pain that occurs at night and awakens the child; pain that is distant from the umbilicus; pain accompanied by fever, dysuria, or hematuria; joint pain or swelling; significant vomiting; a change in bowel movement habits; weight loss; or slowed growth. Constipation, with or without abdominal pain, may also be the result of cystic fibrosis, neurological dysfunction, and hypothyroidism, which should be ruled out in cases of constipation that do not respond to standard interventions. Given Jasmine's history of increased cow's milk intake, her habit of having a bowel movement only 2–3 times per week, and mild tenderness in left lower quadrant, the mostly likely diagnosis is constipation.

What is your plan of treatment, referral, and follow-up care?
Initial management of constipation requires a "cleanout," which can be achieved using oral or rectal medications, including enemas, osmotic laxatives, stimulant laxatives, and polyethylene glycol. Polyethylene glycol (PEG) and stool softeners are safe and effective for long-term treatment and should be considered in patients with recurrent functional constipation. PEG is especially useful in the pediatric population, as it is tasteless and can be dissolved easily in any beverage.

Because much of the management for constipation involves behavior modification and lifestyle changes, it is important to take the time to educate families. Jasmine's parents should be educated about constipation, including management guidelines and when to seek medical care. While there is limited support for dietary and exercise interventions for constipation, these lifestyle changes are healthy choices for all patients and may offer some relief for select patients. Jasmine's parents should be encouraged to provide her with a low-fat, high-fiber diet and ensure that she gets plenty of regular exercise. Jasmine's mother should be told to decrease Jasmine's cow's milk intake to no more than 24 oz per day since excessive intake of cow's milk has been associated with constipation. Adequate water intake may help prevent constipation as well.

In preschool-aged children with a history of constipation, toileting is often met with fear and frustration. Scheduled toileting can help to normalize toilet time as a relaxing and painless activity. Jasmine's parents should be instructed to have her sit on the toilet for 15 to 20 minutes at a time, 2 to 3 times a day, even if she does not have a bowel movement. Due to the gastrocolic reflex, timing this toileting for 15 to 20 minutes after the completion of meals may prove helpful. During toilet time, Jasmine should sit with both feet firmly on the floor and should be encouraged to relax. A parent should be present with Jasmine during toilet time to provide reassurance and to observe bowel movements. Information obtained about the size and shape of Jasmine's stools can provide both her parents and her health care provider information about the success or failure of her treatment. A reward system (such as a sticker chart) for successful toileting efforts and bowel movements may help to encourage future success, while failures should simply be ignored.

Based upon the history and physical exam, there is no indication for referral at this time. It is important that Jasmine and her parents follow up with her health care provider by telephone in 1 to 2 weeks to assess the effectiveness of the recommended interventions. This time will also allow Jasmine's parents to express any questions, concerns, or frustrations that may have arisen regarding her symptoms and treatment. The family should follow up in the office in 1 month or sooner if necessary. Prolonged constipation that does not respond to treatment or recurrent abdominal pain that appears to be unrelated to functional constipation, may require a referral to a pediatric gastroenterologist.

Does this patient's psychosocial history affect how you might treat this case?
Treatment for constipation does not vary significantly based on psychosocial history; but it is important to bear in mind a family's access to fresh produce, as well as their dietary preferences, when offering nutritional recommendations. Furthermore, constipation may be more prevalent during periods of transition, such as starting school, the arrival of a new sibling, or moving to a new home. When these transitions exist, interventions may require more time before they are successful. Parents should be encouraged in their efforts, allowed to air frustrations, and offered regular support from health care providers.

What if the patient lived in a rural setting?
Residence in a rural setting should not affect the treatment of Jasmine's constipation. However, if a more serious etiology were suspected and access to health care were limited by location, more aggressive diagnostics at the time of presentation may be warranted.

Are there any demographic characteristics that might affect this case?
Constipation is a very common complaint in childhood. In fact, it is estimated that 3%–5% of pediatric health care visits are the result of constipation. The prevalence of constipation is equal among girls and boys during childhood, but it occurs more frequently in females than in males following puberty. While constipation occurs throughout infancy, childhood, and adulthood, it appears to be more prevalent during weaning and toilet training, and also in school-aged children. Many children with constipation have a family member who also has constipation.

Are there any standardized guidelines that you should use to assess or treat this case?

The Rome III diagnostic criteria, created by the Rome Foundation offer guidelines for the diagnosis and treatment of functional abdominal pain, including functional constipation, in children (Rasquin et al., 2006). American Academy of Pediatrics—Medical Specialty Society (2005) has also developed guidelines for diagnosing and treating chronic abdominal pain in the pediatric population. The North American Society for Pediatric Gastroenterology and the University of Michigan also offer guidelines for managing pediatric constipation.

REFERENCES AND RESOURCES

American Academy of Pediatrics—Medical Specialty Society (2005). Chronic abdominal pain in children. *Pediatrics, 115*(3), 812–815.

Constipation Guideline Committee of the North American Society for Pediatric Gastroenterology (2006). Evaluation and treatment of constipation in infants and children: Recommendations of the North American Society for Pediatric Gastroenterology, Hepatology and Nutrition. *Journal of Pediatric Gastroenterology and Nutrition, 43*(3), e1–e13.

Daher, S., Tahan, S., Sole, D., Naspitz, C., Da Silva-Patricio, R., Neto, U., & De Morais, M. (2001). Cow's milk protein intolerance and chronic constipation in children. *Pediatric Allergy & Immunology, 12*, 339–342.

Rasquin, A., Di Lorenzo, C., Forbes, D., Guiraldes, E., Hyams, J. S., Staiano, A., & Walker, L. S. (2006). Childhood functional gastrointestinal disorders: Child/adolescent. *Gastroenterology, 130*, 1527–1537.

University of Michigan Health System (2008). *Functional constipation and soiling in children*, Ann Arbor, MI: University of Michigan Health System. Sep. 15.

Case 3.6 Lesion on Penis

By Mikki Meadows-Oliver, PhD, RN and Katharine Swan, MSN, RN

SUBJECTIVE

Two-year-old Lionel presents to the office with his mother and maternal grandmother with a complaint of a red area on his penis. Lionel's mother, Susan, states that when she was changing his diaper 2 days ago, she noticed that Lionel's foreskin was red. She states that she has been putting a diaper rash cream on the area but that it has not helped to relieve the redness. She feels that the area of redness is getting larger and that the area is now painful. Lionel has no fever, cough, runny nose, vomiting, or diarrhea.

Diet: Lionel's nutrition history reveals that he has a balanced diet with enough dairy, protein, fruits, and vegetables. His appetite is good and has not changed in the past 2 days.

Elimination: Lionel is voiding well, but Susan thinks that he may have some pain when he urinates. She states that diaper changes seem to cause him pain when she cleans the area of redness with the baby wipes. He has one bowel movement daily, and Susan denies that he has constipation or diarrhea.

Sleep: Lionel sleeps approximately 11 hours at night and takes one nap daily. He has no trouble falling asleep or staying asleep.

Past medical history: Lionel was born at 40 weeks' gestation via vaginal delivery with vacuum assist. Since birth, Lionel has been healthy and has had no injuries or illnesses requiring visits to the emergency department. Lionel passed his developmental screening at his last well-child visit. He does not currently attend a day care or preschool program. He has no chronic illnesses and is currently taking no medications.

Social history: Lionel lives at home with his mother and maternal grandmother. Lionel's father is involved but does not reside in the home. His mother is currently not working outside of the home. The family has a cat. There are no smokers in the home.

Family medical history: Lionel's mother (21 years old) has a history of having leukemia as child. She is followed periodically by the oncologist. Lionel's father (23 years old) has a history of asthma. Lionel's maternal grandmother (age 39 years) has a history of multiple sclerosis. His maternal grandfather (40 years old) has a history of Type I diabetes. Lionel's paternal grandfather (41 years old) has no known history of health problems. His paternal grandmother (40 years old) has a history of asthma.

Clinical Case Studies for the Family Nurse Practitioner, First Edition. Edited by Leslie Neal-Boylan.
© 2011 John Wiley & Sons, Inc. Published 2011 by John Wiley & Sons, Inc.

Medications: Lionel is not currently taking any over-the-counter, prescription, or herbal medications. His mother does apply diaper rash cream to genital area during diaper changes. Lionel has no known allergies to medication, food, or the environment. He is up to date on required immunizations.

OBJECTIVE

Lionel's vital signs are taken, and his weight in the office is 17 kg. His temperature is 37.0°C (temporal). He is alert, playful, and interactive. When crying, he is easily consolable. He appears well hydrated and well nourished. There is no cyanosis of his skin, lips, or nails. There is no diaphoresis noted, and Lionel has good skin turgor on examination.

HEENT: Lionel's head is normocephalic. His red reflexes are present bilaterally; and his pupils are equal, round, and reactive to light. There is no ocular discharge noted. Lionel's external ear reveals that the pinnae are normal, and there is no tenderness to touch on the external ear. On otoscopic examination, the tympanic membranes are gray bilaterally, in normal position with positive light reflexes. Bony landmarks are visible, and there is no fluid noted behind the tympanic membranes. Both nostrils are patent. There is no nasal discharge, and there is no nasal flaring. Lionel's mucous membranes are noted to be moist. He has 18 teeth present. There are no visible caries or other lesions present in the oral cavity.

Neck: Lionel's neck is supple and able to move in all directions without resistance. There is no cervical lymphadenopathy noted.

Respiratory: Lionel's respiratory rate is 24 breaths per minute, and his lungs are clear to auscultation in all lobes. There is good air entry, and no retractions or grunting are noted on examination. No deformities of the thoracic cage are noted.

Cardiovascular: Lionel's heart rate is 96 beats per minute with a regular rhythm. There is no murmur noted upon auscultation.

Abdomen: Normoactive bowel sounds are present throughout, and Lionel's abdomen is soft and nontender. There is no evidence of hepatosplenomegaly.

Genitourinary: Uncircumcised male genitalia with erythema and mild edema on the foreskin. The affected area is mildly tender to touch. A portion of the glans is visible; and there is no discharge, erythema, or swelling noted. His testes are descended bilaterally. There is no erythema or edema of the scrotum. He has shotty lymph nodes present in the inguinal area.

Neuromusculoskeletal: Good tone and full range of motion in all extremities; extremities are warm and well perfused. Capillary refill is less than 2 seconds, and his spine is straight.

CRITICAL THINKING

Which diagnostic or imaging studies should be considered to assist with or confirm the diagnosis?
___Bacterial culture
___Gram stain
___Microscopic examination
___Potassium hydroxide (KOH)
___Urinalysis

What is the most likely differential diagnosis and why?
___Balanitis
___Phimosis
___Paraphimosis
___Balanoposthitis

What is your plan of treatment, referral, and follow-up care?

Does this patient's psychosocial history affect how you might treat this case?

What if the patient lived in a rural setting?

Are there any demographic characteristics that might affect this case?

Are there any standardized guidelines that you should use to assess or treat this case?

RESOLUTION

Diagnostic tests: To rule out a microbial cause, a swab of the skin under the foreskin and of any discharge should be analyzed for culture and sensitivity. Gram staining may be used to identify the causative microorganism and guide treatment. Dark field microscopy may be ordered to observe the presence of spirochetes, specifically *Treponema pallidum*. A potassium hydroxide test may be performed to look for hyphae if candida is suspected. In addition, a urinalysis should be performed for the detection of microorganisms from the bladder, urethra, meatus, or glans penis and to rule out a urinary tract infection and diabetes.

What is the most likely differential diagnosis and why?
Balanoposthitis:
Conditions to consider in the differential diagnosis of erythema and swelling of the foreskin include balanitis, phimosis, paraphimosis, and balanoposthitis. Balanitis refers to the inflammation of the glans penis. The foreskin is not swollen in balanitis, thus it may occur in both circumcised and uncircumcised males. Balanitis often presents in conjunction with diaper dermatitis. In phimosis, the foreskin cannot be retracted due to adhesion between the prepuce and glans penis, which becomes chronically swollen. This condition is physiologic at birth and should resolve between 3 and 6 years of age. Paraphimosis is a less likely diagnosis for Lionel, but it is one that should be considered for patients with swollen foreskin. In this condition, the foreskin is retracted past the coronal sulcus. Venous stasis results in swelling and pain of the foreskin.

Balanoposthitis refers to any infection of the foreskin. *Staphylococcus* and *Streptococcus* are the most common bacterial causes of posthitis. *Candidiasis* is a common fungal origin of posthitis and often occurs in conjunction with fungal diaper dermatitis. In addition, patients may develop irritant nonspecific balanoposthitis from poor hygiene, especially related to smegma or prolonged contact with wet diapers. Based on the history and physical examination, Lionel has most likely developed a form of balanoposthitis.

What is your plan of treatment, referral, and follow-up care?
In addition to Lionel's diagnosis of balanoposthitis, he will likely have a concurrent diagnosis of physiologic phimosis. Because there is no discharge present, it is likely that the cause of Lionel's balanoposthitis is irritation from his diaper. The best treatment for Lionel at this time is a daily bath with a weak salt solution to alleviate inflammation and the application of bacitracin antibiotic ointment to the affected area 2–3 times daily. Lionel's parents should also be instructed to permit him to be without a diaper for 5–10 minutes after each diaper change to allow air to the area and to allow his diaper area to fully dry. His parents should also be told not to try to retract the foreskin fully as this may result in paraphimosis. Lionel's parents should be further educated to reinforce proper hygiene of the genital area. Lionel's family should follow up by phone in 2 days to report progress and healing. They should return to the office if his condition worsens or if there is no improvement in 48 hours after beginning the salt baths and bacitracin treatment. Health care providers should be aware that circumcision is not a preventative treatment of balanoposthitis in children younger than 3 years old. For chronic or recurrent balanoposthitis, a referral to a pediatric urologist should be considered.

Does this patient's psychosocial history affect how you might treat this case?
Though Lionel's father is involved in his care, his father does not reside with Lionel. Because there is no male figure directly caring for Lionel, it is important to educate the mother and grandmother

in male genitourinary health. Proper hygiene of the glans penis and foreskin should be discussed, emphasizing that Lionel's foreskin will not likely be fully retractable at 2 years of age and that they should not forcibly retract the foreskin under any circumstances.

What if the patient lived in a rural setting?

Care of balanoposthitis would not change in a rural setting. Education regarding hygiene should be emphasized as before. For patients living in agricultural settings, hand hygiene after contact with animals should be discussed.

Are there any demographic characteristics that might affect this case?

When considering ethnicity, balanoposthitis has been noted to occur twice as often in African-Americans and Hispanics. The difference in occurrence rates compared to Caucasians is likely related to different circumcision rates between the ethnic groups. Age is not necessarily a factor in the development of balanoposthitis. This condition can occur in males at any age, and the etiologies will vary depending on the age of the patient.

Are there any standardized guidelines that you should use to assess or treat this case?

The European Association of Urology has issued guidelines on the treatment of balanoposthitis and other pediatric urological conditions (Tekgul et al., 2009).

REFERENCES AND RESOURCES

Gargollo, P., Kozakewich, H., Bauer, S., Borer, J., Peters, C., Retik, A., & Diamond, D. (2005). Balanitis xerotica obliterans in boys. *The Journal of Urology, 174*, 1409–1412.

Kiss, A., Kiraly, L., Kutasy, B., & Merksz, M. (2005). High incidence of balanitis xerotica obliterans in boys with phimosis: Prospective 10-year study. *Pediatric Dermatology, 22*, 305–308.

Lisboa, C., Ferreira, A., Resende, C., & Rodrigues, A. (2009). Infectious balanoposthitis: Management, clinical and laboratory features. *International Journal of Dermatology, 48*, 121–124.

Tekgul, S., Riedmiller, H., Gerharz, E., Hoebeke, P., Kocvara, R., Nijman, R., . . . Stein, R. (2009). Guidelines on paediatric urology: Phimosis. *Paediatric Urology*, Arnhem, The Netherlands: European Association of Urology, European Society for Paediatric Urology, 6–8, 18–22.

Section 4

The School-Aged Child

Case 4.1 Skin Rash

By Emily Croce, RN, MSN, CPNP

A 4-year-old female, Abby, comes to the clinic for evaluation of a rash. She is accompanied to the visit by her mother. According to her mother, Abby first developed a small, red papule between her nose and her upper lip a few days prior to the appointment today. Her mother thinks that she might have scratched or picked at that area. A few more papules appeared that became fluid-filled vesicles for a brief amount of time. The fragile roofs of these vesicles quickly sloughed off. The newly eroded skin developed overlying honey-colored crusts. The patient complains that the rash is sometimes pruritic, so she has been scratching the area. Abby's mother feels that the rash is spreading due to Abby's manipulation of the area. Abby has been afebrile and has maintained a normal appetite and activity level by report.

Diet: Adequate and varied.

Elimination: Voids every 3–4 hours. Normal bowel movements daily.

Past medical history: Abby is a healthy 4-year-old with no significant medical history. She does not have any chronic medical problems and has not had surgery.

Family history: One of Abby's cousins has a similar rash on her arm. Otherwise noncontributory.

Social history: Abby and her mother live in a 4-bedroom duplex with her 2 siblings, a grandmother, a grandfather, an aunt, an uncle, and 3 cousins. There are no pets in the home. Abby's mother works part-time doing housekeeping for a nearby hotel. She reports that she earns minimum wage.

Medications: Abby does not take any medications regularly. Her mother has not given her any oral medications to treat this problem. Her mother did apply some over-the-counter 1% hydrocortisone cream to the area but does not feel that it helped.

Allergies: Abby is not allergic to any medications. There are no suspected allergies to soaps, detergents, foods, or other environmental factors.

Clinical Case Studies for the Family Nurse Practitioner, First Edition. Edited by Leslie Neal-Boylan.
© 2011 John Wiley & Sons, Inc. Published 2011 by John Wiley & Sons, Inc.

OBJECTIVE

General: Alert, well-nourished female in no apparent distress. She appears nontoxic and is coloring pictures calmly during the exam.

Vital signs: Heart rate 96, respiratory rate 16, temperature 98.8°F, height 40 inches, weight 42 lb (19 kg).

HEENT: Moist mucous membranes without ulcerations; nares patent bilaterally without drainage. Conjunctivae clear without erythema or discharge.

Lymphatic: No cervical, supraclavicular, or occipital lymphadenopathy.

Cardiovascular: Regular heart rate and rhythm; no murmur.

Respiratory: Regular respiratory rate with clear and equal air movement bilaterally.

Skin: Mildly erythematous, confluent plaque of eroded skin inferior to nares and superior to upper lip. Honey-colored crusts overlying the affected area.

CRITICAL THINKING

Which diagnostic or imaging studies should be considered to assist with or confirm the diagnosis?
___Bacterial culture
___Bacterial culture of the nares
___Examination of Tzanck smear
___Fluorescent antibody testing of smears
___Fungal culture
___Gram stain:
___Potassium hydroxide (KOH) examination
___Viral culture

What is the most likely differential diagnosis and why?
___Atopic dermatitis
___Herpes simplex virus (HSV)
___Impetigo

What is the appropriate treatment plan for this diagnosis?

What would the appropriate treatment plan for this diagnosis be if the patient were febrile and/or showing other signs of systemic illness?

What is the appropriate plan for follow-up care?

Are any referrals needed?

Should the patient stay out of school and/or day care during treatment? If so, for how long?

What, if anything, should be recommended to unaffected household members?

RESOLUTION

Diagnostic tests:

- Bacterial culture: Positive for *Staphylococcus aureus* +/− *Streptococcus pyogenes*
- Bacterial culture of the nares: Negative or positive for *Staphylococcus aureus*

- Examination of Tzanck smear: Negative
- Fluorescent antibody testing of smears: Negative
- Fungal culture: Negative
- Gram stain: Gram-positive
- KOH examination: Negative
- Viral culture: Negative

What is the most likely differential diagnosis and why?
Impetigo:
Impetigo is the most common bacterial skin infection in children. It occurs most commonly between 2 and 5 years of age, although it can appear at any age. Impetigo is caused by a superficial bacterial invasion of the epidermis via breaks in the normal skin barrier. Although *Streptococcus pyogenes* was once the leading cause of impetigo, the incidence of *Staphylococcus aureus* has risen steadily since the 1980s, and the majority of cases of childhood impetigo are now caused by *Staphylococcus aureus*. Methicillin-resistant *Staphylococcus aureus* (MRSA) accounts for up to 80% of all cases of impetigo in some areas of the country. Most of these strains are community acquired and often affect healthy children with normal immune function, whereas historically MRSA is typically seen in hospitalized patients. Children are most often infected by direct contact with infected individuals, but fomites also pose a risk of infection spread.

Classic impetigo begins as erythematous macules or papules that quickly evolve to become vesicles with fragile roofs. The vesicles easily rupture, and the fluid inside dries to form honey-colored crusts on the eroded skin. Impetigo most often occurs on exposed areas of skin more susceptible to trauma, such as the face and extremities. The incidence is greatest in the summer months. Superficial breaks in the epidermis predispose an individual to develop impetigo. For that reason, impetigo frequently occurs overlying insect bites, atopic dermatitis, and other conditions that lead to skin abrasions. The differential diagnosis includes atopic or other forms of dermatitis, herpes simplex infections, a kerion caused by dermatophyte infection, varicella, Sweet's syndrome, scabies, pemphigus foliaceus, insect bites, ecthyma, discoid lupus erythematosus, and candidiasis.

Another form, bullous impetigo, accounts for approximately 30% of all cases of impetigo. Superficial vesicles also occur in bullous impetigo, but they rapidly enlarge to create bullae with sharp margins and no surrounding erythema. The bullae also rupture and develop honey-colored crusts as in classic impetigo. It is more common in neonates and represents a localized variation of staphylococcal scalded skin syndrome caused by a toxin-producing form of *Staphylococcus aureus*. Bullous impetigo typically occurs in areas prone to friction and moisture such as the diaper area, axillae, and neck folds. The differential diagnosis includes second-degree burns, fixed drug eruptions, immunobullous diseases such as immunoglobulin A dermatosis, bullous pemphigoid, epidermolysis bullosa, and erythema multiforme. Bullous impetigo can be mistaken for cigarette burns, so child abuse is sometimes included in the differential diagnosis.

Although a bacterial culture and Gram stain are useful tools in diagnosing impetigo, the diagnosis can often be made clinically. Bacterial cultures will typically show *Staphylococcus aureus* with or without *Streptococcus pyogenes*. In rare instances, *Streptococcus pyogenes* impetigo can lead to poststreptococcal glomerulonephritis. Bacterial cultures are more useful when nephritogenic strains of *Streptococcus pyogenes* or drug resistance are suspected in a patient. In one study, carriage of *Staphylococcus aureus* was reported in the nasal passage of up to 42% of children between 7 and 19 years of age. A higher incidence has been reported in patients who actually have impetigo. Decisions to treat an individual should not be made based on presence or absence of *Staphylococcus aureus* in the nasal passage, because a large percentage of unaffected individuals will test positive; and, conversely, an individual with impetigo may not be a nasal carrier. Other sites of the body may less commonly be colonized with *Staphylococcus aureus*.

Rare complications of impetigo include sepsis, osteomyelitis, arthritis, endocarditis, pneumonia, cellulitis, lymphadenitis, toxic shock syndrome, poststreptococcal glomerulonephritis, and generalized staphylococcal scalded skin syndrome. If an individual has recurrent MRSA infections, it may be useful to treat the patient and household members with intranasal mupirocin twice daily for 5 days a few times per year in an attempt to reduce the risk of nasal carriage.

What is the appropriate treatment plan for this diagnosis?

Impetigo is usually self-limiting, localized, and heals without scarring, even without treatment. Small patches of impetigo will typically respond to topical antibiotics such as mupirocin applied twice daily for 5–7 days or retapamulin applied twice daily for 5 days. There is now documentation of mupirocin-resistant strains of staphylococci. Although most topical antibiotics cause at least partial clinical improvement, they may prolong the carriage state of the bacteria on the skin surface. Healthy children with impetigo that is widespread or recalcitrant to topical therapy may require oral antibiotics. Preferred oral antibiotics include antistaphylococcal penicillins, amoxicillin-clavulanate, cephalosporins, and macrolides. Erythromycin is not typically recommended due to widespread resistance in North America. If MRSA is recovered from a culture, bacterial sensitivities should guide drug selection. If *Streptococcus pyogenes* is cultured, penicillins are preferred.

What would the appropriate treatment plan for this diagnosis be if the patient were febrile and/ or showing other signs of systemic illness?

Infants and children with extensive disease, signs of progressive cellulitis, and systemic symptoms may need hospitalization for parenteral antibiotic therapy and close observation.

What is the appropriate plan for follow-up care?

A follow-up appointment in 7–10 days to assess response to treatment may be helpful. However, the high rate of cure and low rate of complications related to impetigo may render follow-up unnecessary except in recalcitrant cases.

Are any referrals needed?

Not typically, but some serious or special cases (as mentioned above) may need hospitalization.

Should the patient stay out of school and/or day care during treatment? If so, for how long?

Children should be treated for a minimum of 24 hours before returning to school or other group settings such as day care in order to avoid spread.

What, if anything, should be recommended to unaffected household members?

It is important to emphasize good hygiene to the patient and family members in order to prevent further autoinoculation and spread to previously unaffected contacts. Good hand washing with antibacterial soap and disinfection of fomites is useful.

REFERENCES AND RESOURCES

Cohen, B. A. (2005). *Pediatric dermatology* (3rd ed.). Philadelphia, PA: Elsevier Mosby.

Cole, C., & Gazewood, J. (2007). Diagnosis and treatment of impetigo. *American Family Physician*, 75(6), 859–864.

Durupt, F., Mayor, L., Bes, M., Reverdy, M.-E., Vandenesch, F., Thomas, L., & Etienne, J. (2007). Prevalence of *Staphylococcus aureus* toxins and nasal carriage in furuncles and impetigo. *British Journal of Dermatology*, 157, 1161–1167.

Silverberg, N., & Block, S. (2008). Uncomplicated skin and skin structure infections in children: Diagnosis and current treatment options in the United States. *Clinical Pediatrics*, 47(3), 211–219.

Weston, W. L., Lane, A. T., & Morelli, J. G. (2007). *Color textbook of pediatric dermatology* (4th ed.). Philadelphia, PA: Mosby Elsevier.

Case 4.2 Eye Irritation

By Anna Tielsch Goddard, CPNP-PC

SUBJECTIVE

Tim was sent to the nurse practitioner in the school based health center (SBHC) when his teacher noticed that his eyes were red. Tim is a 13-year-old male in the ninth grade who reports that when he woke up this morning he thought his right eye was a little red and that he has been scratching it all day. He has not used any eye drops or medications today. He reports no double vision but that his eyes are "hurting a little." He said that he had more morning "eye crusties" than usual this morning when he woke up, but no tearing or discharge. He reports that no one is sick at home but that his best friend also had reddened eyes and stayed home from school. Tim does not have glasses or wear contacts. He denies any other symptoms including upper airway congestion or history of seasonal allergies. He does not have asthma or eczema.

Diet: Tim has a normal appetite and eats a varied diet.

Elimination: Tim denies any abdominal pain, nausea, vomiting, or diarrhea. He does not have any irregular voiding patterns or problems going to the bathroom.

Past medical history: He has had nosebleeds in the past, such as when he was hit with a baseball in gym class, but does not experience regular epistaxis. He did not have a cold this past winter, but his brother had the H1N1 virus. Tim has never had any surgical procedures or stayed in the hospital overnight.

Family history: Family history is negative for cancer, heart disease, and diabetes. Tim's grandfather has early onset dementia and rheumatoid arthritis. He does not think that anyone he is related to has asthma or seasonal allergies, but he is unsure. His grandmother has high blood pressure and dyslipidemia and had a stroke several months ago. Tim reports that his grandmother "sees a doctor for her heart." He is not related to anyone with any bleeding or clotting problems or history of anemia. There are no known family members with epilepsy or a history of seizures. Family history is negative for Crohn disease and ulcerative colitis as well as any immunodeficiencies. He has both an aunt and uncle who are alcoholics. He reports that his aunt also has a "disease of the liver," which he thinks is cirrhosis. He is unaware of anyone he is related to with mental illness or retardation, learning disabilities, or any physical disabilities. His grandmother and mother both smoke but "only outside and not in the house."

Clinical Case Studies for the Family Nurse Practitioner, First Edition. Edited by Leslie Neal-Boylan.
© 2011 John Wiley & Sons, Inc. Published 2011 by John Wiley & Sons, Inc.

Social history: Tim lives at home with his mother and 5-year-old brother in an apartment behind the school. He uses the SBHC and the emergency room for his medical care, as the family does not have insurance. He denies tobacco or substance use. He is not sexually active. His mother works part-time as a gas station attendant while he is at school. He sometimes takes care of his younger brother after school before she gets home from work. He has never met his biological father and does not have any contact with him.

Medications: Tim is currently not on any medications and denies use of vitamins or alternative health care remedies.

Allergies: He does not have any known drug allergies and has "never been diagnosed with seasonal allergies."

Additional review of systems (ROS): Further ROS reveals no change in weight or exercise intolerance, and he is generally in a good state of health. He does not have any rashes, itching, skin lesions, or skin changes. He reports that he gets headaches once in awhile but not on a normal basis and does not have a headache today. There is no history of vertigo, lightheadedness, or any recent injuries. He does not regularly see a dentist, but he receives dental cleanings from the school's visiting dental hygienist and has had all of his cavities filled.

Tim does not have any complaints of neck, joint, or muscle pain or tenderness. He reports that he has never been told that he has a heart problem or murmur and that he has never seen a cardiologist. He only gets short of breath when he runs the 2 mile during gym class and does not have a history of wheezing. He has never had to use an inhaler for any illness in the past and is not currently on any breathing medications.

OBJECTIVE

General: Tim is polite and dressed appropriately for the season.

Vital signs: Within normal limits of 118/72 blood pressure in the right arm; 62 pulse at rest; 16 respirations per minute; 98.7F measured temporally.

HEENT: On examination, the eyes are erythematous bilaterally with yellow crusting at the ends of his eyelashes and across his lower lid; normal visual acuity of 20/20 on the Snellen test; the pupils are equal and round, reactive to light, with accommodation showing normal papillary reflexes. The eyes are aligned equally bilaterally. Ocular motility is normal bilaterally. Ophthalmoscopic examination reveals normal red reflexes and optic discs without hemorrhage of any vessels. The patient's upper eyelids and lacrimal sacs are within normal limits. The hyperemia is throughout the conjunctivae bilaterally with no injection of vessels. Visual fields are normal in all four quadrants. Tim's cornea and lens appear within normal limits with no sign of abrasion.

Tim has a normal hairline and scalp with no alopecia or crusting in the hair. He had passed his hearing test at his last examination and external ear and pinnae are normal on examination. Otoscopic examination reveals normal tympanic membranes with no erythema or bulging and all ossicles visible bilaterally. Nasal septum is vertically aligned with normal turbinates and no internal erythema visible. Nasal mucosa is normal. Tim reports no pain or discomfort during palpation of the frontal and maxillary sinuses. Examination of the oral pharynx shows normal tonsil size of 0/4 with no exudates or drainage. Oral mucosa is moist with intact palate and normal uvular size and location. Tim has several cavities in his mouth and fillings in both of his mandibular molars. No mouth breathing is noted.

Skin: No rashes, scars, or lesions on his skin. Trachea is midline with no lymphadenopathy, normal shoulder shrug, and full range of neck motion in all directions. His neck is easily moveable without resistance in all directions. His spine is straight with no curvature. There are no palpable nodes in the cervical, supraclavicular, or axillary areas.

Respiratory: Lungs are clear in all fields bilaterally with no signs of wheezing, shortness of breath, rales, or crackles.

Cardiovascular: S1/S2 with no murmur, thrill, or irregular beats. PMI is at the fifth intercostal space at the midclavicular line. No fourth heart sound with rub is heard. There are no masses or nipple discharge on examination of the chest. Patient has equal radial, femoral, and anterior tibial pulses bilaterally. No cyanosis, clubbing, or edema is noted.

Abdomen: Symmetrical without any distention. Bowel sounds heard in all four quadrants of examination are normal and not hyperactive; no organomegaly or hepatomegaly. Rectal exam and examination of genitalia were deferred.

Neuromuscular: Normal muscle strength (5/5) in all extremities; normal bicep, ankle, and knee reflexes; normal toe-to-heel walking; and a negative Romberg test. Cranial nerves II–XII are grossly intact. Motor and sensory examinations of all extremities are within normal limits. Deep tendon reflexes are normal bilaterally.

CRITICAL THINKING

Which diagnostic or imaging studies should be considered to assist with or confirm the diagnosis?
___Gram stain of discharge
___Bulbar conjunctiva biopsy
___Slit lamp examination
___Wood lamp examination
___Dilation of pupil using mydriatic medications
___Dilation tonometry

What is the most likely differential diagnosis and why?
___Viral conjunctivitis
___Bacterial conjunctivitis
___Allergic conjunctivitis
___Blepharitis
___Keratitis
___Iritis

What is your plan of treatment?

What is your plan for follow-up care?

Are any referrals needed?

What if the patient were over age 65 or under age 13?

What patient and family education is important with red eye diagnoses?

Are there any standardized guidelines that you should use to assess or treat this case?

RESOLUTION

Diagnostic tests: Diagnostic testing is not generally needed in diagnosing conjunctivitis. Laboratory tests to identify bacteria and sensitivity to antibiotics should only be done in severe cases such as in patients who are immunocompromised, contact lens wearers, or neonates, or when initial treatment fails (Hovding, 2008). Would you perform any of the following diagnostic tests?

1. *Gram stain of discharge.* If the history and physical examination suggests bacterial conjunctivitis but there is no response to topical antibiotics, a gram stain of discharge swabs for bacterial culture will be necessary.
2. *Bulbar conjunctival biopsy.* Biopsy of the conjunctivitis is not indicated for red, itchy, dry eyes.
3. *Slit lamp examination.* A slit lamp examination is used for inspection of anterior eye structures and ocular adnexa and would not be indicated for conjunctivitis differentiation. The slit lamp allows a small beam of light that can be varied in width, height, incident angle, orientation, and color to be passed over the eye. This light beam is narrowed into a vertical slit during examination. Examination of the anterior eye structures is not indicated for erythematous conjunctiva.
4. *Wood lamp examination.* Fluorescein staining before a slit lamp examination or with a Wood lamp (using ultraviolent light) may reveal corneal abrasions or herpes simplex infection. A Wood lamp exam would be indicated if the patient had reactive miosis, possible foreign body, or severe eye pain but none of these were reported or indicated in the history and review of symptoms.
5. *Dilation of pupil using mydriatic medications.* Excessive pupil dilation, or mydriasis, can be induced with a mydriatic medication such as tropicamide to examine the retina and deep structures of the eyes. The history, review of systems, and initial physical examination does not indicate that the provider would need to examine the retina. This procedure is usually reserved for the ophthalmologist.
6. *Dilation Tonometry.* Dilation tonometry measures the intraocular pressure of the aqueous humor of the eye used to determine the intraocular pressure when evaluating glaucoma. This patient did not report throbbing, acute onset eye pain or halos around light, which would lead the practitioner to consider a diagnosis of acute angle glaucoma. There was no reduction in visual acuity, poor reaction to light, or tender eyeball that would indicate dilation tonometry would be indicated.

What is the most likely differential diagnosis and why?
Bacterial conjunctivitis:
Acute bacterial conjunctivitis presents abruptly with red eyes, usually bilateral, mild discomfort or pruritus, and purulent drainage. Diagnosis is based on the patient's history and physical symptoms as laboratory investigation is not generally necessary. Patient report of purulent discharge, which may be described as "extra sleep crusts" or "glue" upon awakening is highly predictive of bacterial conjunctivitis when accompanying red eyes. Mucopurulent discharge is present and mild discomfort may exist but pain is usually absent. Topical antibiotic therapy is indicated because it reduces symptoms, shortens duration and contagiousness, and reduces risk of complication. Bacterial conjunctivitis should be differentiated from viral and allergic conjunctivitis as well as other acute causes of red eyes (Cronau, Kankanala, & Mauger, 2010; Hovding, 2008; Leibowitz, 2000).

Bacterial conjunctivitis is the most common form of conjunctivitis in primary care. It is often called "pink eye" due to the pink appearance of the eye, which results from subconjunctival blood vessel congestion. Symptoms may persist for 3 weeks or more without treatment. *Staphylococcus aureus* infection is often the cause in adults, whereas *Streptococcus pneumonia* and *Haemophilus influenzae* infections are the more common causes in children (Hovding, 2008; Leibowitz, 2000).

Viral conjunctivitis usually presents with upper respiratory symptoms such as cough, rhinorrhea, or nasal congestion. This is usually caused by adenovirus and is highly contagious. Enlarged preauricular nodes and history of upper respiratory tract infection would cause the practitioner to consider a viral cause of infection. Treatment includes cold compresses, artificial tears, and education (Hovding, 2008; Leibowitz, 2000; Sethuraman & Kamat, 2009).

Allergic conjunctivitis is associated with atopic disease such as allergic rhinitis, eczema, and asthma, as well as allergic rhinosinusitis. Itching of the eyes and bilateral tearing are the most apparent features of allergic conjunctivitis. Avoiding exposure to allergens and using artificial tears are effective methods to alleviate symptoms (Sethuraman & Kamat, 2009).

Subconjunctival hemorrhage usually presents unilaterally with localized erythema and adjacent conjunctiva free of inflammation and no discharge. These are usually painless and do not affect vision. Subconjunctival hemorrhage is caused by minor trauma (which includes prolonged coughing, vomiting, or the Valsalva maneuver), fragile vessels, bleeding disorders, anticoagulation therapy, and hypertension. They usually resolve in 2–3 weeks, and failure to resolve warrants referral (Leibowitz, 2000; Sethuraman & Kamat, 2009).

Blepharitis is the acute or chronic inflammation of the eyelid often associated with conjunctival inflammation. Caused by infectious agents, including staphylococci bacteria, allergic disorders, and dermatologic diseases, the corneal surface becomes dry and causes microscopic erosions of the corneal epithelium, mild visual distortion, and photophobia. The patient will usually present with crusting of the eyelid margins, swollen eyelids, and erythematous eyes. Corneal involvement and loss of eyelashes may also occur. Treatment includes warm compresses and a topical antibiotic. Severe blepharitis indicates an ophthalmology referral (American Academy of Ophthalmology Cornea/ External Disease Panel, Preferred Practice Patterns Committee, 2008; American Academy of Pediatrics, American Association of Certified Orthoptists, American Association for Pediatric Ophthalmology and Strabismus, American Academy of Ophthalmology, 2003; Sethuraman & Kamat, 2009).

More serious causes of red eyes include acute glaucoma, keratitis, and iritis. Clinical symptoms that usually suggest a more serious cause include moderate to severe eye pain, extreme redness, ciliary injection, and reduced visual acuity. If a serious eye disease is suspected, then immediate referral should be made to an emergency eye clinic or to ophthalmology for a same day assessment (AAO, 2008).

What is your plan of treatment?
Bacterial and viral conjunctivitis are usually self-limiting, but a topical antibiotic is recommended. Cultures should be reserved for treatment failure as they are expensive and impractical in the case of bacterial or viral conjunctivitis (AAO, 2008). Initial treatment recommendations are broad-spectrum antibiotic such as a combination of polymyxin B sulfate and trimethoprim sulfate, 0.3% gentamicin, 0.5% erythromycin, and 0.3% tobramycin drops or ointments. These antibiotics are effective against gram negative and positive organisms. Studies have shown no difference in effectiveness of different ophthalmic antibiotics. The antibiotic choice should be based on the cost effectiveness and local bacterial resistance patterns of the area (Leibowitz, 2000). Prescription of ointment or drops is a matter of patient choice. Drops are usually preferred because ointment can cause blurred vision. Some schools will require proof of treatment before readmitting students to school (Cronau et al., 2010).

What is your plan for follow-up care?
Patients should be counseled to practice strict hand washing and avoid sharing personal items. Bacterial and viral conjunctivitis are highly contagious and are spread through direct contact with contaminated fingers, medical instruments, or personal items (Cronau et al., 2010). Treatment is supportive with cold compresses, ocular decongestants, and artificial tears. As previously discussed, topical antibiotics are rarely necessary but may decrease time away from work, day care, or school. If the patient's symptoms do not resolve, the clinician should re-evaluate for possible reinfection or other causes of red eyes (AAO, 2008; Sethuraman & Kamat, 2009).

Are any referrals needed?
Referral to an ophthalmologist is indicated if the patient has any of the following: visual loss; moderate or severe pain; severe, purulent discharge; corneal involvement; conjunctival scarring; lack of response to therapy; recurrent episodes; or history of herpes simplex virus (HSV) eye disease or is immunocompromised (AAO, 2008; Cronau et al., 2010). Suspected ocular herpetic infection also warrants an immediate ophthalmology referral. Chronic bacterial or viral conjunctivitis should also be referred to an ophthalmologist (Cronau et al., 2010).

What if the patient were over age 65 or under age 13?
Erythematous conjunctiva in a neonate indicates smears for cytology and gram stains to rule out infectious neonatal conjunctivitis (AAO, 2008). *Chlamydia trachomatis* is the most common cause of conjunctivitis infection in the neonate and is acquired from the infected genital tract during birth. Presentation is usually seen 4–10 days after birth and consists of mucopurulent unilateral or bilateral discharge. Diagnosis is confirmed by culture and can differentiate for *Neisseria gonorrhoeae*. *N. gonorrhoeae* usually presents in the first week of life with purulent discharge, chemosis, and lid edema. Complications lead to blindness. Neonates with either infection should be hospitalized, may need a

septic workup, and IV cefotaxime for *N. gonorrhoeae* or topical erythromycin for *C. trachomatis* (Sethuraman & Kamat, 2009).

Cultures of conjunctiva are indicated in all cases of suspected infectious neonatal conjunctivitis (AAO, 2008). Smears for cytology and special stains are recommended in cases of infectious neonatal conjunctivitis, chronic or recurrent conjunctivitis, and suspected gonococcal conjunctivitis in any age group (AAO, 2008). The clinician must be alert to the possibility of child abuse in cases of potentially sexually transmitted ocular disease in children. STD and suspected child abuse must be reported to local health authorities and other state agencies (Sethuraman & Kamat, 2009). Hyperacute bacterial conjunctivitis is also associated with *Neisseria gonorrhoeae* in sexually active adults, which has a sudden onset and progresses rapidly leading to corneal perforation (Cronau et al., 2010).

Caution should be taken with prescription of myelotoxic drugs in pregnant women in their third trimester because of the possibility of "gray baby syndrome". Gonococcal conjunctivitis is treated with a single IM dose of cefotaxime. Ceftriaxone (Rocephin) should be avoided due to possibility of hyperbilirubinemia (Sethuraman & Kamat, 2009). Chlamydial conjunctivitis is treated with oral antibiotics such as erythromycin.

What patient and family education is important with red eye diagnoses?

The clinician should educate the family and patient about the pathophysiology of bacterial conjunctivitis, risk factors, potential complications, treatment benefits, and complications. The practitioner should advise the family when to seek medical attention for new or worsening symptoms. The patient should be advised to avoid wearing contact lenses until the infection is resolved. Contact lenses that were worn during the infection should be replaced and new lenses and lens case should be used. Other family members including close contacts of the patient should use good hygiene and hand washing processes (AAO, 2008; Cronau et al., 2010).

The practitioner should stress that all family members in the house should use good hand and eye hygiene and avoid close contact with the infected individual.

Are there any standardized guidelines that you should use to assess or treat this case?

The American Academy of Ophthalmology formed a panel to discuss preferred practice patterns of conjunctivitis and created a national guideline which can be found at National Guideline Clearinghouse at http://www.guideline.gov. The guideline reviews the initial evaluation and aspects of a comprehensive medical eye evaluation including history and physical examination. These guidelines emphasize the importance of a referral to an ophthalmologist with any visual loss, moderate or severe pain, severe purulent discharge, corneal involvement, conjunctival scarring, lack of response to therapy, recurrent episodes, history of HSV, or history of being immunocompromised (AAO, 2008).

The American Academy of Pediatrics along with the American Association of Certified Orthoptists, the American Association for Pediatric Ophthalmology and Strabismus, and the American Academy of Ophthalmology, released a policy statement published in *Pediatrics* on the eye examination in infants, children, and young adults by pediatricians that reviews the eye examination and vision assessments done in children (AAP, 2008).

REFERENCES AND RESOURCES

American Academy of Ophthalmology Cornea/External Disease Panel, Preferred Practice Patterns Committee (2008). *Conjunctivitis*. San Francisco, CA: American Academy of Ophthalmology (AAO).

American Academy of Pediatrics, American Association of Certified Orthoptists, American Association for Pediatric Ophthalmology and Strabismus, American Academy of Ophthalmology (2003). Eye examination in infants, children, and young adults by pediatricians. *Pediatrics, 111*(4), 902–907.

Cronau, H., Kankanala, R. R., & Mauger, T. (2010). Diagnosis and management of red eye in primary care. *American Academy of Family Physicians, 81*(2), 137–144.

Everitt, H. A., Little, P. S., & Smith, P. W. (2006). A randomized controlled trial of management strategies for acute infective conjunctivitis in general practice. *British Medical Journal, 333*(7563), 321.

Granet, D. (2008). Allergic rhino conjunctivitis and differential diagnosis of the red eye. *Allergy and Asthma Proceedings, 29*(6), 565–574.

Hovding, G. (2008). Acute bacterial conjunctivitis. *Acute Ophthalmologica, 86*(1), 5–17.

Leibowitz, H. M. (2000). The red eye. *The New England Journal of Medicine, 343*(5), 341–345.

Marlin, D. S. (2009). Conjunctivitis, bacterial. In WebMD's eMedicine Sepcialties. Retrieved from http://emedicine.medscape.com/article/1191730-overview

Sethuraman, U., & Kamat, D. (2009). The red eye: Evaluation and management. *Clinical Pediatrics, 48*(6), 588–600.

Case 4.3 Cough and Difficulty Breathing

By Nancy Cantey Banasiak, MSN, PNP-BC, APRN

SUBJECTIVE

Emily presents to the clinic with her mother with complaints of cough and difficulty breathing. Two days prior, Emily developed a nonproductive cough (which is worse at night), clear rhinorrhea, and a fever with a maximum temperature of 102°. The mother has treated the fever with Tylenol 320 mg every 4 hours, as needed, when the temperature was greater than 101°.

Diet: Emily's appetite is fair with a fluid intake of 32 oz/day of juice/milk/water. She also reports normal eating habits without abdominal pain or diarrhea.

Elimination: Urine output: Voiding 4 times yesterday. No vomiting or diarrhea. Her mother complains that everyone in the house is sick with the same symptoms.

Past medical history: Past medical history is positive for obstructive sleep apnea 4. Birth history was uneventful. She was born full term weighing 3200 g by NSVD (normal sanguineous vaginal delivery). Pregnancy and delivery were uncomplicated with Apgar scores of 8 (1 minute) and 9 (5 minutes). EB also has a history of bronchiolitis at 8 months of age, which did not require medication or hospitalization.

Family history: Mother (age 36) healthy, atopic dermatitis, seasonal allergies; father (age 35) healthy, asthma, seasonal allergies; sibling (age 4) healthy; sibling (age 2) healthy; MGM (age 80) hypertension, breast cancer, basal cell skin cancer; MGF (age 81) hypertension, diabetes mellitus type 2; PGM (age 76) hypertension, obesity; PGF (age 72) deceased, hypertension, stroke.

Social history: Emily is a 6-year-old female in the first grade who lives with her mom, dad, and 2 siblings in a house in the city. They have 4 pets: 2 dogs, 1 cat, and 1 turtle. The parents work outside the home and have private health insurance. Emily and her siblings attend an after-school program until her mom picks them up after work. Emily attends regular medical and dental appointments, and they deny tobacco or alcohol use in the home. She plays soccer, ice hockey, and lacrosse.

Medications: Emily is currently on no medications and has no known allergies to medications, food, or the environment. Immunizations are up to date.

Clinical Case Studies for the Family Nurse Practitioner, First Edition. Edited by Leslie Neal-Boylan.
© 2011 John Wiley & Sons, Inc. Published 2011 by John Wiley & Sons, Inc.

HEENT: History of watery eyes, sneezing, and clear rhinorrhea, especially in the spring. Her mother also complains that "when she gets a cold, it lasts longer than normal."

Skin: She does not have any rashes or skin lesions.

OBJECTIVE

General: Emily is alert, well hydrated, active, and cooperative.

Vital signs: Temperature 38°, pulse 72, and respirations 28 per minute with a blood pressure of 100/52 in the left arm. The O2 saturation is 94%, and weight is 25 kg.

Skin: No lesions, rashes, or scars; and the patient is not cyanotic.

HEENT: Normocephalic with no evidence of trauma or lesions. Eyes show no signs of drainage; sclera white, with pink conjunctiva. Otoscopic examination reveals tympanic membranes gray bilaterally with positive light reflex and normal pinnae. The nose has clear rhinorrhea; no nasal polyps with pink turbinates. Examination of the throat shows a cobblestone appearance in the posterior pharynx, uvula midline, tonsils size 0/4 with no exudate or erythema, moist mucous membranes; and the trachea is midline.

Respiratory: Bilateral inspiratory and expiratory wheezing; mild intercostal retractions; mild shortness of breath; no rales, crackles or nasal flaring.

Cardiovascular: No murmur; normal S1/S2; 2+ brachial and femoral pulses; no cyanosis, clubbing, or edema noted.

Lymphatic: There is no lymphadenopathy on examination.

Abdomen: Soft, nontender abdomen; nondistended; + bowel sounds; no hepatosplenomegaly during palpation.

Genitourinary: Normal female genitalia.

Neurological: Grossly intact.

CRITICAL THINKING

What diagnostic or imaging studies should be considered to assist with or confirm the diagnosis?
___Oxygen saturation
___Chest X-ray
___Nasal pharyngeal culture

What is the most likely differential diagnosis and why?
___Foreign body aspiration
___Bronchiolitis
___Asthma
___GERD

What is the plan of treatment?

What is the plan for follow-up care?

Are any referrals needed at this time?

Are there any standardized guidelines that you should use to assess or treat this case?

RESOLUTION

Diagnostic tests: The nasal pharyngeal culture was positive for respiratory syncytial virus (RSV). Oxygen saturation is 94%, which is an indication of poor exchange of oxygenation. Chest x-ray was negative for pneumonia; and there is no peribronchial cuffing, which is more often seen in bronchiolitis. There was no mediastinal shift or collapsed lung seen with foreign body aspiration.

What is the most likely differential diagnosis and why?
Asthma:
Asthma is the most prevalent chronic illness facing American children today. The diagnosis of asthma is based on the exclusion of alternative diagnoses, as well as the history of recurrent and transient obstructive symptoms, the patient's subjective experience of symptoms, and objective clinical manifestations. These criteria will vary among patients and in the same patient over time. The important signs and symptoms needed to diagnose asthma include (1) recurrent wheeze, (2) improvement of symptoms after treatment with a bronchodilator, (3) recurrent cough or shortness of breath (4) impaired peak flow performance when compared to the expected value based on height and age, and (5) exclusion of alternative differential diagnoses.

A differential diagnosis still requires consideration in any patient who is wheezing, including one with a known diagnosis of asthma and a history of exacerbations. Several conditions may lead to a presentation similar to acute asthma. Some of these include congestive heart failure, vocal cord dysfunction, gastroesophageal reflux, acute bronchitis or bronchiolitis, pulmonary emboli, or the presence of a foreign body.

After the diagnosis of asthma has been made, the severity of the patient's asthma can be classified, based in part on the frequency of symptoms, findings on physical exam, and severity of exacerbations. Severity ranges from intermittent to severe persistent, depending on the frequency of asthma symptoms, nighttime symptoms, and impairment of lung function. Accurate classification of asthma severity is critical because treatment goals and pharmacological management are based on the individual's asthma classification. Because individuals may manifest different symptoms over time, periodic reevaluation, repeat classification of severity, and adjustment of the patient's care plan are necessary.

Information gathered during the initial asthma assessment will serve as baseline data, by determining the patient's respiratory status and the severity of the current exacerbation. After an intervention is implemented, repeat assessments are recommended. These serial assessments can be compared against the baseline data so that trends in the patient's response to treatment can be revealed.
Next, the health care provider can assess the severity of the current exacerbation through auscultation of the lung fields, noting the movement of air and presence of abnormal breath sounds. Medicinal treatment should be started as soon as the diagnosis of asthma exacerbation is confirmed.

What is the plan for follow-up care?
Patients should not leave the health care setting without receiving educational information, a written care plan, a follow-up appointment to take place within 3 days of the exacerbation, and a clear understanding of how to contact the provider should their condition deteriorate. It is recommended that children who have experienced an exacerbation should follow up with their health care provider 2–3 days after the acute episode to (1) monitor the response to treatment, (2) encourage continued patient compliance with their medication regimen, (3) prevent a relapse in symptoms, and (4) provide an educational review of information discussed during previous visits.

Are any referrals needed at this time?
No. The provider should consider a referral to a pulmonologist, allergist, or EENT if symptoms cannot be managed using standard approaches or if the provider thinks that there may be additional factors that complicate the case.

Are there any standardized guidelines that you should use to assess or treat this case?

The following approach to acute asthma treatment is based on the findings of the National Heart, Lung, and Blood Institute Expert Report Panel (2007). This information is meant to serve as a guide to exacerbation treatment. Strict adherence to general guidelines should never supersede individual response to therapy, which is monitored through patient report of symptoms, continuous skilled assessment, and accurate data collection. Adjustments may need to be made initially and ongoing during treatment depending on the patient's prior exacerbation history, present respiratory abilities, and response to treatment. The lowest and simplest dosing regimen that effectively controls the individual's acute asthma should be selected to encourage patient compliance.

An asthma exacerbation should be treated with an early intensification of an inhaled beta$_2$-agonist and the administration of oxygen and an oral or systemic steroid when medically necessary. The inhaled beta$_2$-agonists, known as quick-relief or rescue medications, should be given to all patients regardless of the severity of their exacerbation. Exacerbation therapy should begin with up to 3 treatments of a short-acting beta$_2$-agonist, given at 20-minute intervals over an hour. The minimum dose should be 2.5 mg, or 0.15 mg/kg of body weight. The alternative is to give 2–6 puffs of albuterol, 90 mcg/puff by metered dose inhaler (MDI) with a spacer attachment. However, if no improvement is demonstrated after the initial treatment, the exacerbation severity can be classified as moderate or severe; and a steroid should be given in conjunction with the bronchodilator. The recommended child dose for an oral steroid such as prednisolone is a loading dose of 2 mg/kg of body weight, followed by 2 mg/kg of body weight divided twice a day (maximum dose of 60 mg/day). Additionally, an inhaled beta$_2$-agonist should be given every 4 hours as needed for wheezing.

After the treatment goals have been met, the patient can continue therapy and monitoring independently at home with a short-term intensification of their treatment. For most patients, this means an increase in the frequency of beta$_2$-agonist use and the addition of a systemic steroid.

REFERENCES AND RESOURCES

Baena-Cagnani, C., Rossi, G. A., & Canonica, G. W. (2007). Airway remodeling in children: Where does it start? *Current Opinion in Allergy and Clinical Immunology, 7*(2), 196–200.

Banasiak, N. (2007). Childhood asthma part one: Initial assessment, diagnosis and education. *Journal of Pediatric Health Care, 21*(1), 44–48.

Banasiak, N. C. (2009). Childhood asthma practice guideline part three: Update of the 2007 national guidelines for the diagnosis and treatment of asthma. *Journal of Pediatric Health Care, 23*(1), 59–61.

Banasiak, N., & Bolster, A. (2008). Pediatric asthma. *RN, 71*(7), 26–31.

Boluyt, N., van der Lee, J. J., Moyer, V. A., Brand, P. L. P., & Offringa, M. (2007). State of evidence on acute asthma management in children: A critical appraisal of systematic reviews. *Pediatrics, 120,* 1334–1343.

Hanania, N. A. (2009). Asthma control: A new perspective on the management of asthma. *Current Opinion in Pulmonary Medicine, 15*(1), 1–3.

Horner, C. C., & Bacharier, K. B. (2009). Diagnosis and management of asthma in preschool and school-age children: Focus on the 2007 NAEPP Guidelines. *Current Opinion in Pulmonary Medicine,* 52–56.

Meadows-Oliver, M., & Banasiak, N. C. (2005). Asthma medication delivery devices. *Journal of Pediatric Health Care, 19*(2), 121–123.

National Asthma Education & Prevention Program (2007). *Expert panel report 3: Guidelines for the diagnosis and management of asthma* Bethesda, MD: National Institute of Health.

Parsons, J. P., & Mastronarde, J. G. (2009). Exercise-induced asthma. *Current Opinion in Pulmonary Medicine, 15*(1), 25–28.

Robinson, P., & Van Asperen, P. (2009). Asthma in childhood. *Pediatric Clinics of North America, 56,* 191–226.

Stewart, L. J. (2008). Pediatric asthma. *Primary Care: Clinica in Office Practice, 25*(1), 25–40.

Case 4.4 Obesity

By Elaine Gustafson, MSN, PNP

SUBJECTIVE

Tara, a 12-year-old girl, came to the community health clinic with her mother, who had requested an urgent appointment to discuss a note from Tara's physical education teacher with her nurse practitioner (NP). The note stated that Tara was having difficulty keeping up with her classmates because she became short of breath when participating in activities. Tara denies any other episodes of shortness of breath but reports that she occasionally has to stop and rest when climbing stairs. She has no persistent cough, wheeze, or seasonal allergies. She reports that she has not yet had a period.

Diet history: Tara seldom eats breakfast at home and occasionally will eat cereal from the school breakfast. For lunch she likes pizza or macaroni and cheese but does not eat if these items are not on the school menu. She arrives at her grandmother's house around 3:30 p.m. and has a salty snack and a soda. She eats dinner with her father, either at home or at a local fast-food restaurant.

Sleep history: Tara's mother notes that she snores loudly and sometimes awakens at night. She is currently not taking any medications.

Past medical history: Tara was born after 36 weeks' gestation to a 39-year-old mother. She weighed 4 lb and 14 oz; and, in addition to being preterm, she was small for gestational age. Her mother smoked ½ ppd. Her neonatal history was unremarkable, and she was discharged at 1 week of age weighing 5 lb 2 oz. She was formula fed.

Her past medical history is otherwise unremarkable except for treatment on 2 occasions for right otitis media at ages 1 and 5 and for day surgery at age 18 months to repair a bi-lateral inguinal hernia. There were no complications. She has no history of respiratory illness, asthma, or allergy.

Family history: Positive for type 2 diabetes in Tara's maternal grandmother. Her father is positive for cardiovascular disease and had a mild heart attack at age 48, has high blood pressure, and takes statins for elevated cholesterol. Her maternal grandfather died at age 42 from a heart attack and diabetes. Her paternal grandparents are reportedly alive and well and are living in Puerto Rico.

Social history: Tara is in sixth grade. She is seldom absent and frequently makes the honor roll. She says she likes school but notes that she is shy and has few friends. She does not take part in any extracurricular activities and spends her after-school time helping her grandmother cook or watching

Clinical Case Studies for the Family Nurse Practitioner, First Edition. Edited by Leslie Neal-Boylan.
© 2011 John Wiley & Sons, Inc. Published 2011 by John Wiley & Sons, Inc.

TV. She likes to read. She denies ever using tobacco products, drugs, or alcohol. She admits to feeling sad and lonely at times but denies ever wanting to injure herself. She likes her parents but says they don't always understand her or have time to talk to her.

Tara lives with both parents in a 2-bedroom, third floor apartment near to her school. Her father is employed as a laborer, and her mother works for a cleaning service 5 evenings a week. The family has a stable income. She has 3 older siblings, ages 17, 19, and 21, living out of the home. Her maternal grandmother lives nearby, and Tara often goes to her home after school. Both parents were smokers previously but stopped 5 years ago. They moved to this area from Puerto Rico 20 years ago. Both speak fluent English.

OBJECTIVE

General: Tara is a 12-year-old, Hispanic female who is neatly dressed and cooperative.

Vital signs: She is 5 feet tall and weighs 174 pounds. Her blood pressure is 116/70, pulse is 74, and respirations are 16 breaths/minute. Temperature is normal.

HEENT: PERRLA; EOMs intact. Oral pharynx is positive for 3+/4 tonsils, without lesions or exudate. No dental caries are noted.

Neck: Supple with full range of motion. No lymphadenopathy is present.

Respiratory: Her lungs are clear bilaterally with no wheezes, rales, or rhonchi.

Cardiac: Normal sinus rhythm with no murmur or irregular beats.

Chest: Breast buds are present bilaterally, with no tenderness or discharge.

Abdomen: Soft but protuberant with no masses or hepatosplenomegaly. Normal bowel sounds are heard in all 4 quadrants.

Neuromuscular: Back is straight with no curvature noted on forward bend. She has full range of motion in all extremities. Reflexes are normal.

Skin: Clear except for darkly pigmented areas on her neck.

CRITICAL THINKING

Which diagnostic or imaging studies should be considered to assist with or confirm the diagnosis?
___BMI
___Oral glucose tolerance test (OGGT)
___Insulin resistance
___Cholesterol screen
___Sleep study
___Psychosocial evaluation

What is the most likely differential diagnosis and why?
___Sleep apnea
___Obesity
___Insulin resistance
___Type 2 diabetes
___Exercise intolerance
___Psychosocial issues

Are any referrals needed at this time?

Can the school be of assistance?

What community resources are available to this family?

What type of nutrition support may aid this family?

Are there standardized guidelines to assess and treat the problem of childhood obesity?

RESOLUTION

Diagnostic tests: Lipid profile, oral glucose tolerance test, and insulin levels would provide a basis to determine if she currently has risk factors for hypercholesterolemia, insulin resistance, or type 2 diabetes. Sleep apnea should also be considered due to the history of snoring; however, it is a less common complication in obese children accounting for approximately 7% of cases (Mallory et al., 1989). A sleep study should therefore be considered.

BMI: Body mass index is a surrogate for adiposity. It is a number calculated from a person's weight in kilograms to the square height in meters. It provides an indicator of adiposity and is used to screen for weight categories that may lead to health problems.

Oral glucose tolerance test (OGGT): This is a standard laboratory method to determine how the body metabolizes sugar. It is used to diagnose impaired glucose tolerance, a frequent precursor to type 2 diabetes.

Insulin Resistance: Insulin, made in the pancreas helps the body use glucose for energy. In insulin resistance, muscle, fat, and liver cells do not respond properly to insulin; and, as a result, the body requires more insulin to help glucose enter the cells. The pancreas eventually fails to keep up leading to elevated blood glucose levels and type 2 diabetes.

Cholesterol Screen: Cardiovascular disease risk factors are fairly common among obese children. These include elevated cholesterol levels, high blood pressure, and type 2 diabetes. In a population study of obese children, it was found that obese children are more likely to have risk factors associated with cardiovascular disease than other children (Freedman, Mei, Srinivasan, Berenson, & Dietz, 2007).

Sleep Study: Sleep apnea is a less common complication of obesity in children. It is associated with loud snoring and labored breathing and occurs in only a small percentage of obese children.

Psychosocial Evaluation: Psychosocial issues are a fairly common consequence of childhood obesity. Obese children are frequent targets of social discrimination and stigmatization. This may be a cause of low self-esteem that may hinder academic and social functioning over time.

What is the most likely differential diagnosis and why?
Exercise intolerance due to asthma associated with obesity:
The patient is a 12-year-old, Hispanic female with a primary complaint of shortness of breath with exertion. She denies any other symptoms and is taking no medications. Her physical exam is remarkable only for an elevated BMI of 34, which places her in the obese range at greater than the 95th percentile for her age group, and darkly pigmented areas around her neck called acanthosis nigricans, a known risk factor for insulin resistance. Studies have shown an association between obesity and asthma (Luder et al., 1998). In asthma, the airways become narrow and partially obstructed causing breathing difficulty. Cardiovascular disease risk would be another major consideration in Tara's health assessment. In addition to physical concerns, it is important for the provider to also monitor social and emotional development.

Are any referrals needed at this time?
Referral to a dietitian may be helpful. Referral to an ear, nose, and throat specialist would rule out any mechanical breathing difficulties due to enlarged tonsils or adenoids.

Can the school be of assistance?
A referral to the school nurse to counsel and support Tara between office visits may be beneficial.

What community resources are available to this family?

Tara would likely benefit from participation in an after-school activity. Helping her to research programs at her school, her local Boys and Girls Clubs, or her YMCA may assist her on the way to a more active lifestyle. Use of Internet resources like Let's Move may provide ideas to find ways to be more active at home as well.

What type of nutrition support may aid this family?

Involving the entire family in discussing ways to improve eating habits and activity will likely provide much needed guidance. Calorie and fat content lists from local fast-food restaurants will offer guidance in making better food choices.

Are there standardized guidelines to assess and treat the problem of childhood obesity?

The American Academy of Pediatrics released a policy statement in 2003 by the Committee on Nutrition called *Prevention of Pediatric Overweight and Obesity*. It proposes strategies for early identification with the use of BMI and offers options for dietary and physical activity interventions during regular health care visits (American Academy of Pediatrics, Policy Statement, Committee on Nutrition, 2003). The National Association of Pediatric Nurse Practitioners provides guidelines for assessment of physical and mental health concerns in their Health Eating and Activity Together (HEAT) program.

Pediatric obesity is a multi-faceted problem that requires a many-pronged approach. It is a complex health issue involving metabolism, genes, behavior, culture, environment, and socioeconomic status.

Research has shown that there are long-term, midlife, and socioeconomic consequences to being persistently overweight, especially among women and those in a lower socioeconomic class. These include chronic health problems, no further education beyond high school, and higher odds of receiving welfare or unemployment compensation at age 40 (Clarke, O'Malley, Schulenberg, & Johnston, 2010).

In 2011, the tide appears to be turning; early signs of success in the prevention and control of obesity are now emerging. There has been no significant increase in obesity prevalence since 2003. This encouraging sign is attributed to innovative policies and environmental changes in communities, work sites, and schools.

REFERENCES AND RESOURCES

American Academy of Pediatrics, Policy Statement, Committee on Nutrition (2003). Prevention of pediatric overweight and obesity. Retrieved on August 11, 2010. http://aappolicy.aappublications.org/cgi/reprint/pediatrics;112/2/424.pdf

Centers for Disease Control and Prevention. Childhood overweight and obesity. Retrieved on August 11, 2010, http://www.cdc.gov/obesity/childhood/index.html

Clarke, P. J., O'Malley, P. M., Schulenberg, J. E., & Johnston, L. D. (July 7, 2010). Midlife health and socioeconomic consequences of persistent overweight across early adulthood: Findings from a national survey of American adults (1986–2008) American Journal of Epidemiology Advanced access published online. Retrieved from http://aje.oxfordjournals.org/cgi/content/abstract/kwq156v1

Committee on Environmental Health, Policy Statement (2009). The built environment: Designing communities to promote physical activity in children. *Pediatrics, 123*(6), 1591–1598.

Freedman, D. S., Mei, Z., Srinivasan, S. R., Berenson, G. S., & Dietz, W. H. (2007). Cardiovascular risk factors and excess adiposity among overweight children and adolescents: The Bogalusa Heart Study. *Journal of Pediatrics,* Jan: *150*(1), 12–17.

Let's move: America's move to raise a generation of healthier kids. Retrieved from http://www.letsmove.gov/

Luder, E., Melnik, T., & DiMaio, M. (1998). Association of being overweight with greater asthma symptoms in inner city black and Hispanic children. *Journal of Pediatrics, 132*(4), 699–703.

Mallory, G. B., Fiser, D. H., & Jackson, R. (1989). Sleep-associated breathing disorders in morbidly obese children and adolescents. *Journal of Pediatrics, 115*(6), 892–897.

McConnell, P. (2010). Solving the childhood obesity problem, how schools can be part of the solution, practice roundtable. *ICAN Infant, Child and Adolescent Nutrition, 2*(4), 232–236.

National Diabetes Information Clearinghouse. Insulin resistance and pre-diabetes. Retrieved on August 11, 2010. http://diabetes.niddk.nih.gov/dm/pubs/insulinresistance/

Case 4.5 Sore Throat

By Mikki Meadows-Oliver, PhD, RN and Julie Murray, MSN, PNP

Eight-year-old Samantha presents to the office with a complaint of a sore throat for 2 days. She is accompanied by her mother, Michelle. She has had an intermittent fever and her maximum temperature at home was 101°F (oral). Samantha complains that she has pain when she swallows. She also complains of a headache. Both the throat pain and headache are relieved slightly with the use of over-the-counter pain relievers. Samantha has had no vomiting or diarrhea. She has had no runny nose or cough. She denies drooling or difficulty breathing.

Diet: Samantha's nutrition history reveals that she normally has a balanced diet with enough dairy, protein, fruits, and vegetables. Her appetite has decreased over the past 2 days since the throat pain began.

Elimination: She is voiding well with no complaints of dysuria.

Sleep: Samantha usually sleeps approximately 9 hours at night. She usually has no problems falling or staying asleep but since the throat pain has started, her sleep has been interrupted.

Past medical history: Born via vaginal delivery at 38 weeks' gestation. Since being discharged at 2 days of age, she has had no hospitalizations. Samantha had an emergency department visit at 4 years of age for a broken clavicle that she sustained after falling from the jungle gym at preschool. She has had no injuries or illnesses since that time.

Family history: Samantha's mother (28 years old) has a history of hyperthyroidism. Her father (30 years old) is healthy and has no history of chronic medical conditions. Her maternal grandmother (56 years old) has emphysema. Her maternal grandfather (57 years old) has a history of asthma. Samantha's paternal grandfather (58 years old) has a history of hypertension. Her paternal grandmother (53 years old) has multiple sclerosis.

Social history: Samantha currently attends elementary school. She is in the third grade and is doing well, according to Michelle. Samantha lives at home with her mother who works as an office manager. The family has a pet fish. Samantha attends an after-school program.

Medications: Samantha is currently taking no prescription or herbal medications. She has been taking over-the-counter pain relievers/antipyretics to relieve symptoms associated with her throat pain.

Clinical Case Studies for the Family Nurse Practitioner, First Edition. Edited by Leslie Neal-Boylan.
© 2011 John Wiley & Sons, Inc. Published 2011 by John Wiley & Sons, Inc.

Allergies: Samantha has no known allergies to food, medications, or the environment. She is up to date on required immunizations.

OBJECTIVE

General: Alert, quiet, and cooperative; appears well hydrated and well nourished.

Vital signs: Weight in the office today is 36 kg; temperature is slightly elevated at 38.4° Celsius (oral).

Skin: Clear of lesions and warm to touch. There was no cyanosis of her skin, lips, or nails. There was no diaphoresis noted; skin with elastic recoil.

HEENT: Normocephalic; red reflexes are present bilaterally; and pupils are equal, round, and reactive to light. There is no ocular discharge noted. External ear reveals that the pinnae are normal and that there is no tenderness to touch on the external ear. On otoscopic examination, both tympanic membranes are gray, in normal position, with positive light reflexes. Bony landmarks are visible, and there is no fluid noted behind the tympanic membranes. Both nostrils are patent. There is no nasal discharge and no nasal flaring. Samantha's mucous membranes are noted to be moist when examining her oropharynx. Both tonsils are erythematous and inflamed. There are exudates present bilaterally, as well as palatal petechiae.

Neck: Supple and able to move in all directions without resistance; tender anterior cervical nodes present on both sides of the neck; no erythema of the nodes.

Respiratory: Respiratory rate was 28 breaths per minute, and her lungs are clear to auscultation in all lobes. There is good air entry, and no retractions or grunting are noted on examination. No deformities of the thoracic cage noted.

Cardiac: Heart rate was 112 beats per minute with a regular rhythm. There is no murmur noted upon auscultation.

Abdomen: Normoactive bowel sounds were present throughout; soft and nontender; no evidence of hepatosplenomegaly.

Genitourinary: Normal prepubertal female genitalia.

Neuromusculoskeletal: Good tone in all extremities; full range of motion of all extremities; extremities warm and well-perfused. Capillary refill is less than 2 seconds. Her spine is straight.

CRITICAL THINKING

Which diagnostic or imaging studies should be considered to assist with or confirm the diagnosis?
___Throat culture
___Rapid strep test
___CBC
___Monospot
___LFTs

What is the most likely differential diagnosis and why?
___Viral pharyngitis (type?)
___Bacterial pharyngitis (type?)
___Fungal pharyngitis (type?)
___Peritonsillar abscess
___ GABHS

What is your plan of treatment, referral, and follow-up care?

Does this patient's psychosocial history affect how you might treat this case?

What if the patient lived in a rural setting?

Are there any demographic characteristics that might affect this case?

Are there any standardized guidelines that you should use to assess or treat this case?

RESOLUTION

Diagnostic tests: When evaluating a sore throat, several tests may be helpful to determine the cause of the illness and to decide the treatment plan. If group A beta-hemolytic streptococci (GABHS) is suspected, a rapid strep test and a throat culture should be performed. Both tests are needed because the rapid test provides a preliminary result, while the culture provides the final result after 48 hours. The benefits of using the rapid strep test along with the culture are avoiding unnecessary antibiotic usage and treating the patient in an appropriate and timely manner. If the Epstein Barr Virus (EBV) is suspected, a CBC, monospot, and LFTs should be ordered.

If other viral etiology is suspected, diagnostic testing is not needed. Imaging studies are usually not needed unless a retropharyngeal, parapharyngeal, or peritonsillar abscess is suspected. In that case, a plain lateral neck film may be ordered as an initial screening tool.

What is the most likely differential diagnosis and why?
GABHS:
Several differential diagnoses should be considered when evaluating a sore throat. Viral etiologies cause 40% of cases of sore throats, with enteroviruses, adenoviruses, and EBV being the most common. Bacterial pathogens cause 30% of sore throats, which are usually caused by GABHS, although other pathogens such as *Staphylococcus aureus* or *Haemophilus influenzae* should also be considered. Pharyngitis caused by the fungus *Candida albicans* is another differential diagnosis that should be considered, especially for immunosuppressed individuals. Other more urgent diagnoses such as peritonsillar abscess or retropharyngeal abscess need to be ruled out. Given the patient's history of fever of 101°F, sore throat, and headache, along with the physical exam findings of erythematous tonsils with exudates, palatal petechiae, and cervical adenopathy, the most likely diagnosis is GABHS. In addition to this patient's classic symptoms, many children may also experience nausea or vomiting and/or a scarlatiniform rash.

What is your plan of treatment, referral, and follow-up care?
Penicillin VK is the drug of choice for treating GABHS because it is effective and does not contribute to antibiotic resistance. By using Penicillin VK 20 mg/kg/d in 2–3 divided doses for 10 days, not only will the duration of illness be reduced, but the complication of rheumatic fever will be avoided. In pencillin-allergic patients, azithromycin is an appropriate choice. This medication has higher compliance rates due to the 12 mg/kg/d (500 mg maximum) once daily dosing for 5 days. Whether the pharyngitis is viral or bacterial in origin, the use of antipyretics for pain and fever is beneficial, as are other symptomatic treatments such as increasing liquid intake.

Referral to an Ear, Nose, & Throat (ENT) specialist is only necessary should complications arise. Follow-up care is needed if the patient's symptoms worsen or persist for more than 48 hours while on antibiotics.

Does this patient's psychosocial history affect how you might treat this case?
There is nothing in this patient's psychosocial history that would affect how this case is treated.

What if the patient lived in a rural setting?
No changes in diagnosis or treatment are required if the patient lives in a rural setting. However, if the patient has emigrated from or traveled to a high-risk area for diphtheria, other testing and treatment should be considered.

Are there any demographic characteristics that might affect this case?
There is no racial or ethnic predisposition for the development of GABHS. Regarding age, the majority of children who develop GABHS are between 5–10 years of age. Socioeconomic status is not known to be associated with GABHS.

Are there any standardized guidelines that you should use to assess or treat this case?
American Heart Association (2009). See reference below.

REFERENCES AND RESOURCES

Baltimore, R. (2010). Re-evaluation of antibiotic treatment of streptococcal pharyngitis. *Current Opinion in Pediatrics, 22*, 77–82.

Choby, B. (2009). Diagnosis and treatment of streptococcal pharyngitis. *American Family Physician, 79*, 383–390.

Gerber, M. A., Baltimore, R. S., Eaton, C. B., Gewitz, M., Rowley, A. H., Shulman, S. T., & Taubert, K. A. (2009) Prevention of rheumatic fever and diagnosis and treatment of acute streptococcal pharyngitis. A scientific statement from the American Heart Association: Rheumatic Fever, Endocarditis, and Kawasaki Disease Committee of the Council on Cardiovascular Disease in the Young, the Interdisciplinary Council on Functional Genomics and Translational Biology, and the Interdisciplinary Council on Quality of Care and Outcomes Research. *American Heart Association, Circulation 119*, 1541–1551.

Kim, S. (2009). The evaluation of SD Bioline Strep A rapid antigen test in acute pharyngitis in pediatric clinics. *Korean Journal of Laboratory Medicine, 29*, 320–323.

Case 4.6 Rash and Fever

By Mikki Meadows-Oliver, PhD, RN and Jennifer Mygatt, MSN, RN

SUBJECTIVE

Seven-year-old Angela presents to the office with a complaint of a rash for 2 days. She is accompanied by her mother, Jane. Angela has also had a mildly runny nose and cough for 3 days. She has had a low-grade fever, and her maximum temperature at home was 37.9°C (oral). Angela has had no vomiting or diarrhea.

Diet: Normally has a balanced diet with enough dairy, protein, fruits, and vegetables. There has been no change in appetite since her symptoms began.

Elimination: Voiding well with no complaints of dysuria.

Sleep: Sleeps approximately 9 hours at night and has no problems falling asleep or staying asleep.

Past medical history: She was born via cesarean section at 38 weeks' gestation for a breech presentation. Since being discharged home at 4 days of age, she has had no hospitalizations. Angela had an emergency department visit at 5 years of age for sutures to her head after she fell and struck her head on the corner of a table. She has had no injuries or illnesses since that time

Family history: Angela's mother (34 years old) has a history of migraine headaches. Her father (30 years old) is healthy and has no history of chronic medical conditions. Her 5-year-old sibling has type I diabetes. Her maternal grandmother (68 years old) has type II diabetes. Her maternal grandfather (68 years old) has a history of COPD. Angela's paternal grandfather (58 years old) has a history of skin cancer. Her paternal grandmother (53 years old) has hypertension.

Social history: Angela currently attends elementary school. She is in the second grade and is doing well according to her mother. Angela lives at home with her parents and her 5-year-old sibling. Her father is a graduate student, and her mother is an accountant. The family has a pet rabbit.

Medications: Angela is not currently taking any over-the-counter, prescription, or herbal medications. Angela has no known allergies to food, medications, or the environment. At her last well-child check, her mother refused the annual flu shot and the second varicella vaccination because Angela had a cold. The family did not return to the office to receive these 2 vaccines.

Clinical Case Studies for the Family Nurse Practitioner, First Edition. Edited by Leslie Neal-Boylan.
© 2011 John Wiley & Sons, Inc. Published 2011 by John Wiley & Sons, Inc.

OBJECTIVE

General: She is alert, active, and cooperative. She appears well hydrated and well nourished.

Vital signs: Weight in the office today is 33 kg. Her temperature is slightly elevated at 37.9° Celsius (oral).

Skin: A predominantly maculopapular rash is noted on her back and chest. Two vesicles are noted on the upper right side of her chest. There is no rash noted elsewhere in her body. There is no cyanosis of her skin, lips, or nails. There is no diaphoresis noted. Skin has elastic recoil.

HEENT: Normocephalic; red reflexes are present bilaterally; and her pupils were equal, round, and reactive to light. There is no ocular discharge noted. Angela's external ear reveals that the pinnae are normal and that there is no tenderness to touch on the external ear. On otoscopic examination, both tympanic membranes are gray, in normal position, with positive light reflexes. Bony landmarks are visible, and there is no fluid noted behind the tympanic membranes. Both nostrils are patent. There is no nasal discharge, and there is no nasal flaring. Angela's mucous membranes are noted to be moist when examining her oropharynx. There is no inflammation of her tonsils, and there are no oral lesions noted.

Neck: Supple and able to move in all directions without resistance. There is no cervical lymphadenopathy noted.

Respiratory: Rate is 20 breaths per minute, and her lungs are clear to auscultation in all lobes. There is good air entry, and no retractions or grunting are noted on examination. No deformities of the thoracic cage are noted.

Cardiac: Heart rate is 102 beats per minute with a regular rhythm. There is no murmur noted upon auscultation.

Abdomen: Normoactive bowel sounds are present throughout; soft and nontender. No evidence of hepatosplenomegaly.

Genitourinary: Normal prepubertal female genitalia.

Neuromusculoskeletal: Good tone and full range of motion of all extremities; extremities are warm and well-perfused. Capillary refill is less than 2 seconds. Spine is straight.

CRITICAL THINKING

Which diagnostic or imaging studies should be considered to assist with or confirm the diagnosis?
___Tzanck smear
___Viral culture
___Direct fluorescent antigen testing
___Varicella polymerase chain reaction
___KOH smear
___Throat culture for GABHS
___Nasal swab for influenza

What is the most likely differential diagnosis and why?
___Varicella zoster virus (breakthrough)
___Herpes zoster
___Scarlet fever
___Viral exanthem
___Lyme disease
___Tinea corporis

What is your plan of treatment, referral, and follow-up care?

Does this patient's psychosocial history affect how you might treat this case?

What if the patient lived in a rural setting?

Are there any demographic characteristics that might affect this case?

Are there any standardized guidelines that you should use to assess or treat this case?

RESOLUTION

Diagnostic tests: Diagnostic studies to identify a truncal rash can include tests for viruses, bacteria, or fungi. A Tzanck smear of a vesicle scraping would show multinucleated cells if the rash is due to varicella or herpes simplex virus. Additionally, viral culture and direct fluorescent antigen testing (DFA) can be done to differentiate between the two. DFA is more sensitive and much faster than viral culture. If the rash is found to be varicella, polymerase chain reaction (PCR) will assist in determining whether the rash is a wild-type varicella virus or vaccine-induced varicella. If there is any suspicion of a fungal infection, a potassium hydroxide (KOH) smear test can be performed to assess for the presence of hyphae. However, the description of Angela's vesicular rash does not appear to be fungal in origin. In the presence of a sore throat and rash, a bacterial culture for group A beta-hemolytic streptococcus may be performed. No imaging studies are required.

What is the most likely differential diagnosis and why?
Breakthrough varicella zoster virus (VZV), also known as chickenpox:
Key diagnostic clues are the description of the rash as maculopapular with vesicles; the history of a low-grade fever, cough, and rhinitis; and the absence of cervical lymphadenopathy. Angela did not get her second VZV vaccine, and a single dose is only 70%–90% effective for preventing VZV.

As always, other possible diagnoses must be considered. A truncal rash could be shingles, but it is also caused by VZV and only develops after prior infection with the chickenpox. Furthermore, the distribution would most likely be limited to one dermatome. Since Angela reported a sore throat, scarlet fever associated with strep pharyngitis would be part of the differential. However, the scarlet fever rash is often described as a "sandpaper rash," and lacks vesicles. With Angela's symptoms, the rash could also be a viral exanthema. But in the case of a viral exanthema, Angela would likely have a more generalized truncal rash. Lyme disease, with its classic "bulls-eye" rash, must be considered—but this rash is not vesicular. Finally, tinea corporis would be a possible diagnosis; however, Angela's rash does not have erythematous raised edges or central clearing as is common with tinea infections.

Wild-type chickenpox, caused by the varicella zoster virus, is an easily identifiable disease. It is typically a maculopapular rash with vesicles, characteristically with lesions beginning on the trunk and spreading distally. The lesions may be in different stages of healing. A VZV vaccine was introduced in 1995, but one dose is only 70%–90% effective for preventing VZV. It is currently recommended that children get 2 doses of the VZV vaccine. It has been estimated that approximately 7% of children who received only one dose of the VZV vaccine developed VZV over a 10-year period, while only 2.2% of children who received 2 doses developed VZV. In cases of breakthrough VZV, there are often less than 50 lesions, and many times less than 10 lesions. Furthermore, in breakthrough varicella, the rash may be primarily maculopapular with few, if any, vesicles. Typically, the unvaccinated child who contracts chickenpox will have an average of 300–400 vesicles and perhaps, up to 1000 vesicles. It is important for the health care provider to understand that breakthrough varicella infections present differently, and much less acutely, than classic wild-type VZV. If the history and physical presentation of the rash are consistent with VZV, no diagnostic tests are usually done.

What is your plan of treatment, referral, and follow-up care?
Breakthrough VZV is a self-limiting disease. The management is primarily supportive: diphenhydramine for itching and acetaminophen for fever and pain management. Oatmeal baths can be used to

ameliorate itching. Angela should stay home from school until all of her lesions have dried and crusted. Aspirin should be avoided due to the risk of Reye syndrome in children. Acyclovir will not be helpful in Angela's case because her rash appeared more than 24 hours before she presented to the office. The health care provider should inquire about the vaccination status of Angela's brother and whether her parents have positive VZV titers, indicating immunity to the virus.

Does this patient's psychosocial history affect how you might treat this case?

Angela has no psychosocial characteristics that would alter management of her breakthrough VZV.

What if the patient lived in a rural setting?

If Angela lived in a rural setting, the consideration of tick-borne disease might be higher on the differential. However, living in an urban or suburban environment, excursions into rural places need to be considered.

Are there any demographic characteristics that might affect this case?

If Angela were immunocompromised or had contact with an immunocompromised patient, her VZV would be treated more aggressively.

Are there any standardized guidelines that you should use to assess or treat this case?

While there are no standardized guidelines for the management of VZV, the AAP has developed guidelines for the prevention of varicella (American Academy of Pediatrics Committee on Infectious Diseases, 2007).

REFERENCES AND RESOURCES

American Academy of Pediatrics Committee on Infectious Diseases. (2007). Prevention of varicella: Recommendations for use of varicella vaccines in children, including a recommendation for a routine 2-dose varicella immunization schedule. *Pediatrics, 120,* 221–231.

English, R. (2003). Varicella. *Pediatrics in Review, 24,* 372–279. DOI: 10.1542/pir.24-11-372.

Freeman, A., & Shulman, S. (2006). Kawasaki disease: Summary of the American heart association guidelines. *American Family Physician, 74,* 1141–1150.

Case 4.7 Incontinence

By Vanessa Reid, MSN, APRN, CPNP

SUBJECTIVE

An 11-year-old Caucasian female, Kara, enters your school-based health clinic with a request to use your phone to call her mother. "I had an accident," she says. She calls her mother and asks for a change of clothes. While she waits in your office, you talk to her about her "accident."

Kara seems appropriately embarrassed and tells you that she has never wet her pants at school. However, she did have 2 episodes of nocturnal enuresis during the past 2 weeks. When Kara's mother arrives, she tells you that it seems that her daughter has had a "weak bladder" for the past couple of weeks or so. She affirms urinary urgency and increased frequency but denies dysuria or hematuria.

Kara states she also has stomachaches, as she does during this visit. She denies any vomiting or diarrhea, back/flank pain, rashes, or respiratory symptoms. Her mother denies that Kara has had any fevers at home, although Kara tells you she has felt sick several times during this month.

Diet: Typically, Kara will have breakfast and lunch at school (i.e., muffins or Pop-Tarts® with fruit and juice for breakfast and a chicken patty sandwich or slice of pizza with fries, fruit, and 2% milk for lunch). She usually has a peanut butter and jelly sandwich for a snack after school and has dinner at home. A typical dinner meal includes chicken, rice or potatoes, and a vegetable. Kara drinks one glass of milk or juice and a glass of water with her meals. She usually drinks plenty of water throughout the day, including a glass before bed.

Elimination: Kara tells you that she has a bowel movement once every day without complication or difficulty. Her mother says Kara has never had a problem with bowel movements; only her urinary pattern changed.

Sleep: She goes to bed at 8:30 p.m. and is awake for school at 6:30 a.m. during the week. Her schedule is different on the weekends. She normally sleeps through the night and does not take any naps during the day.

Past medical/surgical history: Surgical history includes a tonsillectomy at age 7.

Family history: Family medical history includes hypertension (mother) and asthma (brother). Kara's mother is unsure of the father's family medical history.

Social history: Kara's parents separated, and her father moved out a month ago. She has a 6-year-old brother and a 4-year-old sister. The 4-member family lives on the second floor of a 2-family home in

Clinical Case Studies for the Family Nurse Practitioner, First Edition. Edited by Leslie Neal-Boylan.
© 2011 John Wiley & Sons, Inc. Published 2011 by John Wiley & Sons, Inc.

a neighborhood of multifamily homes built around 1980. Since the separation, Kara and her siblings have spent 2 weekends with her father and his new girlfriend. Kara's mother works 2 jobs, and the downstairs neighbor helps with caring for the children until she gets home. No public assistance programs are utilized. Kara's school performance has declined since her parents' separation. She has not had any disciplinary problems, but her academic performance has suffered.

Medications: Kara takes no medications and has no known allergies. She has not seen her primary care provider or dentist since she was 8 years old.

OBJECTIVE

General: No apparent distress. Cooperative but without direct eye contact with provider.

Vital signs: Height: 60 inches; weight: 60 lbs; BP: 104/60; HR: 80 bpm; RR: 16 rpm; temperature: 98.6.

HEENT: PERRLA; pearly gray TMs bilaterally. Throat: pink, without exudates or petechiae; tonsils absent.

Neck: No masses; thyroid midline and size within normal limits.

Cardiovascular: RRR, no murmurs; pulses equal at +2; brisk refill.

Chest: CTA throughout. Breast development Tanner I.

Abdomen: + BS × 4; no HSM; soft; no rebound tenderness or masses.

Genitourinary: Within normal limits; Tanner I.

CRITICAL THINKING

Which diagnostic or imaging studies should be considered to assist with or confirm the diagnosis?
___Albumin
___ALT
___AST
___Basic metabolic panel
___BUN
___C-peptide
___Calcium
___CBC w/ Diff
___Comp metabolic panel
___Creatinine
___Fasting plasma glucose
___Free T3
___Free T4
___HbA1c
___IGF
___Insulin
___Insulin tolerance
___OGTT
___Phosphorus
___Plasma ADH
___Potassium

___Random plasma glucose
___Sodium
___T3
___T4
___T3 uptake
___Total T3
___TSH
___Two-hour plasma glucose
___Ultrasound, abdominal
___Ultrasound, renal
___Urinalysis
___Urine culture

What is the most likely differential diagnosis and why?
___Urinary tract infection (UTI)
___Diabetes mellitus
___Hyperthyroidism
___Normal urinary function

What is the plan of treatment?

Are any referrals needed at this time?

RESOLUTION

Diagnostic tests: Comp metabolic panel (collected after 12-hr fast, at 0800 hrs):
Na: 140 mmol/L; K: 3.9 mmol/L; Cl: 100 mmol/L; CO_2: 24 mmol/L; Gluc: 187 mg/dL; Ca: 9.7 mg/dL; BUN: 12 mg/dL; Creatinine: 0.6 mg/dL; Total protein: 6.8 g/dL; Alb: 4.1 g/dL; AST: 22 U/L; Alk phos: 205 U/L; Bilirubin, Total: 0.8 mg/dL; ALT: 23 U/L.
HbA1c: 8.4
Urine culture: No growth in 48 hours.
Urine dipstick (clean-catch): pH = 6; Specific gravity = 1.015; Protein: neg; Glucose: pos; Ketones: neg; Nitrites: neg; Leukocyte esterase: neg; Blood: neg; Bilirubin: neg
TSH: 2.6 uIU/mL.
Two-hr plasma glucose: 243.

What is the most likely differential diagnosis and why?
Type 1 (insulin-dependent) diabetes mellitus:
Kara's negative urine culture rules out the possibility of a UTI, and her normal TSH level makes it very unlikely that she has hyperthyroidism (Ross, 2008). The glucose-positive urine dip, elevated fasting glucose, 2-hour glucose, and HbA1c all support a diagnosis of diabetes mellitus. Sometimes, children with Type 1 diabetes mellitus are asymptomatic and diagnosed after an incidental finding during a physical exam. Other times, a diagnosis may result from the child's presenting to the emergency department in diabetic ketoacidosis or after presenting with the classic new-onset symptoms of polyuria, polydypsia, and polyphagia. Appetite is increased initially, but the elevated catabolism and hypovolemia lead to weight loss (Levitsky & Misra, 2010).

A urinalysis and a random blood glucose can be done quickly and conveniently in the office. It is important to remember that glucosuria may suggest diabetes but is not diagnostic in and of itself. Other disorders that affect renal function, such as Fanconi syndrome, may cause glucosuria as well (Brazy, 2006). The following are criteria for a diabetes diagnosis as set forth by the American Diabetes Association (2010): 1. HbA1c ≥6.5 % OR 2. Fasting plasma glucose ≥126 mg/dL OR 3. Two-hr plasma glucose ≥200 mg/dL during an oral glucose tolerance test, using a glucose load of 75 g of anhydrous glucose dissolved in water. Any of these three criteria must be confirmed by a repeat test for confirmation if no unequivocal hyperglycemia is present. If classic symptoms of hyperglycemia or hyperglycemic crisis are present, then a random plasma glucose ≥200 mg/dL is sufficient for a diagnosis (American Diabetes Association [ADA], 2010).

Diabetes in general is a metabolic disorder that results from defective insulin action, insulin secretion, or a combination of both (ADA, 2010). The hallmark of Type 1 diabetes mellitus is an absolute insulin deficiency. The autoimmune destruction of pancreatic beta cells prohibits the insulin production. The difference between Type 1 diabetes and Type 2 is that the insulin deficiency is relative, rather than absolute, in Type 2. Insulin resistance leads to an initial increase in insulin production. Eventually, the pancreas is unable to keep up with the increased insulin requirements; hence, there is a relative insulin deficiency (Cooke & Plotnik, 2008). In many instances, people with Type 2 diabetes are overweight because the extra weight, especially increased abdominal girth, plays a major role in insulin resistance. However, the rise of childhood obesity and adult-onset Type 1 diabetes have blurred the definitions of "juvenile diabetes" and "adult-onset" diabetes, which were used synonymously to describe Type 1 and Type 2, respectively. The clinician should be careful to refrain from making assumptions about type based on body habitus or age of presentation. It is also important to consider that both types may exist in the same person (McCulloch, 2009).

Diabetes mellitus must be properly typed in order to be effectively managed. After initial testing, additional laboratory assessments may be needed to aid in solidifying a diagnosis. Although the presence of serum antibodies to pancreatic islet cells, glutamic acid decarboxylase (GAD), the 40K fragment of tyrosine phosphatase (IA2), and/or insulin strongly suggests Type 1 diabetes, the absence of such antibodies does not exclude a Type 1 diagnosis (Levitsky & Misra, 2010). Measuring C-peptide is helpful since it is secreted along with insulin in a one-to-one molar ratio. Dissimilar to insulin, there is little first-pass liver clearance, but it still indicates a direct relationship to endogenous insulin secretion. C-peptide measurements under standardized conditions are an acceptable assessment of beta-cell function (Palmer et al., 2004).

What is the plan of treatment?
Education is key. Glucose monitoring, ketone monitoring, insulin administration, how to operate an insulin pump, and how to recognize signs/symptoms of hypoglycemia are just a few of the instructional points which usually have to be reiterated. It is crucial to also provide appropriate mental health services for the child and the family. Kara's new diagnosis requires lifestyle changes and development of coping and management strategies which affect family function, thereby placing Kara and her mother at increased risk for depression (Jaser, Whittemore, Ambrosino, Lindemann, & Grey, 2008).

Are any referrals needed at this time?
Kara was referred from the school-based health center to a diabetes clinic that employs a multidisciplinary approach to education and management of diabetes. In Kara's case, it is a good idea to refer her for mental health counseling, since she is coping with her parents' separation, also. She has additional medical and mental health support at school through the school-based health center, school nurse, and school psychologist. The broader the support base, the better the outcome.

REFERENCES AND RESOURCES

American Diabetes Association (2010). Diagnosis and classification of diabetes mellitus. *Diabetes Care, 33*, S62–S69.

Brazy, P. C. (2006). Fanconi syndrome. Retrieved from http://www.merck.com/mmhe/sec11/ch146/ch146f.html

Cooke, D. W., & Plotnik, L. (2008). Type 1 diabetes mellitus in pediatrics. *Pediatrics in Review, 29*, 374–385.

Davidson, M. B. (2001). How do we diagnose diabetes and measure blood glucose control? *Diabetes Spectrum, 14*(2), 67–71.

Gassner, H. L., & Gitelman, S. E. (2003). Case study: Type 1 and type 2, too? *Clinical Diabetes, 21*(3), 140–141.

Halvorson, M., Yasuda, P., Carpenter, S., & Kaiserman, K. (2005). Unique challenges for pediatric patients with diabetes. *Diabetes Spectrum, 18*(3), 167–173.

Jaser, S. S., Whittemore, R., Ambrosino, J. M., Lindemann, E., & Grey, M. (2008). Mediators of depressive symptoms in children with type 1 diabetes and their mothers. *Journal of Pediatric Psychology, 33*(5), 509–519.

Levitsky, L. L., & Misra, M. (2010). Epidemiology, presentation, and diagnosis of type 1 diabetes mellitus in children and adolescents. In *UpToDate Online18.1*. Retrieved from http://www.uptodate.com/online/content/topic.do?topicKey=pediendo/16769&selectedTitle=1%7E150&source=search_result

McCulloch, D. K. (2009). Classification of diabetes mellitus and genetic diabetic syndromes. In *UpToDate Online 18.1*. Retrieved from http://www.uptodate.com/online/content/topic.do?topicKey=diabetes/24654&selectedTitle=1%7E150&source=search_result

Murray, R. (2002). Recognizing the signs of metabolic syndrome and polycystic ovary syndrome in a caucasian adolescent girl: Differentiating type 2 from type 1 diabetes. *Diabetes Spectrum, 15*(4), 227–231.

Palmer, J. P., Fleming, G. A., Greenbaum, C. J., Herold, K. C., Jansa, L. D., Kolb, H., & Steffesu, W. (2004). C-Peptide is the appropriate outcome measure for type 1 diabetes clinical trials to preserve β-cell function: Report of an ADA workshop, 21–22 October 2001. *Diabetes, 23*, 250–261.

Roper, S. O., Call, A., Leishman, J., Ratcliffe, G. C., Mandleco, B. L., Dyches, T. T., & Marshal, E. S. (2009). Type 1 diabetes: Children and adolescents' knowledge and questions. *Journal of Advanced Nursing, 65*(8), 1705–1714.

Ross, D. (2008). Diagnosis of hyperthyroidism. In *UpToDate Online 18.1*. Retrieved from http://www.uptodate.com/online/content/topic.do?topicKey=thyroid/18839&selectedTitle=1%7E150&source=search_result

Case 4.8 Disruptive Behavior

By Patricia Ryan-Krause, MS, RN, MSN, CPNP

SUBJECTIVE

This mother presents with 6-year-old Jack with concerns about his increasingly disruptive behavior at home. She reports that Jack has always been a difficult child to manage, often is irritable, angers easily, and resists any changes in routine. He argues constantly with his 8-year-old sister about simple activities. He grabs her toys, interferes with her play, and has begun to be more physically aggressive with her. Jack argues with his mother and grandmother when any limits are put on his behavior. He is uncooperative regarding the simplest of requests like coming to the table for meals, turning off his video games, or staying in the yard. Jack has had a few good relationships with children in the neighborhood. His mother has attempted to discipline Jack thorough a variety of methods, such as talking, screaming, time out, losing TV and video game time, and occasional spankings. His mother reports that no methods work. She is exhausted by the attention she spends on his behavior and is frustrated facing discipline issues every day from breakfast to bedtime. She is confused because her daughter has never demonstrated these types of issues, and she used basically the same parenting strategies with her daughter as she did with Jack. His mother has not spoken with Jack's first-grade teacher to see if similar behaviors are occurring in school.

Diet: Jack has been a healthy child. He had some initial feeding issues as an infant with excessive irritability causing multiple formula changes. Since then he has had no food allergies or intolerances and eats a fairly well-balanced diet with the exception of excessive juice consumption.

Elimination: No difficulties.

Sleep: Jack has had difficulty establishing nighttime sleep patterns. He continues to have difficulty with sleep onset, wakes frequently, and goes into his mother's bed.

Past medical history: Jack was the second child born to a 27-year-old mother by vaginal delivery after an uneventful full-term pregnancy. He weighed 7 lbs 9 oz and had no problems in the newborn nursery (no temperature instability, no jaundice, and no respiratory issues). He was discharged home with his mother on cow's-milk formula at 48 hours of age. Jack experienced a head injury with a loss of consciousness at the age of 3 years, His head CT was normal, but he was admitted to the pediatric unit for overnight observation. He has not had any obvious sequelae from this incident. Jack has had no respiratory, cardiac, neurologic, or allergic problems.

Clinical Case Studies for the Family Nurse Practitioner, First Edition. Edited by Leslie Neal-Boylan.
© 2011 John Wiley & Sons, Inc. Published 2011 by John Wiley & Sons, Inc.

Family history: Jack's mother has history of Hashimoto thyroiditis and depression and is medicated for both of these conditions. She is fairly adherent to her medication regime. She was an average student, graduated from high school, and works as a cashier. His 33-year-old father has a history of substance abuse, depression, and hypertension. He was incarcerated briefly for selling drugs and now declines all medications. He did not complete high school, has a history of delinquency and attention problems, and currently works intermittently in construction. The maternal grandparents both have well-controlled hypertension and hypercholesterolemia. The paternal grandparents' histories are unknown to the father since he has not had contact with them in 15 years. Jack's sister is healthy and doing average school work.

Social history: Jack's mom is single and lives on the second floor of a 1940s 2- family house with the maternal grandparents on the first floor. The household consists of his mother, an 8-year-old sister, 2 dogs, and several cats. His mother and the children have frequent contact with the father, but he is not a regular part of the household. Both parents smoke while with the children. Jack attended daycare full-time until school entry but now returns home to the care of his grandparents after school. Toward the end of his time in daycare, his mom reports that she had received a few calls about Jack's behavior, specifically some difficulties participating in group activities and following directions.

Medications: Takes no medications.

OBJECTIVE

General: Alert, active, responsive to most requests with good articulation, some fidgeting with instruments.

Vital signs: Height: 46 inches (115 cm); weight: 45 lbs (20.9 kg); heart rate: 92; respiratory rate: 18; blood pressure: 98/62.

HEENT: Normocephalic; PERRL full EOMs, normal convergence, normal discs; gray TMs with good light reflexes and landmarks. Nose is normal, midline septum, boggy turbinates. Throat reveals large tonsils, no erythema, and uvula midline.

Neck: Supple; FROM; thyroid not palpable; no LAD.

Cardiac: RRR; S1/S2; no murmur; pulses full and equal.

Respiratory: Clear breath sounds throughout.

Abdomen: Soft, no mass, no HSM.

Genitourinary: Normal male, circumcised, testes descended ×2.

Musculoskeletal: FROM all extremities; symmetric movement.

Neurologic: Normal tone, strength, coordination, reflexes and cranial nerves II-XII grossly intact.

Skin: Clear, dry patches on elbows and knees.

CRITICAL THINKING

Which diagnostic or imaging studies should be considered to assist with or confirm the diagnosis?
___CBC
___Thyroid studies
___Lead screening
___Vision screening

___Hearing screening
___Vanderbilt ADHD screening for school and parent
___Learning disability evaluation
___Pediatric Symptom Checklist

What is the most likely differential diagnosis and why?
___Normal active behavior of early childhood
___Hearing impairment
___Attention deficit hyperactive disorder (ADHD)
___Learning disability
___Oppositional defiant disorder
___Conduct disorder
___Depression

What is the plan of treatment?

What is the plan for follow-up care?

Are there any demographic factors that might affect this case?

Are there any standardized guidelines that you should use to assess or treat this case?

RESOLUTION

Diagnostic tests: Selected lab evaluations help to convince parents that the child is physically healthy and that other conditions may be important to consider. A CBC and lead screening assures that there is no anemia, infection, or elevated lead level. Hyperactive thyroid would be very unlikely to present this constellation of symptoms and need not be obtained unless the mother is very concerned because of her own thyroid disorder. Vision and hearing screening are essential to assure that Jack has intact sensory systems so he is able to respond appropriately to directions and facial cues.

Jack's hearing screen was normal. Vanderbilt ADHD screening indicated no concerns with inattentiveness or combined type ADHD. Information gathered from the school suggested that Jack started the year as a capable student who has begun to lag behind his peers, especially in reading and social skills. Jack's mother completed The Pediatric Symptom Checklist. Scoring revealed that Jack has trouble obeying his teacher, is often irritable and angry, fights with other children, does not listen to rules, does not understand other people's feelings, blames others for his troubles, teases others, and refuses to share.

What is the most likely differential diagnosis and why?
Oppositional defiant disorder:
To arrive at a working diagnosis, much more information needs to be gathered from Jack's teacher and from standardized screening tools and possibly school assessments of learning issues. Based on the test results and further history from his mother and teacher, it appears that Jack meets the DSM-IV diagnostic criteria for Oppositional Defiant Disorder (ODD). This diagnosis is more likely than depression. Jack's behavior is more extreme than his peers, and it interferes with his social and academic development. Jack also has numerous risk factors for this disorder including financial problems in the family, family instability, a parent with a substance abuse disorder, parents with a history of ADHD, lack of positive parental involvement, and inconsistent discipline.

What is the plan of treatment?
Discuss the diagnosis with his mother and father. Reinforce that this is a manageable condition and that primary care will provide support to the family in their efforts to make change. Discuss that early intervention is critical and has the greatest possibility of preventing ODD from progressing to conduct disorder. Address parental concerns and assure them that effective, consistent discipline can make significant improvements.

- Recommend parent-focused discipline literature such as *1-2-3 Magic* by Thomas Phelan.
- Refer for parent-management training such as Russell Barkley's Parent Management Training or Ross Greene's Collaborative Problem-Solving.
- Refer to Conduct Clinic, if available in community or university setting.
- Refer for family therapy or individual play therapy for Jack.
- Consider social skills training if peer relationships deteriorate.
- Encourage close communication with his teacher to assure consistent approaches to behavior changes.
- If comorbid ADHD develops at a later time, stimulant medications may be helpful.

What is the plan for follow up care?
Follow up in the primary care setting to reinforce strategies learned in therapy and to offer continued support for family efforts. Encourage the grandparents' participation in visits so they will utilize the same approaches as the parents are learning,

Are there any demographic factors that might affect this case?
This condition can occur in any socioeconomic or racial group. Risk factors are noted above.

Are there any standardized guidelines that you should use to assess or treat this case?
American Psychiatric Association (2000). See reference below.

REFERENCES AND RESOURCES

American Psychiatric Association (2000). Diagnostic and statistical manual of mental disorders, 4th text revision DSM IV-IV TR, 4th edition, APA, Washington, DC.

Barkley, R. A. (1997). *Defiant children*. New York, NY: The Guilford Pres.

Greene, R. W., Ablon, J. S., & Goring, J. C. (2003). A transactional model of oppositional behavior: Underpinnings of the Collaborative Problem Solving approach. *Journal of Psychosomatic Research, 55*, 67–75.

Jellinek, M. S., Murphy, J. M., Little, M., et al. (1999). Use of the Pediatric Symptom Checklist (PSC) to screen for psychosocial problems in pediatric primary care: A national feasibility study. *Archives of Pediatrics & Adolescent Medicine, 153*(3), 254–260.

Case 4.9 Nightmares

By Mikki Meadows-Oliver, PhD, RN and Allison Grady, MSN, RN

SUBJECTIVE

Six-year-old Dexter presents to the office with his mother, Deborah, with complaints of frequent nightmares. Deborah states that Dexter will be asleep and will suddenly sit upright with his eyes open and start to scream loudly. She says that Dexter looks terrified and that he sweats and breathes fast during these episodes. Deborah says that while Dexter is screaming, she is unable to wake, console, or comfort him. The screaming episodes typically last about 5 minutes each and happen 3–4 times weekly. Deborah states that after the screaming stops, Dexter returns to sleep and does not remember the screaming episodes when he awakens in the morning. Dexter does not have any problems falling asleep. He sleeps approximately 10 hours each night but does not have a set bedtime or a regular bedtime routine. He sleeps in his own bed and shares a room with his younger brother.

Diet: Balanced diet with sufficient sources of dairy, protein, fruits, and vegetables.

Elimination: Dexter is voiding well with no complaints of dysuria. He has 1 bowel movement daily and denies constipation or diarrhea.

Past medical history: Born via vaginal birth at 40 weeks' gestation. The mother's pregnancy was without problems. She had no infections, falls, or known exposures to environmental hazards. She did not drink alcohol, take prescription medication (other than prenatal vitamins), use tobacco products, or use illicit drugs. There were no problems for Dexter during his neonatal period. Since birth, he has had no injuries or illnesses requiring visits to the emergency department. He has no chronic illnesses.

Family history: Dexter's mother (27 years old) and father (26 years old) are both healthy and have no history of chronic medical conditions. His three-year-old sibling also has no history of chronic medical conditions. His maternal grandmother (54 years old) has a history of asthma. His maternal grandfather (55 years old) has a history of high cholesterol. Dexter's paternal grandmother (52 years old) has a history of hypertension. His paternal grandfather (52 years old) has a history of hypertension and had a stroke at age 47 years.

Social history: Dexter lives at home with his mother, paternal grandmother, paternal uncle, and his younger brother (3 years old). His mother works as a restaurant waitress. Dexter's father is incarcerated. The family has no pets. There are no smokers in the home.

Clinical Case Studies for the Family Nurse Practitioner, First Edition. Edited by Leslie Neal-Boylan.
© 2011 John Wiley & Sons, Inc. Published 2011 by John Wiley & Sons, Inc.

Medications: Dexter is not currently taking any over-the-counter, prescription, or herbal medications. He has no known allergies to medication, food, or the environment. He is up to date for required immunizations.

OBJECTIVE

General: Alert, cooperative, and active; appears well hydrated and well nourished.

Vital signs: Weight in the office was 28 kg. Temperature was 36.9°C (temporal).

HEENT: Normocephalic. Red reflexes are present bilaterally; and pupils are equal, round, and reactive to light. There is no ocular discharge noted; external ear reveals that the pinnae are normal and that there is no tenderness to touch on the external ear. On otoscopic examination, the tympanic membranes are gray bilaterally, in normal position, with positive light reflexes. Bony landmarks are visible, and there is no fluid noted behind the tympanic membranes. Both nostrils are patent. There is no nasal discharge and no nasal flaring. Dexter's mucous membranes were noted to be moist when examining his oropharynx. There is no evidence of visible caries or other lesions in the oral cavity.

Neck: Supple and able to move in all directions without resistance. There was no cervical lymphadenopathy present.

Skin: Clear of lesions; no cyanosis of his skin, lips, or nails; no diaphoresis noted; and there is elastic recoil.

Respiratory: Respiratory rate is 20 breaths per minute, and the lungs are clear to auscultation in all lobes. There is good air entry, and no retractions or grunting are noted on examination. No deformities of the thoracic cage noted.

Cardiac: Heart rate is 102 beats per minute with a regular rhythm. There is no murmur noted upon auscultation.

Abdomen: Normoactive bowel sounds are present throughout. Soft and nontender. No evidence of hepatosplenomegaly.

Genitourinary: Normal circumcised male genitalia without erythema or lesions; testes are descended bilaterally.

Neuromusculoskeletal: Good tone and full range of motion in all extremities. Extremities are warm and well perfused. Capillary refill is less than 2 seconds. Spine is straight.

CRITICAL THINKING

Which diagnostic or imaging studies should be considered to assist with or confirm the diagnosis?
___EEG (electroencephalogram)
___Polysomnography
___MRI (magnetic resonance imaging)
___CT (computed tomography) scan
___Skull radiograph

What is the most likely differential diagnosis and why?
___Nightmares
___Nocturnal seizures
___Night terrors
___Sleepwalking (somnambulism)

What is your plan of treatment, referral, and follow-up care?

Does this patient's psychosocial history affect how you might treat this case?

What if the patient lived in a rural setting?

Are there any demographic characteristics that might affect this case?

Are there any standardized guidelines that you should use for this case?

RESOLUTION

Diagnostic tests: An EEG may reveal altered consciousness during night terror episodes. An EEG will also help to diagnose nocturnal seizures. Polysomnography can help to diagnosis parasomnias such as sleepwalking, nightmares and night terrors. An MRI may show if a brain lesion is causing the problem of night awakening and screaming. A CT Scan and skull radiographs are usually not helpful in the testing for sleep disturbances.

What is the most likely differential diagnosis and why?
Night terrors:
Nightmares happen during REM (rapid eye movement) sleep. Children with nightmares awaken and will recall having vivid dreams. A child who is having a nightmare is fully awake and often will seek comfort from a caregiver. Nocturnal seizures, which occur only during sleep, can cause the victim to cry, scream, walk, run about, or curse. Like other seizures, these are usually treated with medication. With nightmares, the child may also scream and cry. Night terrors (sometimes known as sleep terrors) occur in stage IV of the sleep cycle. Stage IV is also known as slow-wave sleep (SWS) and usually occurs during the first third of the night. Although appearing to be awake, children experiencing a night terror are still in a light sleep. A child suffering from a night terror will be unable to be calmed by a caregiver. Each episode will generally last for less than 5 minutes, although some children experience multiple terrors each night. A child who experiences night terrors will usually have no memory of the event in the morning; while a child with a nightmare may or may not have a memory of the dream, but will almost certainly remember being awake. Night terrors are the most likely diagnosis when taking the history and physical examination into account.

What is your plan of treatment, referral, and follow-up care?
Several factors have been theorized to contribute to night terrors, such as lack of a regular bedtime, a full bladder, and extra noise or lights in the sleeping environment. A treatment plan would encompass education on each of the above aspects. Dexter's lack of a set bedtime may contribute to his being overtired but neither clinical exam nor history suggest that he struggles with daytime fatigue or lack of energy. However, the health care provider should question the mother about this possibility further. A full bladder at the time of a night terror cannot be ruled out and should also be further explored. It should be noted that Dexter shares a bedroom with his younger brother. It is unknown whether the brother uses a nightlight, snores, or otherwise contributes to environmental pollution through music or television.

When providing education, parents should be reminded that the night terror episodes, while disturbing to them, are not remembered by the child. When a child is experiencing a night terror, a parent should check on him to confirm his safety. Although difficult, parents are discouraged from picking up the child or providing other comfort measures. For the child experiencing a night terror, consoling from a parent can cause greater distress and result in full awakening.

The health care provider may suggest that Dexter's mother maintain a sleep diary and observe him throughout several night terror episodes, noting the amount of time after he falls asleep that the night terror begins. After Dexter's sleep-wake pattern is determined, his mother should wake him up approximately 15 minutes before the usual time of the night terror and keep him awake and out of bed for a full 5 minutes. This process should continue for approximately for 5–10 days. By waking up the child before the night terror actually begins, the sleep cycle is consistently disturbed and is then able to be reestablished—typically without the resumption of the night terrors. This may help to break the disruptive sleep pattern that has resulted in the night terrors. Upon awakening the child, the parents can also coax the child to use the bathroom if a full bladder is a suspected contributor to the night terrors.

Prior to sleep, there are other steps that parents can take to reduce the occurrence of night terrors. A consistent bedtime and sleep hygiene routine may reduce the occurrence of night terrors. Dexter's mother can begin by establishing a consistent time for bed along with a regular bedtime routine. Maintaining quiet time without sudden unsettling noises near bedtime may minimize some of the external stimuli that are thought to contribute to night terrors. Since night terrors might be triggered by a full bladder, having Dexter use the toilet prior to bedtime and even during the course of the night might be beneficial in reducing reoccurrence of night terrors. In extreme cases of night terrors, benzodiazepines (known to suppress the stage IV level of deep sleep) have been prescribed, although this is not a standard recommendation. Pharmacological options are controversial and are generally not considered in children under the age of 7 years. Alternative options such as hypnosis, biofeedback, and various relaxation techniques have been used with some success to reduce or eliminate occurrence of childhood night terrors. Calming music or bedtime stories may also assist with the reduction of night terrors.

Followup can be done by telephone in 1–2 weeks to ascertain if the recommendations to reduce the night terrors have been effective. They should also follow up in the office if Dexter exhibits drooling, jerking, or stiffening of the body during the night terror. If the episodes have continued without improvement, consider referring Dexter to a sleep specialist and for a polysomnography test to assist with the diagnosis of a parasomnia.

Does this patient's psychosocial history affect how you might treat this case?
Dexter lives in a home with several family members. With 3 generations of family members in the home, bedtime may not be a quiet time. Including Dexter's grandmother in the treatment plan may also help to reduce or lessen the occurrence of night terrors.

What if the patient lived in a rural setting?
The treatment of night terrors would not vary based on residence in a rural area. However, if Dexter's night terrors continued and he needed to be referred to a specialist, the family might have difficulty accessing specialty services if they do not reside near a major medical center that employs a sleep specialist.

Are there any demographic characteristics that might affect this case?
Children between the ages of 3 and 5 years of age are most likely to experience night terrors with the prevalence decreasing with increasing age. There is no clear indication regarding gender and the occurrence of night terrors. Some studies say that the occurrence is nearly equal. Studies show that 49% of affected children were boys, and 51% were girls. Others studies report that childhood night terrors occur more frequently in boys.

Are there any standardized guidelines that you should use for this case?
The American Academy of Sleep Medicine has issued guidelines regarding night waking, such as night terrors.

REFERENCES AND RESOURCES

Agency for Healthcare Research and Quality. Practice parameters for behavioral treatment of bedtime problems and night wakings in infants and young children. Retrieved from http://www.guidelines.gov/content.aspx?id=15297&search=sleep+disturbances

Guilleminault, C., Palombini, L., Pelayo, R., & Chervin, R. D. (2003). Sleepwalking and sleep terrors in prepubertal children: What triggers them? *Pediatrics, 111,* e17–e25.

Kass, L. (2008). Sleep problems. *Pediatrics in Review, 27,* 455–462.

Morgenthaler, T., Owens, J., Alessi, C., Boehlecke, B., Brown, T., Coleman, J., Jr., & American Academy of Sleep Medicine (2006). Practice parameters for behavioral treatment of bedtime problems and night wakings in infants and young children. *Sleep*, *29*, 277–281.

Nguyen, B., Perusse, D., Paquet, J., Petit, D., Boivin, M., Tremblay, R., & Montplaisir, J. (2008). Sleep terrors in children: A prospective study of twins. *Pediatrics*, *122*, e1164–e1167.

Snyder, D., Goodlin-Jones, B., Pionk, M., & Stein, M. (2008). Inconsolable night-time awakening: Beyond night terrors. *Journal of Developmental and Behavioral Pediatrics*, *29*, 311–314.

Szelenberger, W., Niemcewicz, S., & Dabrowska, A. (2005). Sleepwalking and night terrors: Psychopathological and psychophysiological correlates. *International Review of Psychiatry*, *17*, 263–270.

Section 5

The Adolescent

Case 5.1 Birth Control Decision-Making

By Alison Moriarty Daley, MSN, APRN, PNP-BC

SUBJECTIVE

Keisha, a 16-year-old adolescent, comes to the clinic to discuss her options regarding contraception. She has been in a monogamous relationship with her boyfriend for 3 months and feels she needs to be on another kind of birth control "like the pill or shot—but I heard you can gain weight from them." She and her partner use condoms, "sometimes." Her last menstrual period was 32 days ago, and she experiences regular periods with mild cramps. Menarche was at age 12.5 years. G0P0. Keisha denies vaginal discharge, lesions, dysuria, pruritus, or lower abdominal pain. She has never been tested for sexually transmitted infections (STI) or HIV and states, "I don't have any worries about my boyfriend. He doesn't have anything."

Past medical history: Asthma, mild intermittent; physical exam 4 months ago was within normal limits.

Family history: Noncontributory.

Social history: As above.

Medications: Albuterol MDI 2 puffs every 4 hours, as needed, with spacer.

Allergies: NKDA.

OBJECTIVE

General: No apparent distress.

Vital signs: Weight: 201 lbs.; height: 64 inches; BP: 112/78; HR: 82.

Clinical Case Studies for the Family Nurse Practitioner, First Edition. Edited by Leslie Neal-Boylan.
© 2011 John Wiley & Sons, Inc. Published 2011 by John Wiley & Sons, Inc.

CRITICAL THINKING

Which diagnostic or imaging studies should be considered to assist with or confirm the diagnosis?
___Urine pregnancy test
___Beta pregnancy test
___Urine gonorrhea and chlamydia
___Pelvic examination with wet mount
___Pap smear
___CBC
___Cholesterol

What is the diagnosis at this point?

What are your concerns at this point?

What contraceptive methods would you consider for Keisha?

What contraceptive methods would you not consider for Keisha?

How would you determine which contraceptive method is the best fit?

Given the information provided above, what if any additional questions would you ask?

Describe the relevant side effects of each method of contraception you are considering.

What are some of the most common contraindications for OCP and patch use?

How will you address Keisha's concern regarding weight gain and contraception?

If Keisha is in a monogamous relationship, should she be counseled on condom use?

How would you instruct Keisha to begin OCPs? Is there more than one option for starting OCPs?

Could she receive DMPA today?

RESOLUTION

Diagnostic tests: Urine gonorrhea and chlamydia negative; urine HCG negative.

What is the diagnosis at this point?
Healthy, sexually active teen at risk for pregnancy:

What are your concerns at this point?
Keisha's reported history of unprotected sex and a last menstrual period (LMP) of 32 days ago raise concerns regarding a possible pregnancy and an STI. The clinician should have a discussion with Keisha regarding Keisha's feelings related to a possible pregnancy and should also provide appropriate anticipatory guidance.

What contraceptive methods would you consider for Keisha?
OCPs, Depo Provera , Plan B, intrauterine contraception (IUC), vaginal ring.

What contraceptive methods would you not consider for Keisha?
A patch, because it is less effective in women > 90 kg.

How would you determine which contraceptive method is the best fit?
The clinician should have a careful discussion about what Keisha has heard about various contraceptive methods, what she feels may best fit her needs, her previous experience with contraception, her

ability to take a pill every day, her need/desire for confidentiality, and cost. It is also important to consider how often Keisha is willing to come to the clinic for follow up and how consistent she can be with taking a pill every day or remembering to change the vaginal ring once every 3 weeks. It may also be important to consider how Keisha would feel about the potential of not having a monthly period. Many teens are not comfortable with touching themselves, which may limit their willingness to use the ring. The clinician should also explore Keisha's need to keep her contraceptive method private and how each method may or may not achieve this goal. For example, if she does not want her mother to know she is using contraception, OCPs or the patch may not be ideal because they may be discovered by her mother. DMPA, the vaginal ring, or intrauterine contraception (IUC) would provide more privacy. Amenorrhea or irregular bleeding patterns are common with DMPA and IUC and may cause questions regarding the number of pads or tampons used or not used in a given time frame.

Given the information provided above, what if any additional questions would you ask?
A thorough past medical history, current medical history, and family medical history are essential in determining the existence of any relative or absolute contraindications to contraceptive use.

Describe the relevant side effects of each method of contraception you are considering.

- OCP/vaginal ring: Aches, nausea, vaginal spotting or irregular bleeding, breast tenderness.
- DMPA: Irregular menstrual bleeding/amenorrhea or increased hunger.
- Condoms: Usually none, allergy to latex or spermicide,

What are some of the most common contraindications for OCP and patch use?

- Pregnancy.
- Undiagnosed vaginal bleeding.
- History of liver tumor, benign or malignant.
- Personal history of thromboembolic disease (DVT/PE).
- Thromboembolic disease in first degree relative.
- Arterial cardiovascular disease: stroke, myocardial infarction (MI).
- Complicated valvular disease.
- Currently impaired liver function.
- Hypertension—severe or uncontrolled.
- Systemic lupus erythematosus.
- Breast cancer.
- Migraine with aura/neurologic symptoms.
- Diabetes with vascular complications.
- Postpartum <3 weeks or breast-feeding.

How will you address Keisha's concern regarding weight gain and contraception?
Weight gain is not an inevitable consequence of any contraceptive method. Some women report increased hunger while on DMPA; however, to gain weight, caloric intake must exceed what your body needs to function. A 500 kcal increase per day for 7 days will yield a 1 pound gain in weight. Weights should be taken at the contraception initiation visit and at each follow-up visit. Increases can be identified and suggestions made regarding her diet and exercise patterns.

If Keisha is in a monogamous relationship, should she be counseled on condom use?
Yes, condoms should always be used for protection against STIs and HIV; you cannot be certain if a partner has infection(s) by looking, as many are asymptomatic.

How would you instruct Keisha to begin oral contraceptive pills? Is there more than one option for starting OCPs?

- First day start: OCPs begun on day 1 of the next menstrual cycle.
- Quick start: OCPs begun today regardless of LMP.
- Sunday start: OCPs begun the first Sunday after the beginning of the period.

Could she receive DMPA today?

Begin within first 5 days of the menstrual cycle with a documented negative pregnancy test, or QuickStart if there has been no unprotected sex in the past 2 weeks and if there is a negative pregnancy test today. Keisha has had unprotected sex in the past 2 weeks. A pregnancy test can be done today and repeated in two weeks; if it is also negative, DMPA can be given at that visit. If Keisha gets her period, she can call the clinic and get DMPA in the first 5 days of her cycle. Emphasize the use of emergency contraception in the meantime for any episodes of unprotected sex.

REFERENCES AND RESOURCES

Bonny, A., Harkness, L. S., & Cromer, B. A. (2005). Depot medroxyprogesterone acetate: Implications for weight status and bone mineral density in the adolescent female. *Adolescent Medicine Clinics, 16*, 569–584.

Bonny, A., Ziegler, J., Harvey, R., Debanne, S. M., Secic, M., & Cromer, B. A. (2006). Weight gain in obese and nonobese adolescent girls initiating depot medroxyprogesterone, oral contraceptive pills, or no hormonal contraceptive method. *Archives of Pediatric and Adolescent Medicine, 160*, 40–45.

Clements, A. L., & Moriarty Daley, A. (2006). Emergency contraception: A primer for pediatric providers. *Pediatric Nursing, 32*(2), 147–153.

Cromwell, P. F., Moriarty Daley, A., & Risser, W. (2004). Contraception for adolescents: Part one. *Journal of Pediatric Health Care, 18*, 149–152.

Cromwell, P. F., Moriarty Daley, A., & Risser, W. (2004). Contraception for adolescents: Part two. *Journal of Pediatric Health Care, 18*, 250–253.

Hatcher, R., Trussel, J., Nelson, A. L., Cates Jr, W., Stewart, F. H., & Kowal, D. (2007). *Contraceptive technology* (19th ed.). New York: Ardent Media, Inc..

Lara-Torre, E., & Schroeder, B. (2002). Adolescent compliance and side effects with Quick Start initiation of oral contraceptive pills. *Contraception, 66*, 81–85.

World Health Organization (2004). *Medical eligibility criteria for contraceptive use* (3rd ed.). Geneva: World Health Organization. Retrieved on August 4, 2009. http://apps.who.int/rhl/fertility/contraception/mec.pdf

World Health Organization (2008). Medical eligibility criteria for contraceptive use: Update 2008. Retrieved July 21, 2009 from http://apps.who.int/rhl/fertility/contraception/mec_update_2008.pdf

Case 5.2 Funny Feeling with Urination

By Alison Moriarty Daley, MSN, APRN, PNP-BC

SUBJECTIVE

John, a 17-year-old male patient, comes to the clinic with a complaint of "a funny feeling when I pee." He is sexually active and has not consistently used condoms in the past, because "I don't like them, and my girlfriend is on the pill." John denies any known exposure to a sexually transmitted infection (STI); however, he does not know if he was ever tested in the past. John reports a history of 5 previous partners, 4 without protection. The "funny feeling" began about 1 week ago. He was last sexually active yesterday with his current girlfriend.

Past medical history: Abscess in right axilla 7/08.

Family history: Noncontributory.

Social history: As above.

Medications: None.

Allergies: Penicillin (rash).

OBJECTIVE

General: No apparent distress.

Vital signs: Weight: 151 lbs; height: 71 inches; BMI: 21.1; BP: 118/72; HR: 72.

HEENT: Normocephalic; +PERRL; full EOMs; TMs gray/pearly; oral mucosa is moist and intact; oropharynx is clear.

Neck: Thyroid is firm without masses; no lymphadenopathy.

Respiratory: CTA bilaterally.

Cardiovascular: RRR: S1/S2 II/VI SEM best heard at LLSB no radiation; femoral/radial pulses 2+ bilateral, pink.

Abdomen: Soft, NT/ND; no masses; no HSM.

Clinical Case Studies for the Family Nurse Practitioner, First Edition. Edited by Leslie Neal-Boylan.
© 2011 John Wiley & Sons, Inc. Published 2011 by John Wiley & Sons, Inc.

Genitourinary: Tanner V PH/G, testes ↓↓, no masses; small amount of clear mucoid discharge from the urethra; no lesions; 1-cm round mobile NT right inguinal lymph node.

Wet mount: +WBCs

Skin: Without rashes.

CRITICAL THINKING

Which diagnostic or imaging studies should be considered to assist with or confirm the diagnosis?
__Urine dip
__Urinalysis
__Urine GC/CHL
__Urethral PCR
__HIV-1 antibody
__Venereal Disease Research Laboratory (VDRL)
__Trichomonas antibody culture
__Urine culture
__CBC

Is there any additional information you need?

What is the most likely differential diagnosis and why?
___Chlamydia
___HIV
___Candida albicans
___Gonorrhea

What is the plan of treatment?

How would you counsel this patient regarding the prevention of STIs?

Is he at risk for HIV?

Should he be retested for cure following treatment?

Should you treat his partner(s)?

What health education would you provide to John?

RESOLUTION

Diagnostic tests: Results:

- Urine dip: + Leukocyte esterase may indicate infection.
- Urinalysis: Trichomonads may be visible via wet mount.
- Urine GC/CHL: Diagnostic for gonorrhea and Chlamydia.
- Urethral PCR: Diagnostic for gonorrhea and Chlamydia. However, urine screening is less invasive.
- HIV-1 antibody: Screening indicated for history of unprotected sex.
- VDRL screening: For syphilis.
- Trichomonas culture: Screening for trichomoniasis, often asymptomatic.
- Urine culture: Indicated for diagnosis of UTI.
- CBC: Not indicated.

Is there any additional information you need?
Inquire regarding types of sex (oral, vaginal, and anal), male/female partners, drug/ETOH (alcohol) use, and known or suspected exposure or previous diagnosis of an STI or HIV,

What is the most likely differential diagnosis and why?
Chlamydia:
Clear discharge with minimal dysuria or a tingling sensation is indicative of chlamydia. Chlamydia typically presents a week or more following exposure. Symptoms are often subtle and described as a funny sensation or tingling with urination, an extra drip following urination, or some crusting at the tip of the penis.

What is the plan of treatment?
Azithromycin 1 g by mouth now. Instruct patient to avoid unprotected sex for 6 days.

How would you counsel this patient regarding the prevention of STIs?
Instruct the patient that many infections are asymptomatic. Explain the differences between viral and bacterial infections, signs and symptoms, and when and how to get tested.

Is he at risk for HIV?
Yes. He is at risk for HIV, because he reports a history of 5 partners, 4 without protection, and because he has been diagnosed with chlamydia.

Should he be retested for cure following treatment?
The current STI treatment guidelines for males do not advise retesting for cure. However, he should be reassessed at his next visit and screened, if clinically indicated, if you are concerned about him not taking the medication, or if you are concerned about his re-exposure.

Should you treat his partner(s)?
Yes. He should be encouraged to tell all previous partners and his current partner about the chlamydia. Sex with his current partner should be avoided until 6 days after both are treated. Community resources can be provided to facilitate this process.

What health education would you provide to John?

- Confidentiality agreement.
- Education regarding the prevention of STIs
- Common symptoms.
- Implications regarding viral versus bacterial STIs
- Proper condom use.
- Importance of consistent condom use and STI screening, including HIV.
- Available clinical services and consent laws.

REFERENCES AND RESOURCES

American Academy of Pediatrics (2006). *Red book: 2006 report of the committee on infectious diseases* (27th ed.). L. K. Pickering (Ed.), Elk Grove Village, IL: Author.

Burnstein, G., Eliscu, A., Ford, K., Hogben, M., Chaffee, T., & Straub, D. (2009). Expediated partner therapy for adolescents diagnosed with chlamydia or gonorrhea: A position paper of the Society of Adolescent Medicine. *Journal of Adolescent Health, 45*, 303–309.

Centers for Disease Control (2010). Sexually transmitted diseases treatment guidelines, 2010. *MMWR, 59*(RR-12), 1–110.

del Rio, C., Hall, G., Hook, E. W., III, Holmes, K. K., Whittington, W. L. H., Judson, F. N., & Weinstock, H. S. (2007, April 13). Update to CDC's sexually transmitted diseases treatment guidelines, 2006: Fluoroquinolones no longer recommended for treatment of gonococcal infections. *MMWR Weekly, 56*(14), 332–326.

Case 5.3 Weight Loss

By Alison Moriarty Daley, MSN, APRN, PNP-BC

SUBJECTIVE

Susie, a 14-year-old patient, is being seen today at the request of her mother, who made an appointment for a physical exam because "she is losing too much weight. I want her checked for everything." Susie is accompanied by her mother to the appointment. She is well groomed and somewhat quiet during the introductions to the Adolescent Clinic. Her last physical examination was 2 years ago at a different location and is reported by her mother to have been normal. The mother hands the provider a copy of the school physical form that was completed at the last physical exam. This is Susie's first visit to this clinic.

Past medical history: No hospitalizations, surgery, or chronic illnesses. Sprained right ankle 2 years ago playing soccer, went to physical therapy, and missed 6 weeks of soccer. No pain now. Menarche age 13, had monthly periods for about 6 months, and then began to miss periods; no cramps, "only 1 or 2 times" on day 1 of cycle. Occasional frontal headache, no associated signs or symptoms, lasts "at least an hour" but is relieved with acetaminophen; occurs 1–2 times per week, never upon waking. No trauma.

Family history: Maternal grandmother and mother: Type 2 diabetes; father: hypertension and recent "mild" MI; maternal aunt: cervical cancer.

Social history: Susie is an only child and lives with her mother and father. Her parents moved the family from another town in Connecticut about 1 year ago to coincide with the start of high school. Susie reports that she gets along well with her family, although she still wishes she lived in her former home. She has been doing well in school "mostly As, a few B+s" and has made a few acquaintances at school. Susie plays soccer and states that she enjoys it. Her mother reports that Susie "is quite the runner and runs after soccer practice and on non-practice days."

Medications: Occasional acetaminophen.

Allergies: NKDA; no allergies to foods or the environment.

Clinical Case Studies for the Family Nurse Practitioner, First Edition. Edited by Leslie Neal-Boylan.
© 2011 John Wiley & Sons, Inc. Published 2011 by John Wiley & Sons, Inc.

OBJECTIVE

General: Thin teen dressed in multiple layers, interactive, initially shy and now more talkative.

Vital signs: Height: 63 inches; weight: 100 pounds; BMI: 17.7 (sixth percentile); BP: 90/50; HR:56; RR: 12.

Skin: Cool, mottled, without acne; some white, downy hair on upper back and arms.

HEENT: Normocephalic, +PERRLA, TMs gray pearly, +LR, moist and intact mucous membranes; nose patent without rhinorrhea; oropharynx clear.

Neck: No lymphadenopathy.

Cardiovascular: RRR with clear S1 and S2; no murmur; femoral pulses are equal and +2.

Respiratory: Lungs CTA.

Breast: Tanner IV symmetrical.

Abdomen: Soft, flat, nontender; no HSM.

Genitourinary: Pubic hair; Tanner IV normal female; mucosa pale and pink; no lymphadenopathy, discharge, or odor.

Musculoskeletal: Back straight; FROM ×4 extremities.

Neurologic: Cranial nerves II–XII grossly intact; steady gait and balance; alert and interactive; reflexes +2 and equal.

CRITICAL THINKING

Which diagnostic or imaging studies should be considered to assist with or confirm the diagnosis?
___Urine pregnancy test
___Glucose
___Urinalysis
___CBC
___MCV
___Erythrocyte sedimentation rate
___Electrolytes
___Thyroid function tests
___Thyroid stimulating hormone
___Prolactin
___Testosterone panel
___Sex hormone binding globulin
___Gonorrhea and chlamydia
___HIV

What is the most likely differential diagnosis and why?
___Eating disorder
___Excessive exercise
___Malnutrition
___Malabsorption
___Hyperthyroid
___Depression

Should Susie's mother be in the room or asked to leave? Explain your rationale.

Based on the information you have gathered at this point, are there any additional questions you have for Susie or her mother?

Is her menstrual history a concern or normal given the age of menarche and her current age?

You ask Susie if she is aware of why her mother brought her to the visit today; and she replies, "She is just making a lot out of me losing some weight." How would you reply?

Are there any additional exam findings that are necessary at this point?

Based on the information gathered in the history and physical examination, what will you discuss with Susie and her mother?

When would you like to see her for follow up?

Can she be managed on an outpatient basis?

RESOLUTION

Diagnostic tests: All of the following tests should be done: Urine pregnancy test, glucose, urinalysis, CBC, MCV, erythrocyte sedimentation rate, electrolytes, thyroid function tests, thyroid stimulating hormone, prolactin, testosterone panel, and sex hormone binding globulin.
    Consider urine testing for gonorrhea and chlamydia, and HIV counseling and testing.

What is the most likely differential diagnosis and why?
There are several possible differential diagnoses. The primary diagnosis depends on responses to further questions that should be asked in the history and on the results of the lab work.

Should Susie's mother be in the room or asked to leave? Explain your rationale.
Susie's mother should be asked to leave the room after you have gathered sufficient history. Susie may have questions or information for you that she is not comfortable discussing in front of her mother.

Based on the information you have gathered at this point, are there any additional questions you have for Susie or her mother?

- "When did your weight become a concern? What was her weight at her last physical exam?"
- "You play soccer. Tell me about that. Is it any different this season than last? Has anything changed? Do you enjoy playing?"
- "How are you doing in school? Do you like it? What are your favorite and least favorite subjects?"
- "Do you have friends? Do they all play soccer, too?"
- "Tell me about your periods. How old were you when you got your first period? Do you get it every month? Do you ever miss periods?"
- Questions regarding sexual activity should also be explored without the mother present. "Have you been or are you currently sexually active?"
- "Are you taking any medications? Supplements? Vitamins? Herbal supplements?"
- Do you ever feel sad, depressed, or anxious? Do you have difficulty sleeping? Do you have difficulty concentrating? Do you cry easily?"
- "Do you have headaches, visual changes, constipation or diarrhea, abdominal pain, dry skin, excessive fatigue?"

Is her menstrual history a concern or normal given the age of menarche and her current age?
Menstrual cycles can be irregular for several years following menarche because of anovulation. However, other causes of secondary amenorrhea need to be considered. The most common causes of

secondary amenorrhea, other than weight changes, in an adolescent are pregnancy, side effects of contraception, polycystic ovary syndrome, stress, hypothyroidism, and prolactinoma.

You ask Susie if she is aware of why her mother brought her to the visit today; and she replies, "She is just making a lot out of me losing some weight." How would you reply?

- "Tell me more about that. Have you lost weight?"
- "Your mother said that you run. How many miles per day or per week?"
- "What other activities do you do?"
- "Tell me about your family. Do you get along with everyone? Have there been any changes at home?
- "Describe what your typical breakfast, lunch, and dinner would consist of?"
- "Do you each snacks? If so, what?"
- "Do you ever vomit after eating or take laxatives?"
- "Do you eat in private when no one else is around? If so, tell me about that."

Are there any additional exam findings that are necessary at this point?

- Temperature
- Percentiles for height, weight, and BMI; plot these on a growth curve.
- Pregnancy test
- Urine dip
- Visual fields; fundoscopic exam
- Parotid gland
- Tooth enamel erosion
- Thyroid
- Russell sign
- Palms for carotenemia
- Skin fold thickness and mid-upper arm circumference

Based on the information gathered in the history and physical examination, what will you discuss with Susie and her mother?

Discuss the cause of Susie's weight loss. It is likely the result of an increase in exercise and decrease in caloric intake. Her physical examination was normal. However, she is at the sixth percentile for weight . Laboratory tests will be ordered today to confirm that no other medical problems exist. Provide education on improving daily nutrition, decreasing daily amount of exercise, importance of maximizing bone density during adolescence, and calcium/vitamin D supplementation. A diary or journal can be started to record current weight, diet, and amount/type of exercise.

When would you like to see her for follow up?

Susie's weight, exercise, and eating patterns need to be monitored closely. Susie should return to the clinic in a week for laboratory results, weight check, and further counseling.

Can she be managed on an outpatient basis?

Yes. She is physiologically stable and has family support.

REFERENCES AND RESOURCES

Hacker, K. A., Myagmarjav, E., Harris, V., Suglia, S. F., Weidner, D., & Link, D. (2006). Mental health screening in pediatric practice: Factors related to positive screens and the contribution of parental/personal concern. *Pediatrics, 18*(5), 1896–1906. Retrieved from http://www.pediatrics.org/cgi/content/full/118/5/1896

Neinstein, L., Gordon, C. M., Katzman, D. K., Rosen, D. S., & Woods, E. (2008). *Adolescent health care: A practical guide* (5th ed.). Philadelphia: Lippincott Williams & Wilkins.

Case 5.4 Menstrual Cramps

By Alison Moriarty Daley, MSN, APRN, PNP-BC and Tracey Fender, RN, MSN, CPNP

SUBJECTIVE

Dina, a 15-year-old patient, comes to the school-based health center for her annual examination. Her mother called and spoke to the clinician this morning "very concerned about the number of days Dina has missed from school this year; she is in danger of not being promoted!" The clinician asks Dina how many days she has missed. Dina reports that she missed 5 days in February "because I had the flu and then about 1 or 2 days each month because of my period."

Menarche occurred at age 12.6. Dina usually has monthly periods around the beginning of the month. Each period lasts 5 days; and Dina uses 5 pads or tampons on the heaviest days, fewer on days 4 and 5. The cramps begin typically the day before her period and last until day 2 of her menses. She sometimes also has nausea and threw up last month because "it was so bad." Last normal menstrual period was 1 week ago.

Dina denies any urinary frequency, urgency, dysuria, hematuria, vaginal discharge, pruritus, lesions, pain with sex, or lower abdominal pain other than during the "normal time I have cramps." She has used "some kind of pain reliever in the past but it doesn't work."

Past medical history: None.

Family history: Dina's mother and sister have had heavy menses and dysmenorrhea.

Social history: The clinician learns from Dina that she has been sexually active in the past, but always with condoms. Her last sexual encounter was 1 month ago.

Medications: None.

Allergies: NKDA.

OBJECTIVE

General: No apparent distress; well groomed, pleasant, and cooperative.

Vital signs: Height: 62 inches; weight: 100 pounds; BP: 100/70; HR: 60; RR: 12.

Respiratory: CTA bilaterally.

Clinical Case Studies for the Family Nurse Practitioner, First Edition. Edited by Leslie Neal-Boylan.
© 2011 John Wiley & Sons, Inc. Published 2011 by John Wiley & Sons, Inc.

Cardiac: RRR S1 and S2; no murmurs, clicks, gallops, or rubs.

Breast: Tanner IV symmetrical.

Abdomen: Soft, positive bowel sounds; nontender, nondistended; no HSM

Genitourinary: Pubic hair; Tanner IV normal female; mucosa pale and pink; no lymphadenopathy, discharge, or odor.

CRITICAL THINKING

Which diagnostic or imaging studies should be considered to assist with or confirm the diagnosis?
___Urine HCG
___Pelvic and transvaginal ultrasound
___CBC with differential
___CMP
___Urine pregnancy test
___Cervical swab for GC/CT

What is the most likely differential diagnosis and why?
___Dysmenorrhea
___Endometriosis
___Pelvic inflammatory disease (PID)
___Urinary tract infection (UTI)
___Appendicitis
___Pregnancy—threatened abortion
___Pregnancy—ectopic

What additional information/questions are needed?

What questions would you ask Dina about her menstrual cycle?

What is the plan of treatment?

Are there other options?

Is it common for teen girls to miss school because of their periods?

When would you like to see her for follow up?

RESOLUTION

Diagnostic tests: It would be worthwhile to do a CBC with differential to check if Dina has become anemic and to do a urine pregnancy test to rule out pregnancy, missed, or threatened abortion, and a test for sexually transmitted infection (STI) screening.

What is the most likely differential diagnosis and why?
Primary dysmenorrhea:
Dina is 3 years past menarche, and she is within the age range where symptoms of primary dysmenorrhea first present. The history is consistent with this diagnosis because of the timing with the menstrual cycle.

What additional information/questions are needed?

- Ask Dina how often she participates in sexual activity and whether it is with males, females, or both. Ask whether she uses condoms 100% of the time? Obtain more detailed information about sexual activity to help to determine the risks of STI and pregnancy.

- Does she have a history of sexually transmitted disease or signs and symptoms of sexually transmitted infections? This information will help to rule out infection and/or PID.
- Ask whether she has tried anything for the cramps and whether it worked. Prostaglandin inhibitors and OCPs are the first lines of therapy for primary dysmenorrhea. If a patient is already using these medications without relief of symptoms, consider causes of secondary dysmenorrhea and other diagnoses.
- Has she always had cramps or is this a more recent change? Primary dysmenorrhea typically presents 2 years after the onset of menarche when cycles become ovulatory. It is most common to hear complaints of menstrual pain from adolescents in the age range 14–18 years old. If an adolescent presents with menstrual pain before the age of 14 or first experiences menstrual pain after the age of 19, consider causes of secondary dysmenorrhea.
- Is there a family history of endometriosis? Endometriosis should be considered if Dina has a positive family history of endometriosis in a first-degree relative. The risk of endometriosis increases in the case of relatives with more severe disease.
- Does she have a history of diarrhea, constipation, generalized abdominal pain, or passing gas? Information can help rule out gastrointestinal disorders such as Irritable Bowel Syndrome, lactose intolerance, constipation, and inflammatory bowel disease.
- Does she have a history of psychosocial problems? A positive history of cigarette smoking, trauma, abuse, anxiety, depression, or other somatic complaints has been associated with symptoms of dysmenorrhea.

What questions would you ask Dina about her menstrual cycle?

- What was her age at menarche? Primary dysmenorrhea usually presents within the first 3 years after menarche. During the first 2 years following menarche, cycles are highly irregular and anovulatory. Once ovulation starts to occur, the amount of prostaglandin responsible for the symptoms associated with dysmenorrhea increases.
- What are her number of days of bleeding and the number of hygienic products used in 24 hours? If Dina's cycles last longer than 7 days or if her cycles require frequent changes of feminine hygiene products, consider a workup for bleeding disorders.
- Ask her to describe her symptoms. Complaints of lower abdominal, back, and/or thigh pain within the first 48 hours of menstruation are typical of patients with primary dysmenorrhea. Associated systemic symptoms include nausea, vomiting, mood change, fatigue, and headache. If breast tenderness or bloating is reported consider diagnosis of PMS.
- Ask Dina when she experiences the onset of pain. Symptoms of primary dysmenorrhea usually peak in the first 48 hours of menstrual flow. The first 2 days of menstruation are associated with the highest level of prostaglandin in menstrual fluid. Consider premenstrual syndrome if Dina reports symptoms of pain and discomfort in the luteal phase, day 14 through 28, of the menstrual cycle.

What is the plan of treatment?

Reduce prostaglandin release by starting Dina on NSAID therapy. Treatment can be started before menstruation, with the onset of symptoms, or with the beginning of menstruation. After starting a specific NSAID, wait 2–3 cycles before switching medications if symptoms are not alleviated. Failure of NSAID treatment should not be determined unless they have been tried for longer than 6 months. NSAID treatment helps to lessen symptoms of primary dysmenorrhea in 80% of patients (Table 5.4.1).

Start Dina on OCPs to inhibit ovulation, thereby reducing prostaglandin release. Once started, OCPs should be used for 3–4 months before considering treatment a failure. Success of OCP therapy in relieving the symptoms of primary dysmenorrhea is greater than 90%. A combination of OCPs and NSAIDs should be tried for those who failed individual therapies.

Are there other options?

For the 10% of patients who do not respond to NSAID and OCP therapy, the following is a list of treatments to be considered[2]. Limited research exists for the following alternative therapies.

- Transcutaneous electric nerve stimulation (TENS)
- Laparoscopic presacral neurectomy

TABLE 5.4.1. NSAID Therapy.

Medication	Initial Dose (mg)	Following Dose (mg)
Ibuprofen	400	400 q4-6 hours
Naproxen	500	250 q6-8 hours
Naproxen sodium	550	275 q6-8 hours
Fenamates	500	250 q6 hours
Mefenamic acid	500	250 q6 hours

Source: Table created from data found in Braverman, PK (2008). Dysmenorrhea, p. 676, In L. Neinstein (Ed.) Adolescent health care: A practical guide (5th ed.). New York: Lippincott, Williams & Wilkins.

- Acupuncture
- Omega-3 fatty acids
- Transdermal nitroglycerin
- Thiamine (vitamin B_1)
- Magnesium supplements

Is it common for teen girls to miss school because of their periods?
Yes. Dysmenorrhea is the number one reason for school absences and for refusal to participate in physical activity for adolescent females.

When would you like to see her for follow up?
Follow up in 8 weeks and as needed. A menstrual diary with descriptions of the menstrual pain, medication used and its effect, and any other symptoms will be helpful in determining treatment plan.

REFERENCES AND RESOURCES

American Academy of Pediatrics (2006). Menstruation in girls and adolescents: Using the menstrual cycle as a vital sign. *Pediatrics, 118,* 2245–2250.

Coco, Andrew (1999). Primary dysmenorrhea. *American Family Physician, 60,* 489–496.

Dangal, G. (2005). Menstrual disorders in adolescents. *International Journal of Gynecology and Obstetrics, 4*(1). Retrieved from http://www.ispub.com/journal/the_internet_journal_of_ gynecology_ and_obstetrics/ volume_4_number_1_19/article/menstrual_disorders_in_adolescents-11.html

Montgomery, G. W., Nyholt, D. R., Zhao, Z., Treloar, S., Painter, J. N., Missmer, S. A., . . . Zondervan K. T. (2008). The search for genes contributing to endometriosis risk. *Human Reproduction, 14*(5), 447–457.

Neinstein, L. S. (2008). *Adolescent health care: A practical guide* (5th ed.). Philadelphia: Lippincott Williams & Wilkins.

Case 5.5 Mother's Concern

By Alison Moriarty Daley, MSN, APRN, PNP-BC

SUBJECTIVE

Nathan, a 16-year-old patient, is brought to the office by his mother. She is insisting that Nathan be tested for "drugs . . . all of them, because his grades are terrible and I don't like his friends." You ask his mother to be more specific about her concern regarding drug use. She explains that his grades have slipped in the last 2 months or so and says, "I won't have a son of mine using drugs." His mother denies having any drugs in the house but comments that his teachers say, "He seems zoned out in class and sometimes falls asleep." She has also noticed the same thing but realizes that he has been very busy with school and helping with her recovery from hip surgery. The clinician first interviews Nathan alone,

Nathan denies any complaints other than fatigue. He sleeps 6–7 hours per night and occasionally naps when he does not have football practice after school. He does not have nightmares or wake in the middle of the night.

Past medical history: Broken arm last summer with a surgical repair.

Family history: Father has hypertension. Mother had a hip replacement 8 weeks ago. Older brother has asthma.

Social history: Nathan lives with his mother and 3 older brothers. One has been arrested for marijuana possession "but was let off because it wasn't his. It was in a jacket he borrowed from a friend." Nathan is a junior in high school. He says that he is doing "OK." He has an A in English, Bs in math and history, Cs in Spanish and biology, and a D in Latin. He admits that his grades were better last year. "It's hard to concentrate sometimes because I am tired a lot." He has many friends, some for a long time and other new friends that he met this year. He admits to drinking beer weekly with friends, usually while hanging out. He has drunk to the point of throwing up and blacking out in the past but not recently. He tried marijuana and occasionally smokes a cigarette with one of his friends. "Not really doing any of that now."

Psychiatric: He denies depression or sadness. He reports that "school is harder and I fell behind for awhile, especially when my mother had her surgery." Nathan tells you he took his mother to her physical therapy appointments and picked up her medications from the pharmacy for her. "She had it rough; she was in a lot of pain."

Medications: Denies medication, vitamins, supplements, or over-the-counter medications.

Clinical Case Studies for the Family Nurse Practitioner, First Edition. Edited by Leslie Neal-Boylan.
© 2011 John Wiley & Sons, Inc. Published 2011 by John Wiley & Sons, Inc.

Allergies: No known drug allergies (NKDA).

Following the interview, the clinician speaks to the mother again and comments, "Nathan sounds like he was very helpful taking you to physical therapy and picking up your prescriptions. How are you feeling?" His mother replies that "it wasn't as bad as I thought. I did have some pain but got over it quick. I only used pain medication for a few days."

CRITICAL THINKING

Which diagnostic or imaging studies should be considered to assist with or confirm the diagnosis?
___Toxicology screen
___CBC
___CMP
___TSH

What is the most likely differential diagnosis and why?
__Substance use/abuse
__Alcohol use/abuse
__Depression
__Hypothyroidism
__Sleep disorder

How would you proceed with the visit?

Nathan asks, "If I tell you the truth, will you tell my mother?" How do you respond?

Are there any elements of the history that concern you as the clinician regarding substance use?

After your discussion with Nathan's mother, you ask Nathan if he has ever tried any other drugs. He asks, "Like what?" What would you ask about?

What is your next step?

Can minors seek substance abuse counseling without parental consent?

Under what circumstances would you break the confidentiality agreement?

What other questions would you ask regarding his tiredness?

What aspects of the physical exam to which would you want to pay particular attention?

RESOLUTION

Diagnostic tests: If the patient has not had a CBC or CMP in more than 1 year, then these could also be performed. Consider a TSH if concerned about hypothyroidism. Also consider a toxicology screen with consent from Nathan.

What is the most likely differential diagnosis and why?
Prescription pain medication abuse:
Nathan has had access to his mother's pain medication, and the history points to the likelihood that he has been taking her medicine.

How would you proceed with the visit?
Separate Nathan from his mother. Review the confidentiality agreement and when and how it may need to be broken. Ask Nathan why his mother is concerned and whether her concerns are legitimate. Inquire if they have discussed her concerns at home and how the conversation started.

Nathan asks, "If I tell you the truth, will you tell my mother?" How do you respond?
Consult the local consent laws. Most states allow minors to consent for care related to alcohol and drugs; however, age and service restrictions vary. Adolescent services are confidential unless there is a concern that the teen is hurting himself or another or a concern of abuse. As the clinician you can respond that your role is to assist adolescents to remain healthy and to get the help they need. Reiterate the confidentiality agreement and provide examples for him.

Are there any elements of the history that concern you as the clinician regarding substance use?
The inconsistency in the mother's version of her history regarding her postoperative course, recovery, and experience with pain and Nathan's version differ dramatically. In addition, Nathan admits to alcohol use, binge drinking, tobacco use, and marijuana use.

After your discussion with Nathan's mother, you ask Nathan if he has ever tried any other drugs. He asks, "Like what?"What would you ask about?
It may be helpful to ask first about his peers' drug use and then ask him about what he has tried and used. Ask directly about his past and current use of alcohol, marijuana, and prescription drugs and whether there has been anything else. Take cues from what Nathan reports regarding his friends and what you, as the clinician, know about the prevalence of alcohol and drug use in the community.

What is your next step?
Ask Nathan if he has been taking his mother's pain medication. Determine the frequency and amount and whether there have been any adverse effects. It is also important to ask why he has been taking his mother's pain medications. Ask him what was it like for him while is mother was ill.

Anticipatory guidance regarding substance use should be given in adolescent-friendly and supportive manner. Determine whether he is concerned about his substance use, what happens if he does not use the medication, as well as why and when he takes it. Is he interested in seeking treatment? Why or why not? It is essential to consult with a substance abuse expert to determine the best course of action. Further questioning about anxiety; depression; suicidal ideation, safety, and past attempts need exploration.

Can minors seek substance abuse counseling without parental consent?
Consult local health law to determine the answer to this. Determine adolescent resources within the community and the types of insurance they accept.

Under what circumstances would you break the confidentiality agreement?
The confidentiality agreement made with an adolescent needs to be broken if the clinician determines he is at risk of harming himself or others. This needs to be clearly discussed with him prior to breaking the agreement.

What other questions would you ask regarding his tiredness?
- "What time do you go to bed at night?"
- "Do you feel rested in the morning?"
- "How often do you nap? How long does the nap last? Are you able to go to sleep that night?"
- "Are you able to return to sleep?"
- "Do you have difficulty falling asleep?"
- "Do you use anything to help you fall or stay asleep?"
- "Do you have nightmares?"
- "Do you go to bed at a similar time each night?"
- "Where do you sleep?"
- "Is the TV, radio, computer, or phone on when you are asleep?"
- "How often are you awakened by a phone call or a text message?"
- "Does anyone report you snoring or having long pauses between breaths as you sleep?"
- If his sleep pattern has changed, ask when he first noticed this and any related circumstances.

What aspects of the physical exam would you want to pay particular attention to?
A complete physical examination is indicated to look for organic causes of tiredness.

REFERENCES AND RESOURCES

Boyd, C. J., McCabe, S. E., Cranford, J. A., & Young, A. (2006). Adolescent's motivations to abuse prescription medications. Retrieved from http://www.pediatrics.org/cgi/doi/10.1542/peds.2006-1644

English, A., Bass, L., Boyle, A. D., & Eshragh, F. (2010). *State minor consent laws: A summary*. Chapel Hill, NC: Center for Adolescent Health and the Law.

Patton, G., Patton, G. C., McMorris, B. J., Toumbourou, J. W., Hemphill, S. A., Donath, S., & Catalano, R. F. (2004). Puberty and the onset of substance use and abuse. *Pediatrics, 114*, e300–e306.

Schiffman, R. (2004). Drug & substance use in adolescents. *The American Journal of Maternal Child Nursing, 29*, 21–27.

Case 5.6 Sexual Identity

By Alison Moriarty Daley, MSN, APRN, PNP-BC and Kevy Wijaya, MSN, RN, CPNP

SUBJECTIVE

Samuel, an 18-year-old Asian male, presents alone to the adolescent clinic for a college entrance physical examination. He was last seen in the clinic last year for an annual physical, with no significant health issues. Samuel's immunizations are up-to-date except for the human papillomavirus vaccine. Samuel has a well-balanced diet with adequate intake of fruits and vegetables daily. He drinks two cups of soy milk in the morning and does not drink soda or fruit juice. There are no complaints about elimination. He denies having headache, nausea, vomiting, diarrhea, or fever. He denies blood in the stool, constipation, or diarrhea. There is no blood in the urine or abnormal discharge, but Samuel does admit to having some mild pain when urinating immediately after sex. Samuel sleeps for 7–8 hours each night without any interruption, except on the weekends when he goes out and comes home late.

Past medical/Surgical history: He has no significant past medical history. Past surgical history includes a dental procedure in 2006 and an appendectomy in 2008.

Family history: Samuel does not know his family history.

Social history: Samuel is currently a senior at a local high school. He lives with his mother and his 16-year-old and 13-year-old sisters. His parents divorced when he was in elementary school. His mother is a full-time teacher, and his father is an accountant to whom Samuel occasionally talks. Samuel admits having a great network of friends that "he usually hangs out with."

Medications:

- Methylphenidate 10 mg by mouth every day for attention deficit hyperactivity disorder.
- Escitalopram 10 mg by mouth every day for anxiety.

Allergies: Denies allergies.

Sexual history: During the process of documenting his sexual history, Samuel admits to being sexually active with a male partner and that his last sexual contact was approximately 2 weeks ago. He mentioned that the two met at a bar and had oral and anal sex (protected) that night. He admits to always "playing safe"; but, when asked about his partner, he does not know much about his male partner except the fact that he is attending graduate school here in town. Samuel appears to be anxious and slightly uncomfortable during the interview and said, "My mom does not know that I'm *like this*."

Clinical Case Studies for the Family Nurse Practitioner, First Edition. Edited by Leslie Neal-Boylan.
© 2011 John Wiley & Sons, Inc. Published 2011 by John Wiley & Sons, Inc.

OBJECTIVE

General: Alert, oriented, quiet; in no apparent distress.

Vital signs: Temperature: 98.6F—oral; BP: 118/78 left arm sitting; HR: 68 beats per minute; RR: 18; height: 72 inches; weight: 185 pounds, BMI: 25.1.

HEENT: Head: Normocephalic/atraumatic (NC/AT); hair intact; no alopecia. Eyes: PERRLA; equal ocular movement (EOM) intact; sclera white; conjunctiva clear and noninjected; no ocular discharge. Ears: Tympanic membrane (TM) pearly grey; landmarks visible bilaterally; no effusion, perforation, or bulging noted. Nose: Nares patent, septum midline, no rhinorrhea or epistaxis. Mouth/Throat: Clear, no erythema or exudates; good dentition.

Neck: Supple; full range of motion (FROM); no cervical lymphadenopathy.

Cardiac: RRR; S1 and S2 audible; no murmur, rub, or gallop.

Respiratory: Symmetrical; good air exchange; no abnormal breath sounds, clear to auscultation bilaterally (CTAB).

Abdomen: Normoactive bowel sounds ×4; soft, nontender/nondistended (NT/ND); no hepato-splenomegaly; +femoral pulses.

Back: Spine straight; isolevel scapula and hips.

Genitourinary: Normal circumcised male genitalia; testes descended bilaterally; no masses or pain; Tanner V genitalia/pubic hair; no discharge noted; no hernia present. Anus patent; no lesion; hemorrhoid, or anal fissure.

CRITICAL THINKING

Which diagnostic or imaging studies should be considered to assist with or confirm the diagnosis?
___Urinalysis
___Urine culture
___HIV
___Venereal Disease Research Laboratory (VDRL)
___GC/Chlamydia test through urine or urethra
___Wet mount
___Herpes virus (HSV)

Which differential diagnoses should be considered at this point?
___Urinary tract infection
___Urethritis
___Phimosis
___Sexually transmitted infection (STI)

What problems would you want to address today, and why?
___Dysuria
___Sexual identity
___Medications
___STI screening
___Vaccines
___That he came here alone

What question(s) would be appropriate to ask in order to address the patient's sexual orientation in the most respectful way possible?

Are any referrals needed?

What if Samuel stated that he is feeling depressed and thinking of "ending it all"?

RESOLUTION

Diagnostic testing: A urinalysis, using either dipstick or laboratory testing, should be performed to check for a urinary tract infection. Obtain a urine culture and sensitivity if the urinalysis is positive for infection. Obtain an HIV test and explain about options of HIV testing. Explain that testing is anonymous or confidential. A VDRL is necessary to check for syphilis. Urine testing or a urethral probe can be used to test for GC/Chlamydia. A wet mount should be obtained to check for causes of dysuria. Check for HSV if there is a concern about genital herpes infection.

What problems would you want to address today, and why?

1. Dysuria—You should determine the underlying cause of dysuria as it might be due to conditions such as urinary tract infection, urethritis, phimosis, penile condyloma, herpes simplex virus infection, or contact dermatitis.
2. Sexual identity—Samuel's *"like this"* comment is worth exploring. Discuss sexuality and preferences in a nonjudgmental manner. Offer support and assess whether he feels safe at home or at school. Offer screening for depression, anxiety, and safety as they are immensely important issues in adolescents with sexual identity problems.
3. Screening for STIs—Samuel is currently sexually active with a same-sex partner, possibly more than one partner. He should be screened for sexually transmitted infections.
4. Medications—Samuel is currently on (Methylphenidate 10mg by mouth every day for ADHD and Escitalopram 10mg by mouth every day). Ask why he is on these medications, who prescribed the medications, and how long he has been on them.
5. HPV vaccine—In October 2009, the Food and Drug Administration approved the use of the quadrivalent vaccine in boys and men aged 9–26 years for the prevention of genital warts. Subsequently, the Advisory Committee on Immunization Practices (Centers for Disease Control and Prevention [CDC], 2010) supported the permissive use of the quadrivalent vaccine for this indication and recommended that funding be provided for this purpose through the Vaccines for Children program. Among men having sex with men (MSM) and immunosuppressed men and women, anal HPV infection leads to a high disease burden of warts, AIN, and anal cancer. Male vaccination against HPV has the potential to lead to a substantial reduction in the burden of these diseases, therefore quadrivalent HPV vaccine is recommended. (Palefsky, 2010).

What question(s) would be appropriate to ask in order to address the patient's sexual orientation in the most respectful way possible?

Interviewing an adolescent is a process that requires interest and patience from the health care provider. The interview with an adolescent is important, because it not only allows a provider to collect information, but it also sets the tone for future interactions (Woods & Neinstein, 2008). The confidentiality agreement and reasons why confidentiality would need to be broken (abuse, suicide, homicide) should be explained to the adolescent at the first visit and as necessary.

Establishing rapport with an adolescent patient is vital, yet it is perhaps one of the most difficult parts of the visit. Woods and Neinstein (2008) suggest the following:

1. Always introduce yourself. Tell the adolescent your role and your agenda for this particular visit. Shaking the hand of the adolescent is recommended as it may help ease their anxiety as well as acknowledge that they are the center of the attention in the room at the present time.

2. Explain the "confidentiality agreement" and inform the adolescent of when it may be broken. A confidentiality contract is an agreement that commits you to keeping your conversation private, unless the adolescent is at risk of harming him/herself or others. The key to a successful examination is to establish a sense of confidentiality with the adolescent and honoring it. Emphasize that when there are concerns regarding their safety, you are to share this information to their parents.
3. Start the conversation with easy topics such as things he/she enjoys doing and some general conversational topics. This will enable you to gain insights into the adolescent's personality and mood.
4. Give him/her a chance to talk and voice their opinions.
5. Always treat the adolescent's comments respectfully and seriously. It is important to keep in mind that you should be treating him/her as an adult. The adolescent will appreciate it and it will help to ease his/her anxiety during the visit.

Go further and ask about issues that concern the adolescent. Listening is vital to developing a rapport with an adolescent. Remember always to stay focused on what the adolescent is telling you and to try to understand the adolescent's perspective. As with any routine visits with an adolescent, be sure to emphasize the importance of safe sex practices. Tell patient to always use condoms. Assess the patient's knowledge of STIs, how to prevent them from acquiring and transmitting them, and how to seek help should they become infected with one.

What question(s) would be appropriate to address the patient's sexual orientation in the most respectful way possible?

- "Tell me about your friends!"
- "Are you in a relationship, or do you like one person in particular?"
- "Is your special friend a boy, a girl, or both?"
- "Are you sexually active?"
- "How old were you when you had your very first sexual encounter?"
- "Are you involved with another individual in a sexual relationship?"
- "How many partners have you had sex with?"
- "Do you always have protected sex?"
- "What do you know about sexually transmitted infections (STIs)?"
- "How do you keep yourself free from STIs?"
- "Have you ever been tested for an STI?"

Are any referrals needed?
Lesbian, gay, bisexual, and transgender adolescents may face adverse medical consequences due to physical and psychological changes in lifestyle and risky sexual behaviors. Most sexually transmitted infections are due to unprotected sexual contact. During receptive anal intercourse, the already fragile rectal mucosa is easily damaged causing transmission of pathogens (Meininger & Remafedi, 2008).

Referrals may not be necessary at this time. However, a referral to a mental health professional may be warranted if you suspect the patient is feeling depressed, fears for his safety, or is having suicidal thoughts or ideation. Make sure to assess if the patient has a support system (namely adult supports in the family) and has access to a lesbian, gay, bisexual, transgender (LGBT) group in school or in the community from where he can seek information and help.

What if Samuel stated that he is feeling depressed and thinking of "ending it all"?
Always treat suicidal thoughts or ideation seriously. Kennebeck (2010) suggests that the first step is to find out if he is in danger of acting on his suicidal thoughts. Ask direct, but sensitive questions such as:

- "Are you thinking about hurting yourself?
- "Are you thinking about committing a suicide?"
- "Have you thought about how you would do it?"
- "Do you have the means to do it?"
- "When would you do it?"

Secondly, always be on the lookout for common signs throughout your interaction with the patient. The following may be signs if one is considering suicide (Sherer, 2008).

- Making suicidal remarks such as "I just want to end it all," or "I wish I were dead."
- Being preoccupied with death and dying.
- Abuse of alcohol and illicit drugs
- Change in normal routine or social interaction and being completely out of one's normal character.
- Giving away belongings
- Saying goodbye to people as if he/she was going away for a long time.

If you believe that the patient is at risk of suicide, never leave the patient alone and be sure to seek emergency help by dialing 911 so that the patient can be taken to the hospital emergency room in a prompt manner, as this patient may need to be hospitalized until the suicidal crisis has passed. You will also be required to notify a family member or close friend regarding the matter.

If you believe the patient is not in immediate danger, always offer your support. Encourage the patient to seek treatment, as patients with severe depression or who have suicidal thoughts may not have the courage to seek help on their own. Encourage the patient to communicate with you to express their feelings. Be supportive, respectful, and understanding and express your opinions without placing blame or being judgmental.

REFERENCES AND RESOURCES

Centers for Disease Control and Prevention (2010). FDA licensure of quadrivalent human papillomavirus vaccine (HPV4, Gardasil) for use in males and guidance from the Advisory Committee on Immunization Practices (ACIP). *MMWR Morbidity and Mortality Weekly Report*, *59*, 630–632.

Kennebeck, S., & Bonin, L. (2008). Evaluation and management of suicidal behavior in children and adolescents. *UpToDate*. Retrieved from http://www.uptodateonline.com

Meininger, E., & Remafedi, G. (2008). Gay, lesbian, and transgender adolescents. In Neinstein et al. (Ed.), *Adolescent health care: a practical guide* (5th ed.). Philadelphia, PA: Lippincott Williams & Wilkins.

Palefsky, J. M. (2010). Human papillomavirus-related disease in men: Not just a women's issue. *Journal of Adolescent Health*, *46*, 555–564, 614.

Sherer, S. (2008). Suicide. In Neinstein et al. (Ed.), *Adolescent health care: A practical guide* (5th ed.). pp. 555–564. Philadelphia, PA: Lippincott Williams & Wilkins.

UpToDate. Evaluation and management of suicidal behavior in children and adolescents. http://www.uptodate.com/contents/evaluation-and-management-of-suicidal-behavior-in-children-and-adolescents?source=preview&selectedTitle=6%7E150&anchor=H3#H3

Woods, E. R., & Neinstein, L. S. (2008). Office visit, interview techniques, and recommendations to parents. In Neinstein et al. (Ed.), *Adolescent health care: A practical guide* (5th ed.). pp. 33–43. Philadelphia, PA: Lippincott Williams & Wilkins.

Case 5.7 Missed Periods

By Alison Moriarty Daley, MSN, APRN, PNP-BC

SUBJECTIVE

Shana, a 16-year-old female, comes to the clinic requesting a pregnancy test "because my period is all messed up." Her last menstrual period was 35 days ago, and she thinks it is 5 days late. "It never is." She has a male partner who is 17-years-old. She has been sexually active for approximately 1 year. Shana was on oral contraception for awhile and then ran out and never restarted. She has been off of pills for 2 months and had a period after stopping and then one other 5-day period with cramps. She has had sex both with and without condoms over the course of the last month. The clinician asks her if she wants a baby now; and Shana states, "Not really, but my boyfriend does. If it happens, I mean, I would be okay with it; but I am not trying really."

Past medical history: None.

Family history: Noncontributory.

Social history: Shana is a junior in high school. She lives with her divorced mother. She occasionally sees her father but is close to neither parent. She has no siblings and both of her parents work full-time. She denies substance use of any kind.

Medications: None at this time.

Allergies: NKDA.

OBJECTIVE

Weight: 135; height: 63 inches; BP: 100/64.

General: NAD; pleasant, cooperative, and well groomed.

Respiratory: CTA bilaterally.

Cardiac: RRR S1 and S2; no murmurs, clicks, gallops or rubs.

Breast: Tanner IV symmetrical.

Clinical Case Studies for the Family Nurse Practitioner, First Edition. Edited by Leslie Neal-Boylan.
© 2011 John Wiley & Sons, Inc. Published 2011 by John Wiley & Sons, Inc.

Abdomen: + BS; soft, nontender, nondistended; no HSM.

Genitourinary: Pubic hair; Tanner IV normal female; mucosa pale and pink; no lymphadenopathy, discharge, or odor.

CRITICAL THINKING

Which diagnostic or imaging studies should be considered to assist with or confirm the diagnosis?
___Urine HCG
___HIV testing
___STI screening
___Pap smear
___Urine dipstick

Which differential diagnoses should be considered at this point?

Why is it important to ask Shana what she feels her boyfriend would want if she were pregnant?

What additional questions would you ask Shana?

If she were pregnant today what are her options?

Should you prescribe contraception today?

RESOLUTION

Diagnostic tests: Shana should be given a urine pregnancy test. She should also receive STI screening/testing and HIV counseling and testing because of her history of unprotected sex. A Pap smear should be done within 3 years of the onset of sexual activity or by age 21.

If the pregnancy test is positive and in the absence of symptoms, the pelvic exam may be delayed until the prenatal or pretermination visit. If Shana's pregnancy test is negative today, she should return for a repeat test in 2 weeks if she has had no menses.

Why is it important to ask Shana what she feels her boyfriend would want if she were pregnant?
The perceived desire of the partner is an important influence on future pregnancy. Counseling should be done to help Shana decide what she wants to avoid an unwanted or unintended pregnancy.

What additional questions would you ask Shana?

- "How would you feel about a negative pregnancy test or a positive pregnancy test today?"
- "How do you think your partner would react to a positive or negative pregnancy test?"
- "Do you have any STI signs or symptoms, such as lower abdominal pain, breast tenderness, nausea, vomiting, or fatigue?"
- "Is there a supportive adult with whom you could discuss a positive pregnancy test?"
- "Do you know what your 3 choices are if the test is positive?"
- "What would you do if the test is positive today?"
- "If the test is negative, would you like to restart contraception?" Educate her regarding appropriate options. Discuss what she liked and disliked regarding the OCPs.
- Discuss ways to increase success in preventing pregnancy and sexually transmitted infections.
- Offer STI/HIV testing.

If she were pregnant today what would be her options?
Educate Shana on her options regarding the pregnancy in a nonbiased and adolescent-friendly manner. Those options include continuing the pregnancy, abortion, and adoption.

Should you prescribe contraception today?
Condoms and an advance prescription for Plan B can be provided today. In addition, if she has a negative pregnancy test, a prescription or samples for her choice of hormonal contraception can be given today with clear instructions on how to start if she begins her menstrual cycle prior to her follow-up appointment. If she desires DMPA, she should be instructed to call at the onset of her period so she can begin this method.

REFERENCES AND RESOURCES

Clements, A. L., & Moriarty Daley, A. (2006). Emergency contraception: A primer for pediatric providers. *Pediatric Nursing, 32*(2), 147–153.

Cromwell, P. F., Moriarty Daley, A., & Risser, W. (2004). Contraception for adolescents: Part one. *Journal of Pediatric Health Care, 18*(3), 149–152.

Cromwell, P. F., Moriarty Daley, A., & Risser, W. (2004). Contraception for adolescents: Part two. *Journal of Pediatric Health Care, 18*(5), 250–253.

Neinstein, L. (2008). *Adolescent health care: A practical guide* (5th ed.). Philadelphia: Lippincott Williams & Wilkins.

Case 5.8 Left Knee Pain and Swelling

By Phoebe M. Heffron, MSN, PNP

SUBJECTIVE

Maria is a 14-year-old female who presents with sudden onset left knee pain and swelling which began at soccer practice 10 days ago. Maria reports that the knee "gives out" at times and that the pain has decreased in the last week and a half. She has used ice, ibuprofen, rest, and an ACE bandage with minimal decrease in swelling, though the pain has improved.

Past medical/surgical history: Significant for a previous second degree ankle sprain on the ipsilateral side and Lyme disease at ages 11 and 12 with symptoms of pain and swelling present in the left knee in the first Lyme infection. Maria has not previously had any surgeries.

Family history: Maria's family history includes a maternal grandmother with diabetes, a maternal grandfather with coronary artery disease, a paternal grandfather with rheumatoid arthritis, and a paternal grandfather who died at age 80 from colon cancer.

Social history: Maria lives with her mom, dad, 17-year-old sister, 12-year-old brother, and 2 dogs. She has many friends, is an honors student, plays in the school orchestra, and plays basketball, tennis, and soccer for her school and town recreation leagues. Her family lives in a large house in an upper middle-class town, where her dad (an attorney) works full-time and her mom (who has a master's degree and works at a museum) works part-time. Maria feels very close with her family, denies use of tobacco or any substances, denies depressive symptoms but does see a psychiatric mental health nurse practitioner for some anxiety she experienced following her witnessing a fatal car accident. (She reports that her anxiety is much improved and that she has never required medication for this).

Medications: Cetirizine, as needed for seasonal allergies, and a multivitamin and calcium supplement daily.

Allergies: Seasonal allergies, an allergy to stone fruits and an allergy to penicillin.

Clinical Case Studies for the Family Nurse Practitioner, First Edition. Edited by Leslie Neal-Boylan.
© 2011 John Wiley & Sons, Inc. Published 2011 by John Wiley & Sons, Inc.

OBJECTIVE

General: No apparent distress.

Vital signs: Height: 5 ft 4 inches; weight: 115 lbs; temperature: 98.2; pulse: 76; respirations: 12; BP: 110/72.

Cardiac: RRR S1/S2; no murmurs, clicks, gallops, or rubs.

Respiratory: CTA bilaterally.

Musculoskeletal: Left knee with moderate effusion; no significant ecchymosis. Skin is intact. Leg is in slight external rotation (equal bilaterally). No visible misalignment of patella. No muscle atrophy apparent. Range of Motion (ROM) from about 10–120 degrees, 5+ strength with hamstring and quadriceps testing. Equivocal flexion pinch test. Questionable anterior and posterior joint-line tenderness, both laterally and medially. No tenderness over the patella. Negative sag test; some laxity with varus and valgus testing at 0 degrees, but no laxity with varus and valgus testing at 30 degrees; some laxity with anterior drawer and Lachman testing.

CRITICAL THINKING

Which diagnostic or imaging studies should be considered to assist with or confirm the diagnosis?
___Radiograph
___Urinalysis/urine culture
___Rapid strep test
___Complete blood count with differential
___Blood urea nitrogen/creatinine
___Magnetic resonance imaging (MRI)
___Antinuclear antibody
___Lumbar puncture
___C-reactive protein
___Lyme titer/western blot/ELISA

What is the most likely differential diagnosis and why?
___Lyme disease
___Meniscus tear
___Anterior cruciate ligament (ACL) tear
___Rheumatoid arthritis
___Osgood-Schlatter disease
___Patellofemoral syndrome

What is your plan of treatment?

What is your plan for follow-up care?

Are any referrals needed?

Does the patient's psychosocial history impact how you might treat this patient?

What if this patient was male?

What if this patient was over age 18 or under age 13?

What if the patient was also diabetic or hypertensive?

What if the patient lived in a rural, isolated setting?

What kind of education should you provide to the patient regarding future injury prevention to protect against recurrence or injury to the contralateral side?

Are there any standardized guidelines that you should use to assess or treat this case?

RESOLUTION

Diagnostic tests:

- A radiograph shows a moderate joint effusion.
- The MRI shows a full thickness tear of the ACL with a partial thickness tear of the Medial Collateral Ligament (MCL).
- Antinuclear antibody is within normal limits.
- C-reactive protein is mildly elevated.
- Lyme tests are all negative. (IgG is elevated but IgM is within normal limits indicating a previous—but not current—infection with Lyme disease).

What is the most likely differential diagnosis and why?
Tear of the ACL:
Regardless of the test results, one can be fairly confident that the diagnosis is an ACL tear. It may be harder to determine the certainty of concurrent MCL tear. However, the history of sudden onset knee pain during a high-risk activity with recurrent "giving out" and decrease in pain is classic for an ACL injury. The physical exam is also typical for ACL injury.

What is your plan of treatment?
Recommend that Maria continue rest, ice, compression, and elevation (RICE) therapy until she is seen by the orthopedist. Prescribe crutch use. (Note: Some providers will recommend use of an immobilizing brace, but this practice varies. Know the preference of the orthopedist to whom you are referring the patient.) Instruct Maria about exercises to work on ROM (especially extension) and quadriceps strengthening. Provide educational materials (Heffron & Daley, 2010), including some frequently asked questions with answers and a guide to other useful resources. The orthopedist's plan for Maria is likely to include a recommendation that she undergo ACL reconstruction surgery to repair the torn ligament. The recommendation for the specific type of surgical procedure and graft type will vary both by surgeon but also based on the skeletal maturity—or status of growth plate closure and estimation of remaining growth potential—for the particular patient.

What is your plan for follow-up care?
You should see Maria again after she has seen the orthopedist to review her options and answer any questions. If possible, provide a network of patients who have been through this experience so that Maria can talk to others with similar experiences. Provide psychosocial support throughout the pre-surgery, surgery (if undertaken), and rehabilitation process. Consider talking to Maria's coach(es) about incorporating an ACL injury prevention program into the regular routine for their team(s).

Are any referrals needed?
A referral to orthopedics is warranted. Potentially, a referral to a counselor, psychiatrist, or psychologist (especially one involved in sports psychology and/or experienced with pediatric patients) may be helpful. However, Maria has seen a psychiatric mental health nurse practitioner before, so she may already be comfortable with this professional. A referral for physical therapy may be appropriate, depending on the provider's relationship with the pediatric orthopedist to whom she is referring the patient and the orthopedist's preference for management during the acute post-injury phase.

Does the patient's psychosocial history impact how you might treat this patient?
In this case, there is not any difference in treatment based on psychosocial history; but, given Maria's struggles with anxiety, it is important to make sure that she feels like she is knowledgeable and

empowered to make decisions and manage her care. It is important to gauge the patient's response to the situation and determine the need for a mental health referral.

What if this patient was male?
These injuries are less common in males, but similar treatment considerations regarding skeletal maturity would apply.

What if the patient was over age 18 or under age 13?
If the patient was over age 18, she'd likely be at skeletal maturity; and standard adult reconstruction procedures could be used. If she was under 13, she'd be more likely to have wide open physes; and perhaps delayed surgical reconstruction would be the most appropriate treatment option.

What if the patient was also diabetic or hypertensive?
Standard procedures should be used for any diabetic or hypertensive patient undergoing surgery (i.e., extra insulin to compensate for the stressful situation).

What if the patient lived in a rural, isolated setting?
This might limit access to a pediatric orthopedic specialist but should not otherwise impact the plan or care.

What kind of education should you provide to the patient regarding future injury prevention to protect against recurrence or injury to the contralateral side?
The patient is likely to have many questions. An information sheet may help the patient with an ACL injury based on some commonly asked questions (Heffron & Daley, 2010).

Are there any standardized guidelines that you should use to assess or treat this case?
The major guiding principle in the management of ACL injuries is the importance of skeletal maturity. Skeletal maturity will help determine the appropriate treatment modality for a particular patient with an ACL tear. Different surgical techniques have been developed to try to prevent growth disturbance that may result from the use of standard adult reconstruction procedures; and in adolescents with wide open physes, delayed surgical intervention may be the most appropriate modality.

REFERENCES AND RESOURCES

Griffin, L. Y. (2005). *Essentials of musculoskeletal care* (3rd ed.). Rosemont, IL: American Academy of Orthopaedic Surgeons.

Griffin, L. Y., Albohm, M. J., Arendt, E. A., Bahr, R., Beynnon, B. D., Demaio, M., et al. (2006). Understanding and preventing noncontact anterior cruciate ligament injuries: A review of the Hunt Valley II meeting, January 2005. *The American Journal of Sports Medicine, 34*(9), 1512–1532. Doi: 10.1177/0363546506286866.

Heffron, P. M., & Daley, A. M. (2010). *Anterior cruciate ligament injuries in adolescent girls: The primary care provider's guide.* Unpublished manuscript, New Haven, CT: Yale University School of Nursing.

Magee, D. J. (2008). Knee. In D. J. Magee (Ed.), *Orthopaedic physical assessment.* (pp. 727–843). St. Louis: Saunders Elsevier.

Paletta, G. A., Jr. (2003). Special considerations. Anterior cruciate ligament reconstruction in the skeletally immature. *The Orthopedic Clinics of North America, 34*, (1), 65–77. Retrieved from MEDLINE.

Schachter, A. K., & Rokito, A. S. (2007). ACL injuries in the skeletally immature patient. *Orthopedics, 30*(5), 365–370. Retrieved from MEDLINE.

Section 6

Women's Health Cases

Case 6.1 Headache

By Leslie Neal-Boylan, PhD, CRRN, APRN-BC, FNP

Joan is a 35-year-old woman who presents with a complaint of headaches that have been occurring more frequently over the last 2 weeks. She has never had any problems with headaches before. Rarely, she has had a headache after a stressful day but denies premenstrual headaches or frequent headaches until 2 weeks ago. Her headaches are left sided in the temporal area and are severe (7 out of 10 on a 1–10 scale) and throbbing. They occur 3–5 times each week. She occasionally becomes nauseous but rarely vomits. The headaches tend to last several hours and go away if she is able to get sleep. Joan tries to retreat to a dark and quiet corner when the headaches begin. She sometimes sees "spots in front of her eyes" right before the onset of a headache. Otherwise, she has no trouble with her vision, has had no epistaxis, upper respiratory symptoms, or sinus symptoms. She denies trauma to her head or any neck stiffness. She denies fever, chills, numbness, or weakness.

Past medical history: Joan has been otherwise well and denies any previous surgeries or hospitalizations other than for 3 vaginal deliveries without complications.

Family history: Migraine headaches in her mother and sister. Her uncle had a benign brain tumor that was successfully treated.

Social history: The patient does not smoke, drinks 1 beer 3 times each week, and denies ever using recreational drugs. She is married and works as an administrative assistant in a busy office. She has 1 preteen and 2 teenagers at home, and their behavior sometimes causes her stress. Her husband is supportive and helpful.

Medications: Joan's medications include occasional ibuprofen for "aches and pains." She tried the ibuprofen for the headaches without relief. She takes no other medications. She states that her mother told her that she was allergic to penicillin as a child, but she doesn't know why.

General: Joan is well groomed. Her manner and speech are appropriate and she is articulate. She is in no apparent distress during the visit.

Clinical Case Studies for the Family Nurse Practitioner, First Edition. Edited by Leslie Neal-Boylan.
© 2011 John Wiley & Sons, Inc. Published 2011 by John Wiley & Sons, Inc.

Vital signs: The patient is afebrile. Her blood pressure is 140/90 (which she says is higher than her normal blood pressure). Pulse is 86, and respirations are regular at a rate of 12.

HEENT: The eye exam reveals clear sclera, conjunctiva without injection, and PERRLA. EOMs are intact. There is no AV nicking or papilledema. Optic disks have clear margins. Nasal mucosa is without erythema or drainage. There is no sinus tenderness to palpation. Cranial nerves II–XII are grossly intact.

Cardiac: Unremarkable.

Respiratory: Unremarkable.

Neurologic: Sensation and proprioception are grossly intact, and the Romberg test is negative. Gait is steady. Brudzinski and Kernig signs are negative.

CRITICAL THINKING

Which diagnostic or imaging studies should be considered to assist with or confirm the diagnosis?
___CT scan
___MRI
___CBC
___CMP
___Lipid panel

What is the most likely differential diagnosis and why?
___Migraine with aura
___Migraine without aura
___Cluster headache
___Tension headache
___Meningitis
___Temporal arteritis
___Psychogenic headache

What is the plan of treatment and follow-up care?

Are any referrals needed at this time?

Does Joan's stress impact her diagnosis or treatment?

Is her blood pressure the cause or the result of her headache?

Would your treatment change if the patient were a smoker or on birth control pills?

RESOLUTION

Diagnostic tests: A CT scan is appropriate, and a CBC with differential would be helpful to rule out infection and anemia as causes of the headaches.

What is the most likely differential diagnosis and why?
Migraine with aura
Because these are new onset headaches and also because her family history is significant for an uncle with a brain tumor, it is important to rule out other causes of her headaches, such as a brain tumor or aneurysm. Joan appears to have an aura, because she has noticed "spots" in front of her eyes just before onset. Cluster headaches are more common in men, tend to occur over one side of the head

or one eye, are excruciating and often explosive, and may also involve ipsilateral eye tearing. Patients tend to describe tension headaches as being bandlike and will motion to the temporal areas of the head bilaterally when describing the location of the pain. The headaches usually go away with rest or diversionary activities. Meningeal irritation tends to cause neck stiffness and fever as well as headache, and Brudzinski and Kernig signs tend to be positive. Joan is too young to have temporal arteritis. This is a condition that is typically associated with polymyalgia rheumatica (PMR), a disease of adults over age 50 that presents with shoulder and hip girdle pain. Patients with temporal arteritis tend to have headache, possible jaw claudication, scalp or facial tenderness, and possibly diplopia. Patients who are suspected of having PMR or temporal arteritis should have an ESR done. Typically, the ESR will be very high (over 50) in these cases. High doses of prednisone are typically given to treat both conditions, and a rheumatologist should be consulted as part of the treatment plan.

Joan might have a psychogenic headache but her history does not support this condition. That type of headaches is more often bilateral and does not follow any particular pattern. Joan's headaches are throbbing, unilateral, accompanied by nausea, preceded by an aura, and disappear with sleep. These migraines typically occur in women aged 30 to 50 years, and they often run in families.

There are various migraine triggers, such as hormonal changes (many women have premenstrual migraines), missed meals, certain foods such as chocolate or red wine, weather changes, stress or tension, birth control pills, nitrates, monosodium glutamate, tyramine, caffeine, vasodilation from any source, lack of sleep, glaring or flickering lights, smoking, and alcohol use.

What is the plan of treatment and follow-up care?

Migraine treatment can target suppressive therapy if the patient has several migraines in one week, abortive therapy (at the time of onset) or post migraine. Examples of suppressive therapy include NSAIDs, acetaminophen, SSRIs, topiramate, propranolol, and amitriptyline. Abortive therapies include metoclopramide (an antiemetic), triptans, and ergotamines. Since this patient is having ongoing headaches, topiramate would be a good choice, titrated up carefully. First, a CT scan would need to rule out other causes. Advising the patient to keep a headache diary in order to avoid triggers, as well as to retreat to a dark quiet room at onset of the migraine, would also be helpful. Joan should be seen for followup after 1 week to titrate the medicine as necessary and to review test and lab results.

Are there any referrals needed at this time?

If temporal arteritis is suspected, she should be referred immediately for an ophthalmologic consult to prevent vision loss; but Joan does not need this referral at this time. However, if the CT scan is abnormal or Joan exhibits neurological deficits, she should be referred to a neurologist.

Does Joan's stress impact her diagnosis or treatment?

Joan's level of stress probably does impact her migraines; however, counseling regarding stress reduction and relaxation exercises would be helpful.

Is her blood pressure the cause or the result of her headache?

Joan's blood pressure may be a result of her headache pain. However, followup when she is not in pain is warranted to evaluate her for hypertension.

Would your treatment change if the patient were a smoker or on birth control pills?

If Joan was a smoker or on birth control pills, she would be encouraged to stop smoking (for overall health and because smoking is a migraine trigger). Birth control pills can be a trigger for migraine, and patients with a migraine with aura should discontinue or not start birth control pills. Furthermore, smoking and the use of birth control pills can significantly increase the risk of deep vein thrombosis.

REFERENCE AND RESOURCE

McPhee, S. J., & Papadakis, M. A. (2010). *Current medical diagnosis & treatment* (49th ed.). New York: McGraw-Hill Lange.

Case 6.2 Night Sweats

By Ivy M. Alexander, PhD, APRN, ANP-BC, FAAN

SUBJECTIVE

Susan is a 50-year-old female who presents for her annual physical check up with a complaint of hot flashes and night sweats. Susan reports that some of the night sweats are drenching. She is having difficulty sleeping and is finding it hard to function at work.

Susan says her symptoms have been present for about 4-8 months. They seem to be increasing in intensity and frequency. She says "some days I think I am going crazy! I cannot sleep and I am so easily frustrated and tired all of the time." She expresses embarrassment about sweating at work and says that she sometimes has trouble remembering things and staying focused at work meetings.

Past medical history: No major chronic medical problems, + high blood pressure at the end of her second pregnancy (resolved with the birth), + seasonal allergies.

Surgical history: Tonsillectomy at age 6. Wisdom teeth excisions at age 20.

Family history: Mother—osteoporosis, mild depression. Father—cardiovascular disease (CVD), hypertension, possibly diabetes mellitus. Sister (3 years older)—"terrible menopause symptoms," recently diagnosed with a thyroid problem. Brother (2 years younger)—hypertension. MGM—osteoporosis, depression. PGF—early CVD with myocardial infarction at age 50.

Social history: Susan lives with her husband of 19 years, their two daughters, and the family dog in a private home that they own. She is employed as an editor with a private press agency and enjoys her work. She reports feeling stressed at work lately due to difficulty remembering tasks and missing deadlines as a result. She reports that the most important recent life event was her daughter's graduation from high school. She is happy for her daughter as she was admitted to the university of her choice, but Susan is not looking forward to having her leave home in the fall. She describes her usual day as follows: awakes around 6 a.m., makes breakfast for herself and the family, showers and dresses for work, drives to work and is at her desk by 8:30 a.m. She leaves around 5:30 p.m. and drives home. She makes dinner most evenings and spends time in the evening assisting her younger daughter with homework and doing household chores. She starts getting ready for bed around 10 p.m. She reports walking the dog each day for about 1.5 miles, usually in the evening unless it is too hot.

Diet: Her 24-hour diet recall reveals a bagel with cream cheese and coffee (black) for breakfast, salad with cottage cheese for lunch, grilled fish with potatoes and salad for dinner, and no snacks. She reports that she eats out about once per week and enjoys dessert on occasion.

Clinical Case Studies for the Family Nurse Practitioner, First Edition. Edited by Leslie Neal-Boylan.
© 2011 John Wiley & Sons, Inc. Published 2011 by John Wiley & Sons, Inc.

Substance use: She denies use of tobacco. She reports alcohol use as 1 glass of red wine most evenings. She denies use of recreational/illicit drugs.

Safety: She reports feeling safe at home with her husband and family. She had 1 partner several years ago who threatened her physically, but she has had no contact with him for several years. Since then she has never been hit, slapped, kicked, or otherwise physically hurt by anyone. She denies ever being forced to have sexual activities when she did not want to. She uses a seatbelt and sunblock regularly and has working smoke detectors and carbon monoxide detectors at home. Her husband does have a hunting rifle, which is kept locked with the ammunition stored separately. She denies any concerns for her children or personal safety with regard to the rifle. She denies having any current concerns about HIV.

Medications: OTC antihistamines for allergies PRN; MVI daily; calcium (when she remembers); nasal spray for allergies PRN.

Allergies: NKDA, NKFA, +seasonal allergies

General: Susan describes her overall health as "good, but getting weird lately." She reports a recent weight increase of about 4 pounds. She identifies her usual weight as 145 lbs. She reports fatigue and reduced energy since her hot flashes and poor sleep began. She denies any substantive premenstrual syndrome (PMS) symptoms. "I sometimes crave salty foods or chocolate, but it is not anything big." She denies symptoms of premenstrual dysphoric disorder (PMDD).

Mood: Susan reports her usual mood as "generally good, but I feel crabby when I don't sleep well." Recently she notes increased moodiness, especially after a night of poor sleep. She denies feeling nervous, or anxious but admits to feeling irritable and getting angry more easily than usual when she is tired and having more hot flashes. She says, "I feel depressed. I don't sleep well, and most of the things I used to enjoy doing irritate me now. I feel like I am going crazy." She denies anhedonia and with questioning says that she enjoys reading, eating out with her husband or friends, shopping with her daughters, and doing yoga classes. Susan denies eating disorders, she says "sometimes I eat when I feel irritated, you know, comfort food like chips or chocolate; and it doesn't even make me feel better! But no, I don't think I have an eating disorder."

Cognitive: Susan describes difficulty with concentration and memory, especially at work after a night of particularly poor sleep or several nights of interrupted sleep. She denies problems with cognition, noting that she thinks clearly and can follow the conversation. Her issue is "with remembering what I said I would do. If I don't write it down, it is likely that it will not get done." She does use lists for shopping, puts appointments in a calendar, and carries a notebook to write down tasks when at work.

Systemic: Susan reports that she began having hot flashes about 8 months ago. They have been slowly and progressively getting worse. She does have night sweats as well; sometimes she has to change her pajamas and sheets. She describes the severity of the hot flashes as 4–10 on a 1–10 scale, "sometimes they are tolerable and I just feel hot; other times I am completely drenched with sweat." She reports having hot flashes during the day anywhere from 6 –20 times. Her night sweats occur anywhere from 2–10 times nightly.

HEENT: Susan denies any problems with headaches, unless she forgets her morning coffee; and then she says "I get a headache around 2 p.m., but if I have a cup of coffee then it goes away. Of course then I don't sleep well." Susan reports minor changes in her vision over the past 3 years, requiring her to use reading glasses more and more often. She denies recent changes in hearing, smell, taste, or swallowing. She reports some increased dry eye symptoms and finds that she needs to use eye lubricating drops, especially when she is doing a lot of work on the computer. She has seasonal allergies and experiences sneezing, rhinorrhea, and itchy eyes year round and especially in the early fall.

Respiratory: Susan denies having any cough, wheeze, or shortness of breath in the recent past.

Cardiovascular: Susan denies chest pain, palpitations, dyspnea on exertion, peripheral edema, or a history of blood clots. She says that she has always had cold hands and feet, "Maybe it is Raynaud's.

They get so cold and take a long time to warm up. I am OK if I remember to wear gloves and keep my feet warm."

Breast: Susan reports that she does do self-breast exams, usually each month right after her period. She has forgotten often this past year since she has been missing periods. She denies any concerns or recent breast changes. She denies any discharge, pain, or tingling. She did breast-feed each of her daughters.

Gastrointestinal: Susan reports occasional heartburn after a large or spicy meal that is relieved with Maalox. She denies persistent abdominal pain and reports daily regular bowel movements without constipation or recent changes in color, consistency, or pattern of stools. Specifically, she denies seeing any blood or experiencing fecal incontinence.

Genitourinary: Susan reports some urgency and occasional leakage of small amounts of urine, especially with coughing or laughing. She denies urinary frequency; history of recurrent urinary tract infections, pyelonephritis, or renal stones; and urine dribbling or outright incontinence. She says she does not have dysuria. She reports occasional nocturia of once or twice at night, but is unsure if this wakes her or if she is awake and then feels she needs to urinate before going back to sleep.

Gynecological: Susan reports no abnormal Pap smears or gynecological surgeries. She denies vaginal or vulvar discharge, itching, irritation, soreness, burning, abnormal bleeding, or lesions. She denies pelvic pain or rash. She reports some vaginal dryness, especially noticed with sexual activity.

Pregnancy history: Susan has been pregnant twice. She is P2, G2 with two healthy living daughters aged 15 and 18 years. She reports that she did breast-feed each daughter, the older one for 6 months and the younger one for 8 months.

Menstrual history: Susan reports that her last menstrual period was 6 weeks ago. She reports that the menses was typical and lasted for 6 days with 1–2 days of light flow, followed by 3 days of heavier flow and then 1–2 days of light spotting. She experienced menarche at 13 years of age and after the first few years had pretty regular periods occurring every 28–30 days. Over the past year she has had some missed periods and some with flow that was lighter than her usual pattern. She had one period with light flow that continued for about 2 weeks.

Contraception: Susan reports that she used oral contraceptive pills for contraception in the past. She has not taken any type of hormone for contraception for the past 10 years because her husband had a vasectomy when they decided not to have any more children.

Sexual: Susan reports that she is sexually active with her husband. She is mostly satisfied but notes that it has become harder to get adequately lubricated and that it takes longer to achieve orgasm. She reports she has had 6 lifetime partners and has been monogamous with her husband for over 20 years. She reports that her desire/libido is satisfactory but is less strong than it was 1 year ago. She says this is, "a bummer. We have always had a good sex life and I miss wanting it like I used to." Her arousal is reported as satisfactory, but "it takes longer to get ready than it used to." She usually does achieve orgasm but "it takes longer than it used to and sometimes he is already finished and I am left feeling a bit frustrated." She denies dyspareunia. She reports their usual sexual practices include cuddling and kissing, then foreplay that includes genital manipulation, and then vaginal intercourse with penile penetration. They have used OTC lubricants recently, due to her dryness. She says she feels good and enjoys sex when it happens, but she doesn't initiate activity or wish for it like she used to. She reports their relationship quality as, "Oh, really good. When he finishes before me we laugh about it and talk it over. Sometimes he brings me to orgasm manually, but it can take a long time."

Musculoskeletal: Susan reports that she has noticed some vague joint and muscle pain over the past year. It seems better when she gets regular exercise and does not stop her from her usual activities.

Endocrine: Susan denies polydipsia, polyuria, polyphagia, and symptoms of diabetes mellitus type 2.

Skin/Hair: Susan denies noticing any recent skin changes or lesions of concern. She has noticed some increased acne around her mouth, skin dryness and wrinkles, and dry/thinning hair, especially on her head. She denies hirsutism or facial hair.

Hematologic: Susan denies any bleeding or bruising that doesn't correlate to a specific injury.

Neurologic: Susan reports some numbness and tingling if her hands or feet get too cold, but not otherwise. She denies fainting, dizziness (vertigo), feeling off balance, or having difficulty walking.

Sleep: Susan's usual bedtime routine includes nighttime washing and tooth brushing followed by reading or watching TV for about 30 minutes. She denies use of stimulants except for coffee each morning. She does wake every night with hot flashes/sweats. She is able to fall back to sleep but reports that it can take up to an hour depending on whether she needs to change her pajamas or sheets and how long it takes to feel cool again. She usually goes to bed around 10 p.m. and falls asleep around 10:30 p.m. She gets up for work around 6 a.m. most days. She reports that she usually does not feel refreshed when she wakes up.

OBJECTIVE

Vital signs: BP: 132/80 (L) sitting; P: 78; RR: 10; weight: 152 lbs; height: 5 ft 7 inches; BMI: 23.8.

General: Appears well; in no apparent distress; neatly dressed; appropriate affect.

HEENT: Head: Nontender; without masses; hair thinning slightly in some areas. Eyes: Clear conjunctivae; PERRLA intact; EOMI; fundi sharp optic discs; normal retinal arterioles; no A-V nicking. Ears: Clear external auditory canals; TMs + light reflex and landmarks visible; hearing grossly normal. Mouth/Throat: + normal mucosa, tongue, pharynx, and tonsils; dentition in good repair.

Neck: Supple, without lymphadenopathy. Thyroid nontender, without palpable masses or enlargement. Carotids without bruits.

Respiratory: Clear to auscultation and percussion, anterior and posterior; without wheezes, rales, or rhonchi.

Cardiac: RRR: normal S1 and S2 without murmurs, rubs, or gallops.

Breasts: Without masses, skin changes, or discharge bilaterally; no lymphadenopathy.

Abdomen: Soft, nondistended, nontender; + bowel sounds x 4 Quadrants; without HSM, masses, or bruits.

Gynecological: Vaginal mucosa slightly dry, rugae present; uterus firm and anteverted, nontender, without palpable masses; adnexa nontender, without palpable masses bilaterally; no lesions noted.

Rectal: No lesions or masses noted; + external hemorrhoids; nontender; + normal sphincter tone.

Extremities: Without cyanosis, edema, or clubbing; +2 pulses bilaterally. + FROM throughout, nontender joints without crepitus.

Neurologic: CN II–XII grossly negative; 5/5 motor strength, gait even; DTRs 2+; Romberg negative.

CRITICAL THINKING

Which diagnostic or imaging studies should be considered to assist with or confirm the diagnosis?
__FSH, estrogen, and LH levels
__TSH level

__Fasting lipid panel and fasting blood sugar level
__CBC, BUN/creatinine, CGFR
__LFTs
__Beck Depression Inventory
__PPD
__DXA
__Colonoscopy

What is the most likely differential diagnosis and why?
__Menopausal transition
__Depression
__Thyroid disorders
__Sexual desire disorders
__Tuberculosis
__Untreated DM
__Hypertension
__Other psychiatric disorders

What is your plan of treatment?

What additional patient education is important for Susan?

Are any referrals needed?

Does Susan's psychosocial history affect how you might treat her?

What if Susan were over age 65?

What if Susan also had diabetes or hypertension?

Are there any standardized guidelines that you should use to assess or treat Susan?

RESOLUTION

Diagnostic tests: Diagnostic testing is not needed to diagnose the menopause transition except for ruling out comorbid conditions or identifying medical problems that may exacerbate the woman's menopause transition symptoms and thus affect the plan of care.

1. FSH, estrogen, and LH levels: Hormone levels are not tested to determine menopausal status (North American Menopause Society, 2007). Hormone levels are very volatile during the peri-menopausal years rendering testing at any one point in time useless (North American Menopause Society, 2007). The goal of treatment is symptom management, and hormone levels are not used to monitor efficacy. Thus knowledge of specific hormone levels is unnecessary. Additionally, if hormone levels are tested, the information may falsely suggest that the woman is postmenopausal when she is actually perimenopausal and could still ovulate and become pregnant.
2. TSH level: Testing TSH may be useful to determine if Susan also has a thyroid problem. It will not aid in diagnosing the menopause transition but may guide care as an untreated thyroid disorder can exacerbate symptoms of the menopause transition.
3. Fasting lipid panel and fasting blood sugar level: While it may be reasonable to order a fasting lipid panel for Susan if she has not had one recently, it will not forward the diagnosis of her symptoms. Testing a fasting blood sugar level may be useful in identifying if Susan also has DM. This also will not aid in diagnosing the menopause transition but may guide care as untreated DM can exacerbate symptoms of the menopause transition and may alter the selection of pharmacotherapeutics.
4. CBC, BUN/creatinine, CGFR: These tests are not needed for diagnosing the menopause transition. Knowing her kidney function status may be useful when determining whether to use pharmacotherapeutics to manage her symptoms.

5. LFTs: These tests are not needed for diagnosing the menopause transition. Knowing her liver function status may be useful when determining whether to use pharmacotherapeutics to manage her symptoms.

6. Beck Depression Inventory: Administering the BDS may be useful to determine if Susan also has depression. It will not aid in diagnosing the menopause transition, but it may guide care as untreated depression can exacerbate menopause transition symptoms and may alter the selection of pharmacotherapeutics.

7. PPD: If Susan had a history suggesting exposure to TB, it would be prudent to check a PPD because she is experiencing night sweats. However, most of her history suggests an alternate diagnosis; for example, she is gaining, rather than losing weight and she has no cough or other symptoms suggestive of TB. Thus, it is unlikely that a PPD will provide useful clinical information.

8. DXA: It is too early to order a routine DXA for Susan. Guidelines recommend evaluating all postmenopausal women at age 65 unless they have specific additional risk factors (Dawson-Hughes, 2008; North American Menopause Society, 2010b). DXA test results will not aid in the diagnosis of her symptoms.

9. Colonoscopy: The American Cancer Society recommends that all adults receive colon cancer screening at age 50 or earlier depending on personal history (Smith, Cokkinides, Brooks, Saslow, & Brawley, 2010). Colonoscopy, however, will not aid in the diagnosis of her symptoms.

What is the most likely differential diagnosis and why?
Symptomatic menopause transition
Susan is experiencing several of the most common symptoms (e.g., hot flashes, night sweats, sleep disturbances, weight gain, altered sexual function) as well as several associated symptoms (e.g., altered mood, hair thinning, memory changes) (see Table 6.2.1) (Alexander & Andrist, 2005; North

TABLE 6.2.1. Symptoms Associated with the Menopause Transition.

System	Symptoms
Central nervous system	Anxiety/nervousness, cognitive changes, depression, dizziness, fatigue, forgetfulness, formication, headache, hot flashes/flushes, insomnia, irritability/mood disturbances/"rage," night sweats, poor concentration, sleep disturbances, paresthesia
Eyes	Dry eyes
Cardiovascular	Palpitations
Breast	Mastalgia
Gynecologic and sexual	Dyspareunia, irregular menstrual bleeding, recurrent vaginitis, reduced libido, vaginal atrophy, vaginal dryness, vaginal/vulvar irritation, vaginal/vulvar pruritus
Musculoskeletal	Arthralgia, asthenia, myalgia
Urinary	Dysuria, genitourinary burning, recurrent cystitis, nocturia, stress urinary incontinence*, urinary frequency, urinary urgency
Skin and hair	Acne, dry skin and hair, hirsutism/virilization, skin dryness/atrophy, thinning hair, odor (increased perspiration)

*Data are inconclusive.
Data from: Alexander IM, Ruff C, Rousseau ME, et al. (2003). Menopause symptoms and management strategies identified by black women (abstract). *Menopause.*10(6):601. North American Menopause Society (2007). *Menopause Practice: A Clinician's Guide.* 3rd ed. Cleveland, OH: North American Menopause Society; North American Menopause Society (2008). Estrogen and progestogen use in postmenopausal women: July 2008 position statement of The North American Menopause Society. *Menopause.* Available at: http://www.ncbi.nlm.nih.gov/entrez/query.fcgi?cmd=Retrieve&db=PubMed&dopt=Citation&list_uids=18580541, accessed August 30, 2010; Greendale GA, Lee NP, Arriola ER. (1999). The menopause. *Lancet.* 353(9152):571–580; Jacobs Institute on Women's Health. (2003). Expert Panel on Menopause Counseling. *Jacobs Institute.* Available at: www.jiwh.org/menodownload.htm. Accessed August 30, 2010; Avis NE, Stellato R, Crawford S, et al. (2001). Is there a menopausal syndrome? Menopausal status and symptoms across racial/ethnic groups. *Social Science and Medicine.*52(2001):345–356; McKinlay SM. (1996). The normal menopause transition: An overview. *Maturitas.* 23(2):137–145; and adapted from: Alexander, I & Andrist, L. (2005). Chapter 11: Menopause, in F. Likis & K. Shuiling (Eds), *Women's Gynecologic Health.* Sudbury, MA: Jones and Bartlett.

American Menopause Society, 2007, 2008, 2010a). This diagnosis is usually made based on the history and physical examination. Selected diagnostic studies may be warranted to rule out comorbid conditions that may affect her symptom severity and the management plan (Alexander & Andrist, 2005; North American Menopause Society, 2007).

A thyroid disorder, especially hypothyroidism, must also be considered. Hypothyroidism has many common presenting symptoms that overlap with symptoms of the menopause transition (Norman, 2010; North American Menopause Society, 2007). For example, Susan has described hair loss, fatigue, reduced libido, weight gain, irritability, memory loss, altered menstrual cycles, and reduced libido. These symptoms are all associated with both menopause and hypothyroidism (Norman, 2010; North American Menopause Society, 2007). She has not described cold temperature intolerance, weakness, constipation, hair texture changes, skin texture changes (dry and rough), or muscle aches, which are other symptoms associated with hypothyroidism (Norman, 2010). Additionally, she has described symptoms that are not commonly associated with hypothyroidism but that are commonly associated with the menopause transition, such as hot flashes, night sweats, and sleep disturbances (Alexander & Andrist, 2005; North American Menopause Society, 2007). Given the overlap in symptoms and the potential for untreated hypothyroidism to exacerbate symptoms of the menopause transition, it would be prudent to check a TSH level for Susan.

Like hypothyroidism, a sexual desire disorder is an important comorbid diagnosis to consider for Susan. Reduced libido is common among midlife women; however, a specific sexual desire disorder can also be present. The management of these 2 problems differs, so it is important to distinguish exactly what Susan is experiencing. The most common sexual desire disorder among women is hypoactive sexual desire disorder (HSDD), which affects about 30% of women (Laumann, Paik, & Rosen, 1999). HSDD is defined as "the persistent or recurrent deficiency (or absence) of sexual fantasies/thoughts, and/or desire for or receptivity to sexual activity, which causes personal distress" (Basson et al., 2000). The perception of distress experienced by the woman is a very important part of this diagnosis. While Susan described missing her previous level of desire for sex, she does enjoy sex when it happens; and she does not describe significant distress, noting that it is a "bummer" and that she misses wanting sex like she used to. It is also unlikely that Susan is experiencing sexual aversion disorder as she does not avoid sexual contact with her partner (Basson et al., 2000); conversely, she has noted that she misses their usual level of sexual activity.

Depression is less likely for Susan due to the array of symptoms that she is not experiencing and that are required to make a diagnosis of depression. The 4th edition of the *American Psychiatric Association Diagnostic and Statistical Manual of Mental Disorders (DSM-IV)* specifies criteria for the diagnosis of depression. DSM-IV states that patients must experience symptoms for at least 2 weeks, including a change in functioning with either depressed mood or a loss of interest in things that they used to enjoy. Additionally, there must be at least 5 other symptoms, which can include depressed mood or loss of interest in enjoyable activities/anhedonia, as well as substantive appetite and weight changes, sleep disturbances, suicidal thoughts or ideation, feeling worthless or excessively guilty, fatigue, cognitive changes (forgetfulness, difficulty concentrating), or psychomotor changes (retardation or agitation) (American Psychiatric Association, 2000). When considering depression it is important to note that Susan does not describe enough symptoms to meet the DSM-IV criteria for depression. However, it is also important to recognize that depression often does affect women at midlife and may exacerbate symptoms of the menopause transition (North American Menopause Society, 2007).

Other even less likely differentials might include TB, untreated DM or HTN, and other psychiatric disorders. None of these diagnoses carry enough overlapping symptoms with those described by Susan and commonly associated with the menopause transition to make them likely as her primary diagnosis. DM and HTN could exacerbate her menopause transition symptoms. However, she does not have an elevated BP on examination; and she does not have symptoms suggestive of DM. TB is the least likely of all because the only overlapping symptom is night sweats.

What is your plan of treatment?
Most of Susan's symptoms are related to her hot flashes. Vasomotor symptoms cause sleep disruptions, which in turn affect mood, energy level, memory, and cognitive processes. Once the hot flashes are controlled and sleep is restored the associated symptoms usually will resolve (North American

Menopause Society, 2007). A stepped approach is recommended for managing vasomotor symptoms associated with the menopause transition (Alexander & Andrist, 2005; Nachtigall et al., 2006; North American Menopause Society, 2007, 2008, 2010a). Start by advising Susan about lifestyle and environmental changes that can reduce her symptoms, then explore complementary and alternative medicine therapies (CAM) that might help her, and finally prescribe medications if needed.

Susan likely would benefit from increasing her routine aerobic activity. Her goal should be at least 1 hour each day, but even small increases may be beneficial (Lindh-Astrand, Nedstrand, Wyon, & Hammar, 2004; Thompson, Church, & Blair, 2008). Aerobic exercise helps to decrease hot flash severity and frequency by improving the body's ability to maintain temperature regulation (Alexander, Ruff, & Udemezue, u.d.; Lindh-Astrand et al., 2004; Thompson et al., 2008; Villaverde-Gutierrez et al., 2006). Regular exercise also improves sleep quality, memory, and quality of life; decreases depression; reduces cardiac disease risk; and helps to maintain normal blood glucose levels and weight in midlife women (Alexander et al., u.d.; Gold et al., 2000; Lindh-Astrand et al., 2004; Thompson et al., 2008; Villaverde-Gutierrez et al., 2006).

Susan also needs to be counseled to avoid hot flash triggers such as caffeine (any type can trigger flashes—cold, hot, solid, liquid), concentrated sugar, and alcohol. Reducing or avoiding use of these substances can reduce both frequency and severity of her vasomotor symptoms (Alexander et al., 2003; North American Menopause Society, 2007). Increasing her consumption of ice water may help to stabilize her core temperature and reduce hot flashes.

Susan can further reduce her symptoms by wearing breathable fabrics like cottons that allow for greater air movement and avoiding synthetics and tight clothing. Wearing layers that can easily be removed when she feels hot and avoiding high necklines and turtleneck shirts may reduce her symptoms and embarrassment at work. Using breathable fabrics for her pajamas, sheets, and blankets is important as well. A fan to circulate the air and keeping the room temperature at a moderately cool level may also reduce hot flashes (Alexander et al., 2003, 2004; North American Menopause Society, 2007).

Several CAM therapies such as relaxation and deep breathing exercises, acupuncture, and selected botanical or herbal preparations may be useful in reducing vasomotor symptoms caused by the menopause transition. Stress and anxiety are triggers for hot flashes (Alexander et al., 2004), so it stands to reason that relaxation and stress-reducing practices, like yoga, prayer, and talking over problems, can decrease hot flashes (Alexander et al., 2004; Carson, Carson, Porter, & Keefe, 2008). Susan can be taught to do paced deep breathing (like yoga breathing: breathe in deeply over a count of 4, hold the breath for a count of 7, then exhale over a count of 9) to reduce hot flashes when they occur or to reduce her stress in general (Freedman & Woodward, 1992; Freedman, Woodward, Brown, Javaid, & Pandy, 1995; Irvin, Domar, Clark, Zuttermeister, & Freidman, 1996). Acupuncture is another CAM therapy that provides stress relief. Although several studies have evaluated acupuncture for vasomotor symptom management, clear evidence supporting its efficacy has been lacking (Lee, Shin, & Ernst, 2009). Even so, Susan could try acupuncture if she is interested; it is a well-accepted and safe practice that promotes relaxation.

Many women are interested in trying botanical and herbal preparations to manage their menopause transition symptoms (Brett & Keenan, 2007; Newton, Buist, Keenan, Anderson, & LaCroix, 2002). Several preparations are commonly used including black cohosh, dong quai, various isoflavones (i.e., soy extracts, red clover, soy supplementation), oil of evening primrose, and ginseng (Ihenacho, 2009; Kupferer, Dormire, & Becker, 2009). Black cohosh is usually well tolerated and has the most evidence supporting its use. It may have some estrogenic activity (Bolle, Mastrangelo, Perrone, & Evandri, 2007; Rice, Amon, & Whitehead, 2007), so if Susan decides to try this she will need to be monitored for endometrial overgrowth. She also needs to be warned to watch for signs of liver problems as case reports have identified hepatitis and liver toxicity in some women (Mahady et al., 2008).

Pharmacotherapeutics—Both nonhormonal and hormonal prescription options are available to help Susan if she is still experiencing moderate to severe symptoms (see Table 6.2.2). Many women wish to avoid the use of hormones, so Susan needs to be carefully questioned about her specific preferences. Additionally, because every medication has contraindications, Susan's medical, family, and personal history must be carefully reviewed to assure that any specific medication being consid-

TABLE 6.2.2. Prescription Options* for Managing Vasomotor Symptoms Associated with the Menopause Transition

Medication Class	Example(s)	General Cautions and Contraindications	Comments
Anticonvulsants	Gabapentin (Neurontin)	Do not take within 2 hours of antacids. CNS depression potentiated by alcohol.	Avoid discontinuing abruptly. Titrate dose up slowly to reduce somnolence.
Anti-hypertensives	Bellergal Clonidine Methyldopa	Tricyclic antidepressants antagonize clonidine. CNS depressants are potentiated by clonidine.	Clonidine is available as a patch. SSRIs/SNRIs and gabapentin have higher efficacy than clonidine. Avoid abruptly discontinuing clonidine. Bellergal and methyldopa are not recommended because of toxicity.
Breast cancer agent (progestin)	Megestrol (Megace)	Use caution in patients with diabetes or a history of a thromboembolic disorder.	May increase requirements for insulin.
Selective serotonin reuptake inhibitors (SSRIs)/ serotonin norepinephrine reuptake inhibitors (SNRIs)	Desvenlafaxine (Pristiq) Fluoxetine (Prozac) Paroxetine (Paxil, Paxil CR) Venlafaxine (Effexor XR)	Avoid use with thioridazine or monoamine oxidase inhibitors. Use caution in patients taking warfarin. Warn patients to avoid using with alcohol. Use caution in patients with diabetes, diseases that alter metabolism, and heart disease.	Avoid discontinuing abruptly. Monitor weight regularly (fluoxetine).
Estrogen**	Conjugated estrogens and conjugated estrogens, B (Cenestin, Enjuvia, Premarin) Estradiol (Alora, Climara, Divigel, Elestrin, Esclim, Estraderm, Estrasorb, Estro-Gel, Evamist, Menostar, Vivelle, Vivelle-Dot) Estradiol acetate (Femtrace, Femring) Estradiol hemihydrate (Vagifem) Esterified estrogens (Menest) Estropipate (Ogen, Ortho-est) Micronized estradiol (Estrace, Estring)	Do not use in patients with unexplained vaginal bleeding. Do not use in patients with cardiovascular disease, liver disease, breast cancer, estrogen-dependent cancer, pregnancy, or thromboembolism.	Available in multiple delivery forms: oral pill; transdermal patch, mousse, cream, gel, spray; injectable; vaginal cream, tablet, ring. Also available in combination with progestogens or methyltestosterone in varied forms. Use the lowest dose that controls symptoms for the shortest period of time possible. Wean off with slowly decreasing doses.

*Consult a prescribing reference to obtain complete information regarding doses, cautions, contraindications, and side effects. The use of nonhormonal medications to manage vasomotor symptoms associated with the menopause transition is off label. Nonhormonal medications are less effective than estrogen for managing vasomotor symptoms.

**Progestogen is used to prevent endometrial hyperplasia and endometrial cancer for any woman who is taking estrogen and has her uterus.

Data From: North American Menopause Society (2007). *Menopause Practice: A Clinician's Guide.* 3rd ed. Cleveland, OH: North American Menopause Society; North American Menopause Society (2008). Estrogen and progestogen use in postmenopausal women: July 2008 position statement of The North American Menopause Society. *Menopause.* Jun 20 2008; North American Menopause Society (2007). The role of local vaginal estrogen for treatment of vaginal atrophy in postmenopausal women: 2007 position statement of The North American Menopause Society. *Menopause.* 14(3 Pt 1):355–369; Micromedex. Available at: http://www.thomsonhc.com/hcs/librarian (with membership). Accessed August 30, 2010; ePocrates. Computerized pharmacology and prescribing reference. Updated daily. Available at: www.epocrates.com. Accessed August 29, 2010; Nelson HD, Vesco KK, Haney E, et al. Nonhormonal therapies for menopausal hot flashes:Systematic review and meta-analysis. *JAMA.* May 3 2006, 295(17):2057–2071; Grady D. A 60-year-old woman trying to discontinue hormone replacement therapy. *JAMA.* April 24, 2002, 287(16):2130–2137; Albertazzi P. A review of non-hormonal options for the relief of menopausal symptoms. *Treat Endocrinol.* 2006, 5(2):101–113; Speroff L, Gass M, Constantine G, Olivier S. Efficacy and tolerability of desvenlafaxine succinate treatment for menopausal vasomotor symptoms: A randomized controlled trial. *Obstet Gynecol.* Jan 2008, 111(1):77–87; North American Menopause Society (2009). Hormone Products for Postmenopausal Use in the United States and Canada. *North American Menopause Society.* Available for members at: http://www.menopause.org/htcharts.pdf. Accessed August 29, 2010; Kimmick GG, Lovato J, McQuellon R, Robinson E, Muss HB. Randomized, double-blind, placebo-controlled, crossover study of sertraline (Zoloft) for the treatment of hot flashes in women with early stage breast cancer taking tamoxifen. *Breast J.* Mar–Apr 2006;12(2):114–122; North American Menopause Society. (2010). Estrogen and progestogen use in postmenopausal women: 2010 position statement of The North American Menopause Society. *Menopause,* 17(2):242–255; Gordon PR, Kerwin JP, Boesen KG, Senf J. Sertraline to treat hot flashes: A randomized controlled, double-blind, crossover trial in a general population. *Menopause.* Jul-Aug 2006;13(4):568–575; Stearns V, Beebe KL, Iyengar M, Dube E. Paroxetine controlled release in the treatment of menopausal hot flashes: A randomized controlled trial. *JAMA.* Jun 4 2003, 289(21):2827–2834; and adapted from Alexander, I & Andrist, L. (2005). Chapter 11: Menopause, in F. Likis & K. Shuiling (Eds), *Women's Gynecologic Health.* Sudbury, MA: Jones and Bartlett.

ered is an appropriate option for her. Similarly, common side effects from specific medications must be reviewed to determine if they would help or further increase any of Susan's symptoms. For example, selective serotonin reuptake inhibitors (SSRIs) and serotonin norepinephrine reuptake inhibitors (SNRIs) are known to commonly cause sexual disturbances and anorgasmia. In Susan's case it may be prudent to avoid use of this class of medication since she is already experiencing vaginal dryness, reduced libido, and increased time to orgasm. Systemic estrogen therapy will reduce hot flash frequency and severity as well as improve vaginal dryness among a number of other symptoms. This medication option is reasonable for Susan as she has none of the contraindications that might preclude its use (e.g., no breast cancer, no unexplained bleeding, no heart disease).

Hormone therapy (HT) is the most effective agent for managing vasomotor symptoms as well as multiple other symptoms associated with the menopause transition (Grady, 2002; Nelson et al., 2006; North American Menopause Society, 2008, 2010a). For a woman with her uterus in place, such as Susan, estrogen is taken daily and progesterone is either taken daily to impede endometrial lining buildup or monthly to cause sloughing of the endometrial lining resulting in a withdrawal bleed. Progesterone is used to prevent the development of endometrial hyperplasia and endometrial cancer (North American Menopause Society, 2007, 2008, 2010a).

The combined data from multiple studies, including the Women's Health Initiative, have indicated that HT is safe for women to take for 3–5 years when initiated around the time of transition to post-menopause (North American Menopause Society, 2010a). After 3–5 years of use the risks for developing breast cancer and heart disease may increase. Indeed, most national and international organizations recommend the use of HT for managing symptoms associated with the menopause transition at the lowest dose that effectively controls symptoms and for the shortest time period possible. Women should have regular heath screenings while taking HT, such as mammograms and blood pressure measurements.

Susan needs to be counseled about sexual health and vaginal dryness. HT can take up to 6 weeks to become effective and SSRIs/SNRIs will not help with vaginal dryness. Susan may need to use vaginal lubricants or vaginal estrogen therapy either until the full effect of systemic HT is realized or for the duration of therapy with SSRI/SNRIs and beyond.

In addition, Susan needs to have counseling about midlife health risks such as osteoporosis and heart disease. If she takes HT it will help to protect her from bone loss. She will also need to ensure she is getting adequate daily intake of calcium (1200–1500 mg) and vitamin D (800–1000 IU); has regular exercise that includes aerobic, resistive, and weight bearing activities; avoids smoking or excessive use of alcohol or caffeine; and has regular DXA screening tests when appropriate. If she elects to use a nonhormonal medication or when she stops taking the HT she may also require medication to prevent or treat osteoporosis.

Regular exercise will also help her to prevent heart disease. Her risks for developing heart disease increase dramatically after menopause and may even exceed the risks carried by men. Susan needs to have regular lipid panel screening tests, follow a heart healthy diet, and maintain a normal weight to identify problems early and keep her risk factors as low as possible.

A gynecologic exam is not required to initiate HT. Routine followup is important with annual bimanual exams, clinical breast exams, and mammography. Followup specific to initiating HT or another medication for symptom management is intended to monitor efficacy while also identifying early any untoward side effects or sequelae. HT takes up to 6 weeks to reach full efficacy. Thus an appointment around 6 weeks after initiation is reasonable to determine whether the initial dose is appropriate and effective and to evaluate for bleeding, increased blood pressure, or other side effects.

The North American Menopause Society (2010a) recommends starting at a low dose and increasing using small increments if symptom management is not achieved. Once symptoms are stabilized, annual reevaluation of the need for therapy and the present dose is recommended (North American Menopause Society, 2007, 2008, 2010a). For Susan, a return appointment at about 6 weeks and again at 1 year is appropriate if she is not having concerning side effects and if her symptoms are manageable. At 1 year it might be reasonable to try skipping some days of therapy or reducing the dose even further to see if her symptoms increase or if she is tolerant to a small increase in symptoms. If not, then return to the prior dose; and if so, then consider reducing the dose further or remain at the lowered dose and reassess in another year.

If Susan's symptoms are not well controlled, or if her libido does not respond to estrogen plus progestin therapy despite an adequate dose, it may be reasonable to add methyltestosterone. Although off label for sexual benefit, this treatment is approved for women who have resistant vasomotor symptoms and has been shown to improve libido and sexual experiences for women (North American Menopause Society, 2005, 2007).

Are any referrals needed?
Referrals are not likely to be needed for Susan unless her symptoms are resistant to usual management options. If this occurs, then referral to a menopause specialist is warranted.

Does Susan's psychosocial history affect how you might treat her?
Several aspects of Susan's psychosocial history can be important when developing a management plan with her. If Susan had depression in addition to experiencing symptoms associated with the menopause transition, she might benefit from the use of an antidepressant agent, despite the possible risks for reduced sexual functioning. Consideration of Susan's insurance medication coverage is also important when selecting an agent. Several generic medications are available among both the hormonal and nonhormonal prescription options. This is taken into account when prescribing an agent for Susan so that the cost of therapy does not become a barrier to her ability to use the therapy she has selected. Additionally, Susan's preference for prescription therapy versus CAM therapy is important. If Susan does not think HT is safe, then she may have increased anxiety if she uses it, or she might take the prescription and never fill it. An open discussion that provides her with ample opportunity to share her concerns and considerations and that provides factual information including both benefits and risks is needed to individualize therapy for Susan and develop an acceptable and beneficial management plan (Alexander & Andrist, 2005; Alexander & Moore, 2007; Wysocki, Alexander, Schnare, Moore, & Freeman, 2003).

What if Susan were over age 65?
The Women's Health Initiative (WHI) study evaluated the use of HT, either estrogen plus progesterone or estrogen alone, and concluded that the risks of use outweighed the benefits. The average age of the women who participated in the WHI study was 62 (Anderson et al., 2004; Rossouw et al., 2002). More recent subanalyses of the WHI data demonstrated that there might be an important effect related to when HT is started. The risks seen in the larger study were not present in younger women when the data were analyzed according to 10-year aged cohorts (i.e., 50–59, 60–69, 70–79) (Chlebowski et al., 2009; Hsia et al., 2006; Rossouw et al., 2007). Thus, if Susan were 65 and presented with similar symptoms, HT would not be a great option for her. Instead, Susan might do better with neurontin or one of the SSRIs/SNRIs, despite the possible sexual side effects.

What if Susan also had diabetes or hypertension?
If Susan had diabetes or hypertension a transdermal delivery method for HT might be preferable to oral. This is because oral HT can alter blood sugar levels and is processed in the liver with a first pass effect. These combined effects can create medication interactions that potentially interfere with diabetes and hypertension management. These effects are reduced with transdermal therapy. There is little to no liver first pass effect with transdermal therapy; and since the delivery is via the skin, hormone levels may be steadier, possibly reducing the effects on glucose levels.

Are there any standardized guidelines that you should use to assess or treat Susan?
The combined data from multiple studies, including the WHI study, suggest that HT is safe for women to take for 3–5 years when initiated at the time of transition to postmenopause (Anderson et al., 2004; Chlebowski et al., 2009; Grodstein, Manson, & Stampfer, 2006; Heiss et al., 2008; Hsia et al., 2006; North American Menopause Society, 2010a; Rossouw et al., 2002; Rossouw et al., 2007; Salpeter, Walsh, Greyber, Ormiston, & Salpeter, 2004). After 3–5 years of use, the risks for developing breast cancer and heart disease may increase. Further, the research indicates that HT is not effective for preventing heart disease or other chronic conditions. Thus, most national organizations and the US Food and Drug Administration recommend the use of HT only for managing symptoms associated with menopause at the lowest dose that effectively controls symptoms and for the shortest time possible (American College of Obstetricians and Gynecologists, 2004; American Society of Reproductive

Medicine, 2004; US Food and Drug Administration, 2003; US Preventive Services Task Force, 2005; Wysocki et al., 2003). Regular health screenings are also recommended while any woman is taking HT, so Susan should be counseled to have an annual mammogram, regular blood pressure screenings, and to report any signs or symptoms of heart disease or any breast changes.

REFERENCES AND RESOURCES

Alexander, I. M., & Andrist, L. A. (2005). Menopause (chapter). In F. L. K. Shuiling (Ed.), *Women's gynecologic health*. Sudbury, MA: Jones and Bartlett.

Alexander, I. M., & Knight, K. (2005). *100 questions and answers about menopause*. Sudbury, MA: Jones and Bartlett.

Alexander, I. M., & Knight, K. (2010). *100 questions and answers about osteoporosis and osteopenia* (2nd ed.). Sudbury, MA: Jones and Bartlett.

Alexander, I. M., & Moore, A. (2007). Treating vasomotor symptoms of menopause: The nurse practitioner's perspective. *Journal of the American Academy of Nurse Practitioners, 19*(3), 152–163.

Alexander, I. M., Ruff, C., Rousseau, M. E., White, K., Motter, S., McKie, C., et al. (2003). Menopause symptoms and management strategies identified by black women (abstract). *Menopause, 10*(6), 601.

Alexander, I. M., Ruff, C., Rousseau, M. E., White, K., Motter, S., McKie, C., et al. (2004, April 1–3). Experiences and perceptions of menopause and midlife health among black women. Paper presented at the Eastern Nursing Research Society (ENRS) 16th Annual Scientific Sessions, Partnerships: Advancing the Research Agenda for Quality Care, Quincy, MA.

American College of Obstetricians and Gynecologists (2004). Vasomotor symptoms. *Obstetrics and Gynecology, 104*(4 Suppl.), 106S–117S.

American Psychiatric Association (2000). *Diagnostic and statistical manual of mental disorders* (4th ed.). Washington, DC: American Psychiatric Association.

American Society of Reproductive Medicine (2004). ASRM Statement on the release of data from the estrogen-only arm of the Women's Health Initiative. *ASRM Bulletin, 6*(23), 1–6.

Anderson, G. L., Limacher, M., Assaf, A. R., Bassford, T., Beresford, S. A., Black, H., et al. (2004). Effects of conjugated equine estrogen in postmenopausal women with hysterectomy: The Women's Health Initiative randomized controlled trial. *Journal of the American Medical Association, 291*(14), 1701–1712.

Basson, R., Berman, J., Burnett, A., Derogatis, L., Ferguson, D., Fourcroy, J., et al. (2000). Report of the international consensus development conference on female sexual dysfunction: Definitions and classifications. *Journal of Urology, 163*(3), 888–893.

Bolle, P., Mastrangelo, S., Perrone, F., & Evandri, M. G. (2007). Estrogen-like effect of a *Cimicifuga racemosa* extract sub-fraction as assessed by in vivo, ex vivo and in vitro assays. *The Journal of Steroid Biochemistry and Molecular Biology, 107*(3–5), 262–269.

Brett, K. M., & Keenan, N. L. (2007). Complementary and alternative medicine use among midlife women for reasons including menopause in the United States: 2002. *Menopause, 14*(2), 300–307.

Carson, K. M., Carson, J. W., Porter, L. S., & Keefe, F. J. (2008). Yoga program decreases hot flashes in breast cancer survivors: Results from a randomized trial (abstract). *International Journal of Yoga Therapy, Supplement 2008* (The Second IAYT Symposium on Yoga Therapy and Research; March 6–9, 2008. LAX Hilton Hotel, Los Angeles, Calif.), 34.

Chlebowski, R. T., Kuller, L. H., Prentice, R. L., Stefanick, M. L., Manson, J. E., Gass, M., et al. (2009). Breast cancer after use of estrogen plus progestin in postmenopausal women. *The New England Journal of Medicine, 360*(6), 573–587.

Dawson-Hughes, B. (2008). A revised clinician's guide to the prevention and treatment of osteoporosis. *The Journal of Clinical Endocrinology and Metabolism, 93*(7), 2463–2465.

Freedman, R. R., & Woodward, S. (1992). Behavioral treatment of menopausal hot flashes: Evaluation by ambulatory monitoring. *American Journal of Obstetrics and Gynecology, 167*, 436–439.

Freedman, R. R., Woodward, S., Brown, B., Javaid, J. I., & Pandy, G. N. (1995). Biochemical and thermoregulatory effects of treatment for menopausal hot flashes. *Menopause, 2*, 211–218.

Gold, E. B., Sternfeld, B., Kelsey, J. L., Browne, C., Mouton, C., Reame, N., et al. (2000). Relation of demographic and lifestyle factors to symptoms in a multi-racial/ethnic population of women 40–55 years of age. *American Journal of Epidemiology, 152*(5), 463–473.

Grady, D. (2002). A 60-year-old woman trying to discontinue hormone replacement therapy. *Journal of the American Medical Association, 287*(16), 2130–2137.

Grodstein, F., Manson, J. E., & Stampfer, M. J. (2006). Hormone therapy and coronary heart disease: The role of time since menopause and age at hormone initiation. *Journal of Women's Health (Larchmt)*, *15*(1), 35–44.

Heiss, G., Wallace, R., Anderson, G. L., Aragaki, A., Beresford, S. A., Brzyski, R., et al. (2008). Health risks and benefits 3 years after stopping randomized treatment with estrogen and progestin. *JAMA*, *299*(9), 1036–1045.

Hsia, J., Langer, R. D., Manson, J. E., Kuller, L., Johnson, K. C., Hendrix, S. L., et al. (2006). Conjugated equine estrogens and coronary heart disease: The Women's Health Initiative. *Archives of Internal Medicine*, *166*(3), 357–365.

Ihenacho. (2009). Herbal medicines for menopausal symptoms. *Drug and Therapeutics Bulletin*, *47*(1), 2–6.

Irvin, J. H., Domar, A. D., CLark, C., Zuttermeister, P. C., & Freidman, R. (1996). The effects of relaxation response training on menopausal symptoms. *Journal of Psychosomatic Obstetrics and Gynaecology*, *17*, 202–207.

Kupferer, E. M., Dormire, S. L., & Becker, H. (2009). Complementary and alternative medicine use for vasomotor symptoms among women who have discontinued hormone therapy. *Journal of Obstetric, Gynecologic, and Neonatal Nursing*, *38*(1), 50–59.

Laumann, E. O., Paik, A., & Rosen, R. C. (1999). Sexual dysfunction in the United States: Prevalence and predictors. *JAMA*, *281*(6), 537–544.

Lee, M. S., Shin, B. C., & Ernst, E. (2009). Acupuncture for treating menopausal hot flushes: A systematic review. *Climacteric*, *12*(1), 16–25.

Lindh-Astrand, L., Nedstrand, E., Wyon, Y., & Hammar, M. (2004). Vasomotor symptoms and quality of life in previously sedentary postmenopausal women randomised to physical activity or estrogen therapy. *Maturitas*, *48*(2), 97–105.

Mahady, G. B., Low Dog, T., Barrett, M. L., Chavez, M. L., Gardiner, P., Ko, R., et al. (2008). United States Pharmacopeia review of the black cohosh case reports of hepatotoxicity. *Menopause*, *15*(4 Pt 1), 628–638.

Nachtigall, L. E., Baber, R. J., Barentsen, R., Durand, N., Panay, N., Pitkin, J., et al. (2006). Complementary and hormonal therapy for vasomotor symptom relief: A conservative clinical approach. *Journal of Obstetrics and Gynaecology Canadian*, *28*(4), 279–289.

Nelson, H. D., Vesco, K. K., Haney, E., Fu, R., Nedrow, A., Miller, J., et al. (2006). Nonhormonal therapies for menopausal hot flashes: systematic review and meta-analysis. *JAMA*, *295*(17), 2057–2071.

Newton, K. M., Buist, D. S., Keenan, N. L., Anderson, L. A., & LaCroix, A. Z. (2002). Use of alternative therapies for menopause symptoms: Results of a population-based survey. *Obstetrics and Gynecology*, *100*(1), 18–25.

Norman, J. (2010). July 7). Hypothyroidism: Too little thyroid hormone. Part 1: Introduction, causes, and symptoms of hypothyroidism. Retrieved August 23, 2010, from http://www.endocrineweb.com/hypo1.html

North American Menopause Society (2005). The role of testosterone therapy in postmenopausal women: Position statement of The North American Menopause Society. *Menopause*, *12*(5), 496–511; quiz 649.

North American Menopause Society (2007). *Menopause practice: A clinician's guide* (3th ed.). Cleveland, OH: North American Menopause Society.

North American Menopause Society (2008, Jun 20). Estrogen and progestogen use in postmenopausal women: July 2008 position statement of The North American Menopause Society. Retrieved from http://www.ncbi.nlm.nih.gov/entrez/query.fcgi?cmd=Retrieve&db=PubMed&dopt=Citation&list_uids=18580541

North American Menopause Society (2010a). Estrogen and progestogen use in postmenopausal women: 2010 position statement of The North American Menopause Society. *Menopause*, *17*(2), 242–255.

North American Menopause Society (2010b). Management of osteoporosis in postmenopausal women: 2010 position statement of The North American Menopause Society. *Menopause*, *17*(1), 25–54; quiz 55–26.

Rice, S., Amon, A., & Whitehead, S. A. (2007). Ethanolic extracts of black cohosh (*Actaea racemosa*) inhibit growth and oestradiol synthesis from oestrone sulphate in breast cancer cells. *Maturitas*, *56*(4), 359–367.

Rossouw, J. E., Anderson, G. L., Prentice, R. L., LaCroix, A. Z., Kooperberg, C., Stefanick, M. L., et al. (2002). Risks and benefits of estrogen plus progestin in healthy postmenopausal women: Principal results from the Women's Health Initiative randomized controlled trial. *Journal of the American Medical Association*, *288*(3), 321–333.

Rossouw, J. E., Prentice, R. L., Manson, J. E., Wu, L., Barad, D., Barnabei, V. M., et al. (2007). Postmenopausal hormone therapy and risk of cardiovascular disease by age and years since menopause. *Journal of the American Medical Association*, *297*(13), 1465–1477.

Salpeter, S. R., Walsh, J. M. E., Greyber, E., Ormiston, T. M., & Salpeter, E. E. (2004). Mortality associated with hormone replacement therapy in younger and older women. *Journal of General Internal Medicine*, *19*(7), 791–804.

Smith, R. A., Cokkinides, V., Brooks, D., Saslow, D., & Brawley, O. W. (2010). Cancer screening in the United States, 2010: A review of current American Cancer Society guidelines and issues in cancer screening. *CA: A Cancer Journal for Clinicians*, *60*(2), 99–119.

Thompson, A. M., Church, T. S., & Blair, S. N. (2008, March 13). Effect of different doses of physical activity on quality of life in overweight, sedentary, postmenopausal women (presentation, abstract). Paper presented at the American Health Association Nutrition, Physical Activity and Metabolism Conference and 48th Annual Cardiovascular Disease Epidemiology and Prevention Conference, Colorado Springs, CO.

Udemezue, C., Alexander, I. M., & Ruff, C. C. (July, 2003). Correlation between lifestyle behaviors and severity of menopausal symptoms in black women. Podium presentation at Yale University School of Nursing, Yale-Howard Scholars Day, New Haven, CT.

US Food and Drug Administration (2003). Guidance for industry. Estrogen and estrogen/progestin drug products to treat vasomotor symptoms and vulvar and vaginal atrophy symptoms-recommendations for clinical evaluation. Retrieved March 5, 2007, from http://www.fda.gov/cder/guidance/5412dft.pdf

US Preventive Services Task Force (2005). Hormone therapy for the prevention of chronic conditions in postmenopausal women. Recommendation statement. Retrieved March 5, 2007, from http://www.ahrq.gov/clinic/uspstf05/ht/htpostmenrs.pdf

Villaverde-Gutierrez, C., Araujo, E., Cruz, F., Roa, J. M., Barbosa, W., & Ruiz-Villaverde, G. (2006). Quality of life of rural menopausal women in response to a customized exercise programme. *Journal of Advanced Nursing, 54*(1), 11–19.

Wysocki, S., Alexander, I. M., Schnare, S. M., Moore, A., & Freeman, S. B. (2003). Individualized care for menopausal women: Counseling women about hormone therapy. *Women's Health Care: A Practical Journal for Nurse Practitioners, 2*(12), 8–16.

SUBJECTIVE

Rachel is a 17-year-old female who presents with complaints of decreased appetite, fatigue, nausea, and abdominal pain for the last 2–3 weeks. She describes the abdominal pain as sharp and focused in the right epigastric area. She denies vomiting, diarrhea, or constipation. Her typical diet consists of pizza, hot dogs, and salads. Rachel denies any association of her symptoms with food or hunger. Her last normal menstrual period was 3 weeks ago, and she has had 2 negative pregnancy tests at home.

Past medical history: She delivered her son 6 months ago vaginally without complications. Her only other medical history includes a kidney infection 4 months ago.

Social history: She smokes 7 cigarettes a day but admits, "I really don't need them. I am bored." Rachel lives with her boyfriend (the father of her child) and his parents. She moved in, far away from her home, only recently. Her parents made her leave their house when she told them she was pregnant, and they have no contact with her. She states that she feels safe at home and is enjoying her baby. Her boyfriend helps with the baby but often goes out at night with his friends and leaves her at home with the baby. She feels a little isolated because everyone works during the day and she has no access to transportation. She is dependent on her in-laws if she needs to go anywhere by car, and they do not often support her need to go anywhere. Otherwise, she walks. She walked here today for her appointment.

Medication: She is not allergic to any medication and only takes birth control pills.

OBJECTIVE

Vital signs: Rachel is afebrile. BP is 120/80. Pulse is 68 and regular.

Eyes: PERRLA. EOMs are intact. Optic disks are sharp.

Cardiac: Cardiac exam reveals regular rate and rhythm.

Respiratory: Respirations are 12, steady, and unlabored. Lungs are clear.

Clinical Case Studies for the Family Nurse Practitioner, First Edition. Edited by Leslie Neal-Boylan.
© 2011 John Wiley & Sons, Inc. Published 2011 by John Wiley & Sons, Inc.

Abdomen: Soft with mild tenderness to palpation (TTP) in the RUQ with a negative Murphy's sign. There is no CVA tenderness.

Genitourinary: A urine dipstick reveals positive protein. A urine HCG is negative.

Rachel is diagnosed this first visit with possible cholecystitis and is given Antivert 12.5 mg for her nausea. Blood is drawn and sent to the lab. Her urine is sent for analysis, and she is told to return in 1 week.

Rachel returns 1 week later. Her blood work reveals fasting blood glucose of 11 mg/dL. Her other blood work is within normal limits. Her urinalysis returns with few bacteria and no protein. Rachel reports that the abdominal pain has worsened and that she now has headaches, as well. She denies a history of migraines or headaches. Her vision is blurry, and she is sensitive to light and sound. Her nausea is still present but decreased.

Her exam remains unchanged.

CRITICAL THINKING

Which diagnostic or imaging studies should be considered to assist with or confirm the diagnosis?
__Abdominal ultrasound
__Abdominal CT scan
__Head CT scan
__KUB x-ray
__CBC
__Metabolic panel
__LFTs
__Insulin level
__C-peptide
__OGGT
__Gastrin level

What is the most likely differential diagnosis and why?
__Cholelithiasis
__Gastroenteritis
__Diverticulitis
__Insulin tumor
__Gastric tumor
__Cholecystitis

What should be the plan of treatment at this point?

Are any referrals needed?

Does the patient's home situation influence your plan?

RESOLUTION

Diagnostic Testing: In addition to urine testing, Rachel should have had a metabolic panel, hepatic function panel, and CBC. Once her fasting blood sugar was noted to be 11 mg/dL, a fasting insulin level, c-peptide, and oral glucose tolerance test (OGTT) should have been ordered. Her first insulin level was 43 uIU/mL (normal ≤ 17), and her c-peptide was 5.1 (normal = 0.8–3.1 ng/mL). These levels are suspicious for an insulinoma. A gastric tumor must also be ruled out as Rachel has abdominal pain. Therefore, a gastrin level was obtained which was normal. Rachel told the clinician that she had not eaten when the test was done. It was necessary to repeat this to be sure that Rachel fasted, and the best way to do this was to have these labs repeated just prior to beginning the OGTT which would also support or refute a diagnosis of an insulinoma. Rachel's fasting levels, including the OGTT turned out to be normal, and both an insulin tumor and a gastric tumor were ruled out.

The abdominal pain required an abdominal ultrasound to confirm or rule out cholecystitis or gallstones. When Rachel mentioned the new onset headache, especially accompanied by the visual change, a CT scan of the head was ordered.

Rachel returns in 2 weeks and states that she did not go for the imaging you suggested because of lack of transportation. She is following a low fat diet per your recommendations and her abdominal pain feels slightly better. Now, she denies any headaches, nausea, and dizziness. On exam, she has RUQ TTP and a positive Murphy's sign.

What is the most likely differential diagnosis and why?
Rachel most likely has cholecystitis. The positive Murphy's sign with RUQ pain and nausea support the diagnosis. Her fatty diet clearly contributes to her condition, even though she denies any associated pattern with food.

What should be the plan of treatment at this point?
Rachel should be assisted to obtain transportation, and the clinician should check if there is a location within walking distance where she can get the tests done. Since Rachel's headaches resolved before she could get the CT scan of her head, it is possible to make a case for holding off on the CT scan (to avoid unnecessary radiation) and instead perform teaching to make Rachel aware of when to go to the emergency room or to report to the clinic if headaches resume.

Rachel still needs the abdominal ultrasound. She should be asked to return to the clinic to review the results and to review her diet progress. It is also advisable to recommend that Rachel stop smoking for the sake of herself and her baby.

Are any referrals needed?
A referral may be needed to a gastroenterologist to further assess the cholecystitis and to establish a baseline for the condition of the gallbladder as surgical options are considered.

Does the patient's home situation influence your plan?
Rachel's home life does play a role in her care. She has trouble getting her in-laws to support her need for transportation or her boyfriend to support her need for socialization. The clinician should coach her and provide support to assist her in helping her in-laws and boyfriend to understand that she needs transportation for her health needs and that of her baby and also to help her make friends in her new location. Rachel is at risk for depression and the consequences of social isolation. This could then put her at high risk for child abuse. The clinician should also offer to speak with the family. It is important that the clinician act as a confidante and support for Rachel while being careful not to malign her family.

REFERENCES AND RESOURCES

Friedman, L. S. (2010). Liver, biliary tract, & pancreas disorders. In S. J. McPhee, & M. A. Papadakis (Eds.), *Current medical diagnosis & treatment* (pp. 598–648). New York: McGraw Hill, Lange.

Stevens, T., & Conwell, D. L. (2009). Pancreatic neoplasms. In W. Carey (Ed.), *Cleveland clinic current clinical medicine* (pp. 503–509). Philadelphia: Saunders.

Case 6.4 Fatigue and Joint Pain

By Leslie Neal-Boylan, PhD, CRRN, APRN-BC, FNP

SUBJECTIVE

Sue is a 22-year-old African-American female who presents with profound fatigue, sore hands and wrists, and frequent episodes of oral and nasal ulcers. She has been told by others that she has a rash across her cheeks when she is exposed to the sun; and she has just begun to notice this herself. Sue describes the fatigue as debilitating, and she finds it difficult to work as a legal assistant. When she is home, she frequently naps; but this never fully relieves her fatigue. Her hands and wrists ache, and this further complicates her ability to do her job as she is expected to type most of the day.

She also reports occasional cold sores since she was a teen, but recently these sores have become worse and harder to heal. She has also developed intermittent sores in the nose. Sue reports intermittent episodes of fever, and she has been using acetaminophen to control these episodes. She states, "I just don't have any energy, and I really don't feel well."

Sue's menses have always been heavy and accompanied by significant dysmenorrhea. The periods started out regular (at age 12) but have gradually become less predictable. Sue is a smoker. She denies chest pain, palpitations, coughing, dyspnea, swelling of her extremities, seizures, headaches, changes in sensation, weakness, changes in bowel or bladder function, dry eyes or dry mouth, eye pain, or changes in vision.

Past medical surgical history: None.

Family history: No connective tissue or inflammatory diseases, heart disease, diabetes mellitus, or respiratory illness.

Medications: Acetaminophen and a birth control pill.

OBJECTIVE

Vital signs: Temperature: 100.6 orally. HR: 68 and regular. RR: 12 and regular. BP: 110/64. Weight: 110 lbs (down from 120 lbs 4 months ago). Height: 5 feet 4 inches.

HEENT: Mild alopecia is noted. TMs are clear and intact. PERRLA; EOMs are intact; sclera and conjunctiva are clear. Aphthous ulcers are noted in the mouth and nose. Dentition is grossly intact. There is mild bilateral anterior cervical lymphadenopathy.

Clinical Case Studies for the Family Nurse Practitioner, First Edition. Edited by Leslie Neal-Boylan.
© 2011 John Wiley & Sons, Inc. Published 2011 by John Wiley & Sons, Inc.

Cardiac: RRR S1/S2; without murmurs, clicks, gallops, or rubs.

Respiratory: CTA bilaterally.

Skin: An erythematous rash is noted across the cheeks, sparing the nasolabial folds. Livedo reticularis is noted on the lower extremities. Nailfold capillaries are positive for loops.

Musculoskeletal: No synovitis or swelling is noted. There is no TTP. There is LROM of wrists and fingers bilaterally due to pain.

Neurologic: Mentation is grossly intact. CNs II–XII are grossly intact. Sensation and proprioception are grossly intact. DTRs are +2. Romberg is negative. Heel-toe is negative. RAMs are negative.

CRITICAL THINKING

Which diagnostic or imaging studies should be considered to assist with or confirm the diagnosis?
__Urinalysis
__Metabolic panel
__CBC with differential
__Lipids
__TSH
__CK
__ESR or CRP
__Rheumatoid factor
__CCP
__ANA with reflex
__Anti-DS DNA
__Anti-SM
__Anti-RO/SSA
__Anti-LA/SSB
__Homocysteine
__C3, C4
__HIV
__Hepatitis B
__Hepatitis C
__X-rays

What is the most likely differential diagnosis and why?
__Rheumatoid arthritis
__Systemic lupus erythematosus
__Vasculitis
__Discoid lupus
__Fibromyalgia
__Osteoarthritis
__Influenza

What should be the plan of treatment?

Are there any referrals needed?

Are there other manifestations of this disease?

Would it change the diagnosis or impact the prognosis or treatment if the patient was taking minocycline? What if the patient had a parvovirus?

What are the potential complications of this disease?

RESOLUTION

Diagnostic Testing: CBC with differential will help determine if the patient has anemia or chronic disease, leukopenia, lymphopenia, or thrombocytopenia, which are all possible with systemic lupus erythematosus (SLE). An increased ESR and/or CRP will indicate active inflammation, but neither informs the clinician regarding disease or flare severity. Lipids may be abnormal due to renal dysfunction or prednisone use. In addition, the CK level may indicate myositis and the homocysteine level can be indicative of atherosclerosis or renal dysfunction. The ANA is positive in most patients with SLE. However, healthy persons can have a positive ANA. The ANA titer is most helpful because it indicates the presence of connective tissue disease. A titer of 1:640 or higher is indicative. The anti-DS DNA and anti-SM (Smith) tests are more specific. APL antibodies (lupus anticoagulant, anti-Beta 2 glycoprotein-1) are present in half of patients with SLE at some point in the course of the disease. These antibodies are associated with an increased risk of blood clots and pregnancy losses. Decreased C3 and C4, while unspecific, are often present and can help signal a flare. X-rays of the hands and wrists will not show erosion as in rheumatoid arthritis.

An elevated serum creatinine, BUN, and /or proteinuria can be indicative of renal dysfunction. A renal biopsy is required to investigate this further. The urine should be examined for hematuria and red blood cell casts (Petri, 2007).

What is the most likely differential diagnosis and why?
Systemic Lupus Erythematosus (SLE)
SLE is most commonly seen in African American women with an onset typically between the ages of 20 and 30 years. However, Caucasian women and men also get SLE, and anyone can get it at a younger age. Only 10% of people with SLE have a family member with the disease. The development of autoantibodies and the presence of low complements are typical of SLE and are chiefly responsible for its symptoms. There is potential for multiorgan involvement (Petri, 2007).

The following environmental factors have been correlated with SLE, both onset and flares: ultra-violet light (UVA and UVB), echinacea, smoking, Epstein Barr virus, silica exposure, and mercury exposure. Risk of developing SLE can be increased by the use of oral contraceptives or hormone replacement therapy. However, only HRT has been found to contribute to flares. Although the disease typically includes relapses and remissions, it can be characterized by continuous symptoms (Petri, 2007).

One must meet 4 of the following 11 criteria to be diagnosed with SLE (Petri, 2007):

- Malar rash
- Discoid rash
- Photosensitivity
- Oral ulcers
- Arthritis
- Serositis
- Renal disorder
- Hematologic disorder
- Immunologic disorder
- Positive ANA

Differential diagnoses (or co-diagnoses with SLE) include Sjögren's syndrome (dry eyes, dry mouth), fibromyalgia (muscle tender points), multiple areas of inflammation of cartilage (polychondritis), and involvement of the eyes (such as scleritis). Elevated liver enzymes are not unusual. Patients with SLE may have cognitive changes, seizures, and stroke; and many have antiphospholipid syndrome (APL). APL can affect a woman's ability to deliver healthy normal children. Nephritis is another possible sequela but is often asymptomatic.

Sue has a malar rash (spares the nasolabial folds), livedo reticularis, nail fold capillary loops (all are very indicative of SLE), alopecia, nasal and oral ulcers, fever, weight loss, fatigue, lymphadenopathy, and polyarthritis.

What should be the plan of treatment?

Sue should be instructed about getting exercise, rest, eating nutritiously, protection of the skin from the sun, and smoking cessation. If she had hypertension or abnormal lipids, those should be well managed to avoid atherosclerosis and renal dysfunction. Sue should receive influenza and pneumonia vaccines to protect her from opportunistic infections. Her bone density should be monitored, especially if steroids are used to help control flares. Topical glucocorticoids are typically used to help cutaneous lupus. However, a referral to a dermatologist is sensible if the patient has cutaneous symptoms.

SLE is initially treated with NSAIDs. These should be accompanied by a proton pump inhibitor to protect the gastrointestinal tract. However, a patient with Sue's symptoms would probably be started on Plaquenil (hydroxychloroquine) as it slows progression of the disease and helps symptoms. It is usually given at doses of 200–400 mg daily. It can cause retinal damage, so it is important for the patient to have a baseline and annual eye examination by an ophthalmologist. Prednisone is often used to control flares and methotrexate is used to supplement Plaquenil (Dall'Era & Wofsy, 2007).

Are there any referrals needed?

Patients who are diagnosed with SLE or discoid lupus should be referred to a rheumatologist. However, it is not always possible to get patients in to see the rheumatologist right away. In the meantime, the rheumatologist can be consulted telephonically and the patient can be started on NSAIDs or Plaquenil.

Are there other manifestations of this disease?

If discoid lupus skin lesions are suspected, it is important to order a skin biopsy. Nerve conduction studies and biopsies can help identify vasculitis and myositis.

Would it change the diagnosis or impact the prognosis or treatment if the patient was taking minocycline? What if the patient had a parvovirus?

Minocycline along with tumor necrosis factor alpha inhibitors can cause drug-induced lupus. Symptoms should resolve after removing the causal agent. Parvovirus, HIV, hepatitis, and malignancy can also cause lupus like symptoms (Petri, 2007).

What are the potential complications of this disease?

Organ damage may occur as a result of the disease itself, prolonged steroid treatment, interstitial pulmonary fibrosis, renal complications, and atherosclerosis. Other complications include pleuritic pain, pleural effusions, pericarditis, pulmonary hypertension, and esophageal abnormalities (Petri, 2007).

REFERENCES AND RESOURCES

Dall'Era, M., & Wofsy, D. (2007). Treatment of systemic lupus erythematosus. In J. Imboden, D. Hellmann, & J. Stone (Eds.), In *Current diagnosis & treatment: Rheumatology* (2nd ed., pp. 210–217). New York: McGraw-Hill Lange.

Petri, M. (2007). Lupus & related autoimmune disorders: Systemic lupus erythematosus. In J. Imboden, D. Hellmann, & J. Stone (Eds.), *Current diagnosis & treatment: rheumatology* (2nd ed., pp. 203–210). New York: McGraw-Hill Lange.

Case 6.5 Muscle Tenderness

By Leslie Neal-Boylan, PhD, CRRN, APRN-BC, FNP

SUBJECTIVE

Zelda is a 32-year-old female who reports tenderness when anyone or anything touches her. She has experienced these myalgias throughout her body for the last 6 months, and the pain is affecting her quality of life. She describes pain in the back of her head, her neck, her upper chest, upper back, her elbows, backside, and knees. The pain occurs on both sides of her body. "My joints feel swollen, and my skin burns." She feels profoundly fatigued and yet is unable to get a full night's sleep. She has trouble falling and staying asleep. She finds that she is often irritable, and this is affecting her relationships. She denies fever, chills, nausea, vomiting, and diarrhea. She denies changes in her hair, skin, or nails or any change in her menstrual period, which occurs every 28 days and last 5 days. Her LNMP was 3 weeks ago. She had unprotected sex 2 weeks ago with an old friend who consoled her after her move here. She denies any joint pain, dry eyes, dry mouth, ulcers, rashes, lesions, or morning stiffness.

Past medical/Surgical history: Hypertension that is controlled; irritable bowel syndrome; and appendectomy age 14 years.

Social history: She moved to this state 2 months ago and had been given opioids by her previous primary care provider. These helped moderately, and she would like some more. "At least they help me get some sleep." Zelda divorced her husband, prompting the move out of state; and she moved here with her two teenagers who are getting into trouble and are confused by the recent changes in their lives. Zelda admits to feeling sad often but denies suicidal ideation. She often feels unfocused and unable to concentrate. She denies use of tobacco, alcohol, and recreational drugs.

Zelda grew up in a broken home. Her father was an alcoholic and was occasionally abusive to her. She has worked since age 15 and currently works in the school cafeteria so she can be around her children and be home when they come home. She receives some financial assistance from her ex-husband.

Family medical history: Mother had rheumatoid arthritis. Father died of colon cancer at age 65 years.

Medications: Lisinopril 10 mg; Percocet 10/325 mg every 6 hours as needed for pain; MVI. The patient has been out of Percocet for 4 weeks.

OBJECTIVE

Height: 5 ft 3 inches; weight: 5 pounds; temperature: 98.7 F oral. HR is 68 and regular. RR is 12 and regular. BP is 124/70.

General: Teary, appears anxious.

HEENT: Head: Normocephalic, mild tenderness to palpation (TTP) of occiput. Eyes: PERRLA, EOMs intact. Nose: No polyps, no erythema. Mouth and throat: No oral ulcers, no erythema, no exudates; tonsils are +2. Neck: TTP, LROM on rotation due to pain; thyroid is nonpalpable.

Cardiac: S1/S2; RRR without murmurs, gallops, clicks, or rubs,

Lungs: Clear to auscultation bilaterally.

Abdomen: Soft, no bruits; positive for bowel sounds; nontender; nondistended. No organomegaly.

Neurologic: Mentation grossly intact; CNs II–XII grossly intact; DTRS +2 UEs and LEs; negative Romberg; negative RAMs; proprioception and sensation grossly intact.

Musculoskeletal: Using 4 kg of pressure, pain was elicited from the cervical spine, trapezius muscles bilaterally, just below the clavicle (2nd rib) bilaterally, elbows bilaterally, gluteals, and knees. There is FROM, and strength is 5/5 throughout. There is no synovitis, and there are no effusions.

Skin: No rashes or lesions noted.

CRITICAL THINKING

Which diagnostic or imaging studies should be considered to assist with or confirm the diagnosis?
__TSH
__CBC with differential
__Metabolic panel
__ESR and CRP
__Rheumatoid factor
__CCP
__ANA
__SS-A and SS-B
__X-rays
__MRIs
__HCG
__Urine dipstick

What is the most likely differential diagnosis and why?
__Rheumatoid arthritis
__Systemic lupus erythematosus
__Fibromyalgia
__ Sjögren's syndrome
__Osteoarthritis
___Thyroid disease
__Pregnancy
__Mononucleosis

What is the plan of treatment?

Are any referrals needed?

RESOLUTION

Diagnostic Testing: If the history or exam raised suspicion for other illnesses, then lab work and diagnostic tests should be pursued to rule out these illnesses. However, other than a suspicion of pregnancy, Zelda does not have any symptoms that would suggest any of these other diseases. Therefore, she should not undergo unnecessary testing. If she has not been tested recently for thyroid disease, this might be considered, although fatigue seems to be her only relevant symptom.

What is the most likely differential diagnosis and why?
Fibromyalgia (FM)
The following data support this diagnosis: Widespread pain for longer than 3 months, occurring bilaterally and above and below the waist, along with tenderness to palpation in 11/18 tender points. Patients with FM also typically have sleep disorders, depression and/or anxiety, stressful or dysfunctional childhoods and current lifestyles, and fatigue. People with FM often have burning pain and perceive that they have joint swelling but do not have it on examination. The inability to concentrate is not uncommon, and these patients often have a coexisting problem such as irritable bowel syndrome, chronic fatigue, or another systemic disease.

What is the plan of treatment?
Zelda should be encouraged to lose weight, to eat more fruits and vegetables, to exercise, and to reduce her stress level. Aquatic therapy can be useful. She will probably benefit from counseling to help her through this period of stress. However, her insurance may not cover it. Cognitive behavioral therapy (CBT) often helps, as can hypnotherapy. Encouraging her to engage in pleasurable activities, both alone and with her children, will help distract her from her difficulties and from her symptoms. Zelda should be taught sleep hygiene activities so she can improve her sleep without sleeping aids, if possible. If a sleeping aid is necessary, use a nonbenzodiazepine and consider a sleep study to fully evaluate the quality of sleep.

Antidepressants can help both the symptoms of FM and the depression Zelda has been experiencing. Cymbalta (Duloxetine), 30–60 mg, is a good option as it helps both physical pain and depression. However, a less expensive alternative that works quite well is the use of amitriptyline (10–15 mg) at bedtime to help with anxiety and sleep alone or in combination with an SSRI taken in the morning. Effexor (venlafaxine), 150–225 mg daily, like Cymbalta, combines norepinephrine and epinephrine, which help decrease all of the symptoms of FM. Anxiolytics may be pursued as adjunct therapy if the patient is anxious, but should be pursued carefully and only for as long as needed.

For a patient who has hyperalgesia or allodynia to a severe degree, Neurontin (gabapentin) or Topamax (topiramate) titrated up at weekly intervals can help. Lyrica or pregabalin started at 75 mg daily and increased, if needed to 150 mg twice each day, will make the patient sleepy and also help relieve symptoms. Savella (Milnacipran) is an alternative to Lyrica. The patient must get used to the drug, as daytime sleepiness can be initially a significant problem. Tramadol (Ultram) may also be used for pain relief but does not relieve the emotional symptoms of FM. Topical capsaicin can help relieve burning pain.

Patients with FM should **not** be given opioid medications or NSAIDs to treat the condition as these have been shown to not help and may worsen symptoms in the long run. Monosodium glutamate and aspartame can also worsen symptoms.

Follow-up care should be provided as necessary to monitor the effects of new medications and other treatment. The patient needs opportunities to be heard and reassured that the provider listens, understands, empathizes with her, and takes her concerns seriously.

Are there any referrals needed?
A referral to a rheumatologist may be considered if the case is not straightforward or if there are confounding factors or symptoms that warrant suspicion of a connective tissue or inflammatory disorder. A referral to an orthopedist may be warranted if the patient is found to have joint pain or swelling with LROM on examination.

REFERENCE AND RESOURCE

Winfield, J. B. (2007). The patient with diffuse pain. In J., Imboden, D., Hellman, & J., Stone (Eds.), *Current diagnosis & treatment: Rheumatology* (2nd ed., pp. 138–145). New York: McGraw-Hill Lange.

Case 6.6 Urinary Frequency

By Leslie Neal-Boylan, PhD, CRRN, APRN-BC, FNP

SUBJECTIVE

Susan is a 32-year-old female who presents with a report of burning pain on urination for the last 2 days. She has been urinating frequently and finds that she has to run to make it to the bathroom in time to void in the toilet. She vaguely remembers similar symptoms once in college but doesn't remember what she was diagnosed with or how she was treated for it. She denies flank pain but does have some mild suprapubic pain. She admits to mild dyspareunia in the last few days. Susan is otherwise well but admits to being thirsty more frequently than usual. Her menses are regular, and her LNMP was 10 days ago. She denies vaginal itching, foul odor, or discharge. Her children were born via vaginal deliveries without complications. Her last pelvic exam and Pap smear were 10 months ago and "everything was normal."

Social history: Susan is a recently divorced mother of 2 young children. Her ex-husband was "fooling around" while they were married, so Susan is worried that she might have a sexually transmitted infection. Since the divorce, Susan has had one new male sexual partner. They began their sexual relationship about 1 week ago and did not use condoms because Susan was on birth control pills and "I trust this new man." She works full-time as a preschool teacher and takes care of her children, ages 7 and 9, by herself and without financial support from her ex-husband. Susan does not smoke but has an occasional (1 per month) glass of wine. She admits to having used marijuana in college.

Family medical history: Notable for diabetes type 2 (mother) and hypertension (father).

Medications: Birth control pills.

OBJECTIVE

General: The patient is in no acute distress and is pleasant and cooperative.

Vital signs: Oral temperature is 98 degrees Fahrenheit. BP is 116/74. HR is 64 and regular.

Respiratory: Respirations are 14 and regular. Lungs are clear bilaterally.

Back: There is no CVAT.

Clinical Case Studies for the Family Nurse Practitioner, First Edition. Edited by Leslie Neal-Boylan.
© 2011 John Wiley & Sons, Inc. Published 2011 by John Wiley & Sons, Inc.

Cardiac: RRR S1/S2; without murmurs, clicks, gallops, or rubs.

Abdomen: Soft, nontender, nondistended, without organomegaly. Bowel sounds are active in all 4 quadrants.

Reproductive: Pelvic exam reveals no inguinal lymphadenopathy; moist pink vaginal mucosa, negative chandelier sign, and pink anterior cervix without friability. Cervical discharge is thin, white, and odorless. Samples are obtained for culture. This patient could also have provided a urine sample to test for gonorrhea and chlamydia. However, given her history with a new partner and an ex-husband who had other partners, as well as the length of time since her last pelvic exam, it is reasonable to do a pelvic exam at this time. A Pap smear may not be taken at this time if there is a question regarding whether it would be reimbursed because it was last done less than 1 year ago. The next Pap should include HPV testing. The bimanual exam reveals no masses or tenderness.

CRITICAL THINKING

Which diagnostic or imaging studies should be considered to assist with or confirm the diagnosis?
__Urine dipstick
__Urinalysis
__Urine culture and sensitivity
__CBC
__CMP
__TSH
__Renal ultrasound
__Abdominal and pelvic ultrasound

What is the most likely differential diagnosis and why?
__Pregnancy
__Acute cystitis
__Interstitial cystitis
__Diabetes mellitus
__Pyelonephritis
__Pelvic inflammatory disease
__Urinary tract infection (UTI)

What is the plan of treatment?

Are there any referrals needed?

Would the diagnosis change if the patient had a fever and flank pain?

Would the most likely diagnosis change if the patient was male?

RESOLUTION

Diagnostic testing: It is important to send Susan's urine out for a complete urinalysis and culture and sensitivity. The pelvic exam was helpful in Susan's case to rule out PID or vulvovaginitis (McPhee & Papadakis, 2010). It is unlikely, but possible, that Susan is pregnant; so a urine or serum HCG is appropriate. The clinician checks a urine dipstick while Susan is in the office. The results are negative except for positive leukocytes and positive nitrites. In addition, she has a family history of diabetes mellitus; so a fasting blood sugar should also be included in her workup. People with DM are often prone to UTIs.

What is the most likely differential diagnosis and why?
Acute cystitis or a UTI
A UTI is characterized by difficulty with voiding and a positive urine culture. The patient is usually afebrile. Urgency, frequency, and pain with voiding are common as is some pain following sexual activity. Some women experience hematuria, as well. A new partner for Susan is a risk factor for a UTI.

Interstitial cystitis is a diagnosis of exclusion (McPhee & Papadakis, 2010), and a negative urine culture is an essential part of the diagnosis. Other causes of urinary urgency must first be ruled out. Pyelonephritis is characterized by flank pain in addition to dysuria, urgency, frequency, and a positive urine culture. Fever and chills are typically present. If the clinician is in doubt about Susan having pyelonephritis, a CBC could be added to the workup, as it will show definite leukocytosis. For this case, none of the other diagnostic tests that are listed are necessary at this time. However, if Susan's symptoms get worse, a renal scan to look for hydronephrosis might be warranted.

What is the plan of treatment?
In Susan's case, the UTI is uncomplicated and could therefore be treated with a short course of antibiotics. Fluoroquinolones and nitrofurantoin (McPhee & Papadakis, 2010) are good choices. Bactrim is used less often now due to bacterial resistance. Phenazopyridine obtained over-the-counter can help relieve pain with urination, but the patient should be warned that the medication will stain clothes orange. Susan should be encouraged to push fluids until she feels better and in the future to help prevent UTIs.

Are there any referrals needed?
No referrals are need at this time, but a referral to a urologist might be in order if the patient has recurrent episodes or is found to have a stone.

Would the diagnosis change if the patient had a fever and flank pain?
Pyelonephritis should be suspected if the patent develops fever or flank pain.

Would the most likely diagnosis change if the patient was male?
If the patient was male, the likelihood of UTI is less and is of more concern when it happens. It is important to determine the etiology of the symptoms in a male to help to determine a plan of treatment. Prostatitis, epididymitis, and sexually transmitted infection are possible causes of urinary symptoms in men.

REFERENCES AND RESOURCES

Abdelmalak, J. B., & Potts, J. M. (2009). Acute and chronic bacterial cystitis. In W. Carey (Ed.), *Cleveland clinic current clinical medicine* (pp. 755–758). Philadelphia: Saunders.

Fang, L. S.-T. (2009). Approach to dysuria and urinary tract infections in women. In A. H. Goroll, & A. G. Mulley (Eds.), *Primary care medicine* (pp. 947–953). Philadelphia: Lippincott.

Goroll, A. H., & Mulley, A. G. (2009). Screening for asymptomatic bacteriuria and urinary tract infection. In A. H. Goroll, & A. G. Mulley (Eds.), *Primary care medicine* (pp. 918–922). Philadelphia: Lippincott.

McPhee, S. J., & Papadakis, M. A. (2010). *Current medical diagnosis & treatment* (49th ed.). New York: McGraw-Hill Lange.

Case 6.7 Insomnia

By Leslie Neal-Boylan, PhD, CRRN, APRN-BC, FNP

SUBJECTIVE

Iris, a 48-year-old female presents with a report of insomnia and impaired concentration. She has not slept through the night for approximately 6 weeks and finds that while she can fall asleep readily, she is too restless to stay asleep. At work (she works as an office manager), she is unable to concentrate and has found herself making simple mistakes. Iris is easily fatigued and states that she frequently feels warm and flushed, but she attributes this to "the time of life." Her menstrual periods have become irregular. Her LNMP was 2 months ago. It lasted 10 days and was slightly heavier than usual. Iris states that she occasionally feels her heart "fluttering" when she feels anxious. She is surprised at this because she has always felt that she coped well with life and was generally happy. "Now, the littlest things seem to bother me and I feel my heart start to flutter. Oh, the change of life. I have dreaded it. Can you give me something for it?"

Iris denies fever, chills, pain, weakness, or tremors.

Elimination: She has not noticed any changes in her weight or loose stools.

Past medical history: Hospitalization for a Cesarean section without complications 15 years ago. She also had a hemorrhoidectomy 7 years ago without complications.

Family medical history: Iris has a husband and one son who are alive and well. Her mother, age 67, has stage 1 Alzheimer's disease and hypothyroidism. Her father has diabetes mellitus type 2 and a history of colon cancer. Both are alive.

Social history: She lives with her husband and son and states that she is happily married and comfortable financially. She stopped using any form of birth control since her periods became irregular 6 months ago. She is a smoker, takes no medications, and has been generally healthy.

OBJECTIVE

The patient appears anxious but is pleasant and cooperative. Her weight is 136 lbs; she comments that this is 10 lbs less than the last time she checked her weight 3 months ago. Oral temperature is 100 degrees Fahrenheit. BP is 148/94. HR is 96 and regular. Respirations are 12 and regular.

HEENT: Hair is shiny and soft. No exophthalmos is observed. There is no lid lag or eye retraction. Sclerae are clear and conjunctivae are without injection. PERRLA and EOMs are intact. CNs II–XII are grossly intact. There is no cervical lymphadenopathy. Trachea is midline. The thyroid is mildly palpable with a bruit. There are no nodules.

Skin: The patient's skin is warm and moist.

Cardiac: HR: 96; RRR: S1/S2; no murmurs, clicks, gallops or rubs. EKG reveals NSR without abnormalities.

Pulmonary: Lungs are clear bilaterally.

Abdomen: Soft without tenderness or distention. No organomegaly, no bruits. Bowel sounds are active throughout.

Neurologic: There are no tremors. Sensation and proprioception are grossly intact. DTRS are +3 in upper extremities and lower extremities. Romberg is negative. RAMs are negative. Gait is steady.

Musculoskeletal: FROM and strength of 5/5 in all extremities.

CRITICAL THINKING

Which diagnostic or imaging studies should be considered to assist with or confirm the diagnosis?
__TSH
__CBC
__CMP
__HCG
__Lipids
__CXR
__Radionucleotide uptake scan with iodine (RAI)
__FSH
__T3
__T4
__Free T4
__Thyrotropin receptor antibody (TRAb)
__Antithydroperoxidase antibody (TPO)
__ANA
__Anti DS DNA

What is the most likely differential diagnosis and why?
__Hyperthyroidism
__Hypothyroidism
__Menopause
__Pregnancy
__Anxiety/depression
__Infection

What should be the plan of treatment?

What is a likely diagnosis if this patient returns with severe tachycardia, confusion, vomiting, diarrhea, high fever, and dehydration?

What if this patient's lab results return and the TSH is low with normal results for free T4 and T3?

Are there any standardized guidelines that should be used to assess and treat this case?

RESOLUTION

Diagnostic testing: A low TSH and elevated T3 and T4 would confirm hyperthyroidism or thyrotoxicosis. Graves disease is an autoimmune disease, so the TRAb and TPO would also be elevated. ANA and antiDS DNA may also be elevated although the patient does not have systemic lupus erythematosus (McPhee & Papadakis, 2010). Iris requires a thyroid RAI and imaging of the pelvis to screen for ovarian problems that rarely accompany hyperthyroidism (McPhee & Papadakis, 2010). The RAI will be high in Graves disease.

What is the most likely differential diagnosis and why?
Hyperthyroidism
Iris's symptoms of palpitations, tachycardia, insomnia, impaired concentration, fatigue, heat intolerance, weight loss, and irregular menses all support the diagnosis of hyperthyroidism. Additionally, the exam finding of soft, shiny hair, hyperreflexia, goiter, and thyroid bruit also support the diagnosis. However, Iris does not yet have some symptoms she might acquire without treatment, such as exophthalmos, lid lag, tremors, and atrial fibrillation. There are many causes of hyperthyroidism, but Graves disease is the most common.

Hypothyroidism would cause other symptoms, such as oversleeping, weight gain, dryness of the skin, hair, or nails, cold intolerance, and dyspnea. The TSH would be high, and the free T4 may be low or normal.

Iris could be pregnant, or she could be going through perimenopause. Lab workup should include an HCG and an FSH. A CBC and a CMP will be helpful to rule out additional causes of her symptoms, such as infection, and to provide a baseline prior to treatment. Thyroid disease often affects lipid levels, so fasting lipid levels should be obtained. Iris may be anxious aside from the thyrotoxicosis, although her history does not appear to support that diagnosis; but screening for depression and anxiety is always helpful.

What should be the plan of treatment?
The clinician should consider an MRI, CT, or ultrasound of the orbits of the eyes to check for exophthalmos if the patient develops a severe or unilateral case (McPhee & Papadakis, 2010). Iris could be given some propranolol to relive her symptoms of nervousness, tachycardia, diaphoresis, and palpitations. Methimazole or propylthiouracil (PTU) can also be used especially if the patient is very young or has a mild case. As symptoms of hyperthyroidism decrease and the free T4 nears the normal range, drug dosages are reduced. Sometimes, methimazole is given first and then is followed the day after with ipodate sodium or iopanoic acid. Radioactive iodine is a very common method for destroying the thyroid, and this treatment does not increase the risk for thyroid cancer or other cancers. Methimazole should be stopped for at least 4 days if the patient is to be started on radioactive iodine treatment. Iris smokes, so she runs the risk of increased likelihood of eye problems after iodine treatment. Followup with TSH and free T4 is critical as the procedure may render the patient hypothyroid requiring thyroid replacement therapy. Thyroid surgery is another option for treatment but is used less often than previously.

Iris will need frequent followup as treatment progresses to monitor symptoms and lab results and to check for complications of the disease. Most likely, Iris will need synthetic or natural thyroid replacement following the destruction of the thyroid gland. Table .6.7.1 is included to help show the differences between hypo- and hyperthyroidism.

What is a likely diagnosis if this patient returns with severe tachycardia, confusion, vomiting, diarrhea, high fever, and dehydration?
If this patient returns with all of these symptoms, suspect thyroid storm. This condition typically requires hospitalization. Methimazole or propranolol is given. Steroids are often used and then tapered as the symptoms improve.

TABLE 6.7.1. Comparison of Hypo- and Hyperthyroidism.

Hypothyroidism	Hyperthyroidism
Can be caused by a rare pituitary gland tumor.	Graves disease is most common; caused by IgG (binds to TSH), initiates production and release of thyroid hormone.
Typical presentation: The body cannot make enough thyroid hormone. The body produces less body heat and consumes less oxygen.	
Other causes: Hashimoto's, surgical removal of the thyroid gland, post Graves disease (after treatment), thyroid irradiation.	Other causes: Toxic adenoma, toxic multinodular goiter, painful subacute or silent thyroiditis, iodine-induced hyperthyroid (amiodarone treatment), oversecretion of pituitary TSH, excess endogenous thyroid hormone production.
TSH is up. Free T4 is down. High lipids. Low sodium.	TSH is low. Free T4 is elevated.
	Radionucleotide uptake and scan with iodine to determine if it is secondary to Graves disease, thyroid nodule. or thyroiditis.
	Hyperactivity of thyroid: Increased uptake on RAI.
	Nodules: Limited areas of uptake on RAI and surrounding hypoactivity.
	Subacute thyroiditis: RAI uptake is patchy and decreased overall.
Treatment: Check pituitary function.	Treatment: Radioactive iodine (if not pregnant). Postpone pregnancy for 6 months after scan. Do not use during lactation. PTU may be used to treat condition (prevents conversion of T4 to active T3).
Give thyroid hormone (lower dosage for elderly).	
Initial dose (for anyone): 125 mcg–150 mcg (0.10–0.15 mg/d). Dose depends on age, weight, cardiac status, duration, and severity of disease. Titrate after 6 weeks and following any change in dose.	Give PTU BID for 7 days (can use in pregnancy or may use Tapazole daily. Side effect of PTU is agranulocytosis.
Use TSH to gauge dose and monitor treatment.	Post ablation: Follow up 6 weeks after treatment and regularly until evidence of early hypothyroidism (based on TSH); then start treatment for hypothyroidism.

What if this patient's lab results return and the TSH is low with normal results for free T4 and T3?

If this patient's lab results return and the TSH is low with normal results for free T4 and T3, then the patient most likely has subclinical hyperthyroidism. However, the patient would be asymptomatic and does not need treatment.

Are there any standardized guidelines that should be used to assess and treat this case?

The American Association of Clinical Endocrinologists has guidelines that can help the clinician make diagnostic and treatment plan choices (http://www.aace.com/).

REFERENCES AND RESOURCES

Birnbaum, S. L. (2009). Approach to the menopausal woman. In A. H. Goroll, & A. G. Mulley (Eds.), *Primary care medicine* (pp. 866–874). Philadelphia: Lippincott.

Fauci, A. S., Braunwald, E., Kasper, D. L., Hauser, S. L., Longo, D. L., Jameson, J. L., & Loscalzo, J. (2009). Thyroid gland disorders. In A. S. Fauci, E. Braunwald, D. L. Kasper, S. L. Hauser, D. L. Longo, J. L. Jameson, & J. Loscalzo (Eds.), *Harrison's manual of medicine* (17th ed., pp. 925–933). New York: McGraw Medical.

Case 6.8 Vaginal Itching

By Leslie Neal-Boylan, PhD, CRRN, APRN-BC, FNP

SUBJECTIVE

Martha is a 24-year-old female who reports vaginal itching for 3 days. She says that she can barely focus on other things because of the itching. She also reports a copious, white vaginal discharge. Her last Pap smear was at age 21 and was negative. She has not received the HPV vaccine series. Martha denies previous episodes and states that she is otherwise healthy. She denies fever, chills, nausea, vomiting or diarrhea. She is sexually active and has been with females and males since she was 15 years old. She states that recently she has been exclusively with females but has only had 2 relationships in the past year. She states that she still feels somewhat confused about her sexual preferences. She admits to dyspareunia and burning with urination. She denies use of vaginal sprays, douches, or powders or the use of new soaps, detergent, or clothing. Martha does like eating sweets. She does admit to wearing a thong regularly.

Past medical history: Tonsillectomy at age 7 years.

Family history: Remarkable for diabetes mellitus and COPD.

Social history: Martha is a college graduate and still lives with her widowed mother. She feels safe and has a good relationship with her mother but has not disclosed her sexual preferences to her mother. Martha does worry about their financial status as she and her mother have low-paying jobs and do not have other financial support. They are currently renting their apartment from a friend. Martha does not smoke and denies substance use.

Medications: None (no antibiotics, steroids, or estrogens).

Allergies: Seasonal in spring.

OBJECTIVE

Vital signs: Martha is afebrile. Her BP is 110/70. Pulse is 64 and regular. Respirations are 12 and unlabored. She is 5 ft 3 inches tall and weighs 120 lb.

General: Martha is pleasant and cooperative but seems anxious about the visit.

Clinical Case Studies for the Family Nurse Practitioner, First Edition. Edited by Leslie Neal-Boylan.
© 2011 John Wiley & Sons, Inc. Published 2011 by John Wiley & Sons, Inc.

Cardiac: Regular rate and rhythm.

Respiratory: Lungs are clear.

Abdomen: Soft, nontender, nondistended, and without organomegaly.

Pelvic exam: Inguinal lymph nodes are without swelling or tenderness; vaginal mucosa is moist, pink, and mildly swollen. There is no foul odor; but there is a white, cottage cheese–like discharge at the introitus. The cervix is pink and without friability. There is a negative chandelier sign. The pH of the discharge is within normal range (3.8–4.2). The wet prep indicates pseudohyphae.

CRITICAL THINKING

Which diagnostic or imaging studies should be considered to assist with or confirm the diagnosis?
___Pap smear
___Cultures for gonorrhea and Chlamydia
___Urine testing for gonorrhea and Chlamydia
___Whiff test
___KOH test

What is the most likely differential diagnosis and why?
___Bacterial vaginosis
___*Candida albicans*
___Trichomonas
___Gonorrhea
___Chlamydia
___Herpes simplex

What is the plan of treatment?

Are any referrals needed?

Is the family history of diabetes relevant to this case?

How can the clinician support the patient regarding her confusion with her sexual identity?

RESOLUTION

Diagnostic testing: The findings of pseudohyphae on the wet mount and a normal pH confirm the diagnosis. Martha is due for a Pap smear, and it might be wise to test her for HPV as well. Her multiple partners warrant a check for sexually transmitted infections. Martha should be asked about these tests before they are done. The testing for STIs (gonorrhea and chlamydia) may be done via a urine sample or through cultures during the pelvic exam.

What is the most likely differential diagnosis and why?
Candida Albicans
The symptom of itching, the curd-like white discharge, the burning with urination, and the dyspareunia support this diagnosis. The vaginal swelling also contributes to the diagnosis. A high intake of sweets can put Martha at risk, as can her multiple partners (or a changed partner) and her use of thongs.

What is the plan of treatment?
Both OTC and prescription remedies are available. Butoconazole 2% cream and Lotrimin are possible treatments. Clotrimazole vaginal tablets or suppositories may be used. Miconazole (Monistat) is

TABLE 6.8.1. Differential Diagnosis.

Condition	Signs and Symptoms
Trichomonas	Foul smelling discharge, usually a fishy odor; vaginal burning sensation; possible postcoital bleeding; itching; dysuria, dyspareunia; may be asymptomatic.
Bacterial vaginosis	Fishy vaginal odor; thin white or gray discharge; postcoital burning; possible itching; may be asymptomatic.
Chlamydia	Possibly mucopurulent discharge; pelvic pain; dysuria, spotting and altered menstruation; postcoital bleeding; may be asymptomatic. Male: Dysuria, cloudy and thick penile discharge.
Gonorrhea	Asymptomatic early; leukorrhea; suprapubic pain, dysuria, dyspareunia, pharyngitis; labial pain and swelling. Later: purulent discharge, rectal pain and discharge; nausea, vomiting, fever; arthralgias and joint swelling; genital lesions and swelling. Male: Dysuria, pharyngitis, white penile discharge that progresses to yellow green, epididymitis, and proctitis.
Herpes genitalis	First episode: Lesions; malaise, fever, dyspareunia, arthralgias and myalgias, fever and lymphadenopathy. Recurrent episodes: Less symptomatic, usually have prodrome of itching, burning, or tingling.

another option and there are others. Martha should also be encouraged to begin and complete the HPV vaccine series.

Are there any referrals needed?

No referrals are needed unless Martha has an intractable case, and she does not require followup unless this infection is unresponsive.

Is the family history of diabetes relevant to this case?

Martha has a family history of diabetes mellitus, so it is worthwhile testing her for DM and monitoring her for prediabetes. *Candida albicans,* especially frequent infections, can be a warning sign of diabetes.

How can the clinician support the patient regarding her confusion with her sexual identity?

Instruction regarding how to avoid recurrent candida infections and how to avoid STIs will be paramount during the visit. Martha could also use some support regarding her sexual confusion at this time in her life. The clinician can work to develop a rapport with Martha and gain her trust so that Martha feels comfortable sharing her feelings. The clinician should provide factual information, resources, and news of community support groups.

REFERENCE AND RESOURCE

Hawkins, J. W., Roberto-Nichols, D. M., & Stanley-Haney, J. L. (2008). *Guidelines for nurse practitioners in gynecologic settings* (9th ed.). New York: Springer.

Case 6.9 Abdominal Pain and Weight Gain

By Geraldine F. Marrocco, EdD, APRN, CNS, ANP-BC

SUBJECTIVE

Patient Annette, a 28-year-old female, presents to the primary care practice for an initial visit. She presents with two major concerns. First, she is concerned because she was told she had gallstones by ultrasound and was advised by another primary care provider (PCP) that she needed her gallbladder removed. She has had several bouts of abdominal pain and some dyspepsia, but no nausea, vomiting or any other gastrointestinal symptoms. She points to an area in her abdomen that has been painful, especially when she eats high-fat foods. She has no other gastrointestinal complaints.

Her second complaint is weight gain. Her diet has not changed over the past few years; however she has noticed a change in the way her clothes fit as well as a 15-pound increase in her weight over the last year. Also over the last year, she has had irregular menses. She often "skips months," and she reports 7 cycles of menstruation over the past year. When she does have her period, "it lasts for over 2 weeks." At one point she did not have a period for 3 months, and she thought that she might be pregnant. Her review of systems is negative except for increased hair growth across the sides of her face, her chin, and the middle of her chest, arms and upper thighs, which she has had since she was an adolescent. She also complains of acne.

Further review of systems reveals no dizziness, no headache, no problems with her vision, no ringing in her ears; she is not short of breath. She has no complaints of cough, no palpitations, no chest pain. She has no genitourinary complaints. She has no musculoskeletal complaints. She has no weakness, no paresthesia, and no numbness or tingling of the extremities.

Past medical history: Noncontributory.

Past surgical history: None.

Family medical history: Her mother has type 2 diabetes and hypertension. Her father died at age 50 due to lung cancer and had a positive smoking history. Her brother is alive and well at age 26, and her sister is alive and obese at age 22.

Social history: She was born in Brazil and reports no tobacco, alcohol, or substance abuse. She drinks 1 cup of coffee daily and lives at home with her mother, brother, and sister in a single-family home in a suburban town. She works full-time as an administrative assistant and is a part-time student finishing a bachelor's degree in science at a state college. She has a network of friends and family

Clinical Case Studies for the Family Nurse Practitioner, First Edition. Edited by Leslie Neal-Boylan.
© 2011 John Wiley & Sons, Inc. Published 2011 by John Wiley & Sons, Inc.

and her hobbies include traveling and theater. She is currently in a sexual relationship with one partner and does not practice any form of contraception. Her LMP was 2 months ago, and her last Pap smear was 2 years ago and negative.

Medication and allergies: She has no medication allergies but reports allergies to pork and cats. She is not on any regular medications but takes Tylenol 2 tablets as needed for headache. Her immunizations are up to date.

OBJECTIVE

Vital signs are within normal limits with a blood pressure of 110/80 and a temperature of 98.2 F. Pulse is 76 and regular, and respiratory rate is 18. Height is 62 inches, and weight is 200 lbs (BMI 36.6). She is a well-developed, obese female who is in no acute distress. She is coherent, alert, and pleasant.

Skin: She has fine, dark hair on her chin and on the sides of her face. There is increased hair growth on her forearms, sternal area, and upper thighs. Acne is present on her forehead and lateral cheeks bilaterally.

Neck: Goiter, thyroid is palpable, nontender; no nodules are palpable or appreciated. Neck is supple and without lymphadenopathy.

Respiratory: Her lungs are clear, and the chest is symmetrical.

Cardiac: Regular heart rate and rhythm. S1 and S2 are present and normal.

Abdomen: Obese and soft; bowel sounds are present; and there is tenderness in the epigastric area. Liver and spleen are nonpalpable.

Musculoskeletal: Extremities are without edema. There is full range of motion and good strength. Carotid, femoral, dorsalis pedis, and post-tibial pulses are all +2.

Neurologic: DTRs are 2+ in the biceps, triceps, brachioradials, patella, and Achilles. Cranial nerves II–XII are grossly intact.

CRITICAL THINKING

Which diagnostic or imaging studies should be considered to assist with or confirm the diagnosis?
___Androgen elevation, testosterone level
___Lipids
___LH
___FSH
___Insulin level
___Urea breath test
___Serum *H. Pylori*
___TSH, free T4
___LFTs
___HCG
___Vitamin D
___HIV
___Urinalysis

___Transvaginal ultrasound
___Abdominal ultrasound
___CBC with differential
___Metabolic panel
___Prolactin level
___DHEA

What is the most likely differential diagnosis and why?
___Gastroesophageal reflux disease (GERD)
___Cholecystitis
___*Helicobacter pylori* infection/peptic ulcer disease
___Polycystic ovarian syndrome (PCOS)
___Hypothyroidism
___Hyperprolactinemia

What is your plan of treatment?

Are any referrals needed at this time?

What if the patient had a positive pregnancy test?

What if the patient was trying to conceive?

Are there any standardized guidelines that you should use to assess or treat this case?

RESOLUTION

Diagnostic testing: CBC with differential normal; hemoglobin A1c: 7.3 (elevated); chemistries normal; LFT normal; *H. pylori* + (abnormal); TSH: 1.34; LH: 9.8 (elevated); FSH: 2.3 (low–normal: 3–20); DHEA: 244; testosterone: 88; bioavailability: 36 (elevated/high normal); HCG: negative; serum prolactin: 102 (elevated); lipids: total cholesterol: 186; triglycerides: 94; LDL: 103; HDL: 46; HIV: negative; vitamin D: 9 (low); urinalysis: normal.

Transvaginal ultrasound: Multiple follicles noted within the uterus which are arranged in a more peripheral pattern as seen in polycystic ovarian disease. She had a retroverted uterus without any abnormality and multiple cysts on the left ovary indicative of polycystic ovarian syndrome.

To rule PCOS in or out, evaluating androgens is recommended, along with a hemoglobin A1c to evaluate insulin resistance. Hypothyroidism can be diagnosed with a TSH level. Serum prolactin and DHEA are needed to rule in or rule out the suspicion of hyperprolactinemia. Since Annette reported being sexually active without a form of contraception, getting an HCG is wise. Other labs for routine health maintenance include a vitamin D level, HIV test, and urinalysis. In addition to laboratory studies, a transvaginal ultrasound is needed to evaluate for the presence of ovarian abnormalities. An abdominal ultrasound can also help pinpoint the cause of the abdominal pain.

What is the most likely differential diagnosis and why?
H. pylori *infection and PCOS*
Since the laboratory studies give a positive result, we can conclude that Annette's abdominal pain is at least in part due to an *H. pylori* infection. The ultrasound reveals that she does have gallstones, though her LFTs are within normal limits and her constellation of symptoms do not suggest an acute gallstone emergency. While her symptoms do still fall under the possible realm of GERD, it is likely that the plan to eradicate the *H. pylori* infection will include gastric acid suppression, therefore alleviating the shared symptoms.

It is now commonly known that greater than 95% of duodenal ulcers and greater than 90% of gastric ulcers are caused by an infection by the bacterium *H. pylori*. Other causes of aggravation of peptic ulcer disease include stress, smoking, alcohol, and coffee. *H. pylori* affects the mucosal defenses by attaching to the epithelium, causing apoptosis and an inflammatory response. This leads to increased gastric acid production, increased pepsin secretion, and a decrease in mucosal defense. Symptoms of peptic ulcer disease include intermittent epigastric pain that can last for days at a time and then be absent for months. The pain is most often relieved by antacids.

Annette's secondary amenorrhea, hirsutism, acne, and obesity reflect a constellation of symptoms associated with PCOS. PCOS affects 5%–7% of women, and many symptoms overlap with those of metabolic syndrome. Since PCOS is a condition of hyperandrogenism, it would explain Annette's increased male-pattern hair growth and her acne. PCOS is a clinical diagnosis based on 2 of the following criteria: (1) oligo or anovulation, (2) hyperandrogenism or hyperandrogenemia, or (3) polycystic ovaries. Lab studies for PCOS would show androgen elevation, decreased sex hormone binding globulin, increased LH, low-normal FSH, and hyperinsulinemia.

PCOS is the most likely diagnosis given the subjective reports of Annette, coupled with the objective laboratory study and ultrasound findings. While the Rotterdam criteria for diagnosis only require 2 of the 3 diagnostic criteria, Annette meets all 3, along with the very common constellation of signs and symptoms. At least 50% of women with PCOS also have marked insulin resistance, which is seen with Annette as demonstrated by her A1c level. Due to the overlap with metabolic syndrome, she will find herself at risk for cardiovascular disease and diabetes mellitus. The condition of PCOS also has repercussions for fertility, as anovulation is among the symptoms. While there is a great deal about PCOS that is still unknown, the common treatment approach is the correction of hyperinsulinemia via either weight loss, medications, or both.

Hypothyroidism can be ruled out due to the normal TSH level. The shared symptoms of hair growth, weight gain, and menstrual irregularities can also be explained by PCOS. Though Annette does not appear to have this disorder, hypothyroidism can be easily treated with exogenous thyroid hormone replacement. Monitoring is required and dose adjustments may be needed to assure a constant euthyroid state, but many individuals with the disease only require daily maintenance medication.

While the lab results show that Annette does in fact have hyperprolactinemia, knowing that it often occurs with PCOS suggests that Annette has both disorders. The treatment approach would be to address the PCOS first and hope that both states are normalized through a streamlined treatment.

1. **Gastroesophageal reflux disease (GERD):** Epigastric abdominal pain exacerbated by high-fat foods is a common complaint of individuals with reflux. Heartburn, regurgitation, and difficulty swallowing often accompany the abdominal pain. The physical exam of someone with GERD can often be negative, while other times dental erosion is seen and epigastric tenderness is noted. Contributing lifestyle factors to GERD include tobacco use, alcohol use, excessive chocolate ingestion, high-fat meals, and high-carbohydrate meals.

2. **Cholecystitis:** The fact that a previous practitioner noted gallstones on an ultrasound suggests that Annette's abdominal pain could be caused by an acute gallbladder infection. Cholecystitis is often hallmarked by dyspepsia, belching, bloating, and sudden onset colicky epigastric pain that is accompanied by nausea and vomiting. An acute gallstone emergency, choledocholithiasis, will present as recurrent pain plus mildly increased LFTs. It is possible to have asymptomatic gallstones, as well, which is often an incidental finding and does not require intervention.

3. **Hypothyroidism:** Annette's unexplained weight gain, along with her goiter, dark hair, and heavy periods suggest the diagnosis of hypothyroidism. Hypothyroidism is fairly common, and occurs much more often in women than men. The disease presents with the symptoms above, along with fatigue, constipation, dry skin, and cold intolerance. On exam, besides a goiter, there may be diminished bowel sounds or delayed deep tendon reflexes. The diagnosis of hypothyroidism can be confirmed by an increased TSH level and a low or normal free T4 level.

4. **Hyperprolactinemia:** Hyperprolactinemia is a possible explanation for Annette's hirsutism, as prolactin stimulates androgen production, and androgen excess is the cause of excess dark hair. Other common features are amenorrhea and galactorrhea. Hyperprolactinemia often appears accompanying PCOS.

What is your plan of treatment?

The protocol for eradicating *H. pylori* includes antibiotics and acid suppression. Antibiotic therapy works to promote ulcer healing, prevent relapse, and decrease the need for long-term acid suppression. In all cases, combination antibiotic therapy is needed due to the high rates of resistance. To suppress acid, proton pump inhibitors (PPIs) are most often used. An appropriate treatment for Annette would be lansoprazole (30 mg twice daily), amoxicillin (500 mg twice daily), and clarithromycin (500 mg twice daily) for 14 days. There are several different combination therapy suggestions ranging from 7–14 day treatments.

The treatment plan for Annette's PCOS should be based mostly on her symptoms. Three reasons for treatment can be considered in her case: (1) regulation of uterine bleeding and reduction in risk for endometrial hyperplasia, (2) the improvement of dermatological complaints including acne and increased dark hair growth, and (3) the correction and prevention of possible metabolic abnormalities, including DM and cardiovascular disease. To address Annette's irregular menstrual bleeding, a hormonal contraceptive method should be considered based on her individual contraceptive needs and comfort level. A common starting place is the combined oral contraceptive pill (COC), but the ring and progestin-only methods such as the implant or the hormonal IUD could also be considered.

To address Annette's complaint of acne and dark hair growth, an androgen receptor blocker could be considered as pharmacotherapy in an extreme circumstance. However, if looking for a more conservative treatment, choosing a combined contraceptive option would improve acne; and a cosmetic route could be chosen for the hair growth (such as bleaching, electrolysis, or laser removal).

The correction of any metabolic abnormalities is also of great concern, and the treatment should begin with a discussion of diet and lifestyle modifications. Many studies have shown that weight loss can lower the level of circulating androgens, thus causing the resumption of normal menstrual patterns and the reduction in insulin resistance. Since Annette's lab studies show a high hemoglobin A1c level, indicative of long-term insulin resistance, starting a hypoglycemic agent would be an acceptable adjunct therapy to lifestyle changes.

To address preventive health practices for Annette, starting her on daily calcium, vitamin D, and fish oil supplementation would also be appropriate.

It would be important to follow up with Annette after her treatment course to see if the *H. pylori* infection was in fact eradicated. If the infection persists, it would be appropriate to continue therapy, most likely changing antibiotics due to suspicion of resistance. If the infection was eradicated but symptoms persist for more than 4 weeks, it would be recommended to refer for a gastrointestinal specialist for endoscopic evaluation.

PCOS is a common condition that can be managed within the realm of primary care, so it would not be recommended that Annette be followed by a specialist. However, to evaluate progress on the treatment options discussed today, the time frame for acceptable follow-up visits would be monthly for the first 3 months and then quarterly until specific treatment goals are reached. At the follow-up visits, diet and exercise journals should be reviewed; and blood tests should be done to evaluate insulin resistance (hemoglobin A1c) and androgen levels (FHS, LH, testosterone). Since this is also Annette's establishment of primary care, it is important to encourage followups for routine gynecology care and other routine health maintenance.

What if the patient had a positive pregnancy test?

If Annette had a positive pregnancy test, the first step would be to establish if this was a planned and/or desired pregnancy. If the pregnancy is either unplanned or undesired, options counseling should be included to discuss keeping the pregnancy, adoption, and termination of the pregnancy. If Annette wanted to continue the pregnancy, she should be offered or referred to prenatal care. Since a common side effect of PCOS is the inability to conceive due to irregular cycles, she has already overcome a hurdle of the condition. The treatment for irregular menstrual bleeding would be a topic to address postpartum. Metformin is category B in pregnancy, so it would be acceptable to treat the insulin resistance concomitantly with the pregnancy. Androgen receptor blockers would be contraindicated during pregnancy.

What if the patient was trying to conceive?

To treat infertility, a fair trial of treatment should be done to evaluate whether regular menstrual patterns return. If difficulty conceiving persists beyond 9 months or a year, referral to a fertility specialist is acceptable.

Are there any standardized guidelines that you should use to assess or treat this case?

There are 3 published guidelines for the diagnosis of PCOS. National Institutes of Health, European Society for Human Reproduction and Embryology/American Society of Reproductive Medicine, and Androgen Excess Society (https://nurse-practitioners-and-physician-assistants.advanceweb.com/SharedResources/Downloads/2010/012510/NP020110_p18table1.pdf). The Rotterdam criteria are most widely used, as they increase the affected population by about 50% and include less severe forms of the condition.

NOTE: The author would like to recognize Amanda La Manna, RN, ANP for her contribution to the editing of this case.

REFERENCES AND RESOURCES

Gibbs, R. S., et al. (2008). *Danforth's obstetrics and gynecology*. Philadelphia, PA: Lippincott Williams & Wilkins.

Goroll, A. H., & Mulley, A. G. (2009). *Primary care medicine: Office evaluation and management of the adult patient*. Philadelphia, PA: Lippincott Williams & Wilkins.

https://nurse-practitioners-and-physician-assistants.advanceweb.com/SharedResources/Downloads/2010/012510/NP020110_p18table1.pdf

National Institute of Health (2011). Health info: Peptic ulcer. http://health.nih.gov/topic/PepticUlcer

Rotterdam ESHRE/ASRM-sponsored PCOS Consensus Workshop Group (2004). Revised 2003 consensus on diagnostic criteria and long-term health risks related to polycystic ovary syndrome. *Fertility and Sterility, 81*, 19–25.

Case 6.10 Contraception

By Leslie Neal-Boylan, PhD, CRRN, APRN-BC, FNP

This grouping of cases is written somewhat differently than the others in this book in order to offer the reader a variety of possible scenarios regarding contraception.

CASE 1

SUBJECTIVE

A 26-year-old woman presents to the clinic because she wants to change her method of contraception. She used birth control pills for 1 year a few years ago but stopped because she didn't feel she needed them as she was not sexually active at the time. She has rarely been sexually active for the last 3 years, and on those occasions she has made sure that her male partners used condoms.

CRITICAL THINKING

What methods of contraception would you discuss with her?
___Condoms with spermicide
___Diaphragm with spermicide
___Birth control pills
___IUD if the clinician can rule out contraindications

What are the major advantages, disadvantages, and effectiveness of each method?

What are the potential contraindications for each of the methods?

What workup should be done before prescribing oral contraceptives? Should a patient be given a prescription on the initial visit for this concern? What aspects need to be considered before making the decision?

Clinical Case Studies for the Family Nurse Practitioner, First Edition. Edited by Leslie Neal-Boylan.
© 2011 John Wiley & Sons, Inc. Published 2011 by John Wiley & Sons, Inc.

The patient asks when she should start her pills and when she will be protected from pregnancy.

What issues regarding the use of a diaphragm or IUD should be addressed?

CASE 2

SUBJECTIVE

A 34-year-old woman is interested in a diaphragm. She has been using the "rhythm method" combined with condoms. She has not had a period for 5 weeks, although her periods are usually every 29 days. When she was in her twenties, she used an IUD but had it removed about 5 years ago during an episode of abdominal pain.

CRITICAL THINKING

1. What issues would you discuss at this office visit?
2. Should the IUD have been suggested to her at the time she used it? Why or why not?
3. What would be the treatment plan?

For cases 3–9 discuss the choice of contraception for the following women. Be prepared to indicate appropriate and inappropriate choices for each case and the rationale for your conclusions.

CASE 3

The patient is an 18-year-old woman who has had 3 abortions. She has one steady partner but frequently has other partners as well. She has been using condoms in the past. She is a smoker but is otherwise healthy.

CASE 4

The patient is a 42-year-old woman with two children. She is married and has one partner. She is a nonsmoker but has a family history of hypertension.

CASE 5

The patient is a 23-year-old woman who has never been pregnant. She has sex every few months, usually with different partners.

CASE 6

The patient is a 36-year-old, obese woman with hypertension and diabetes who asks you if she can start on the pill. She has one steady partner and has 3 children.

CASE 7

The patient is a 14-year-old girl who is sexually active with "usually one partner."

CASE 8

The patient is a 50-year-old woman, who is single, travels a good deal on business. She quit smoking about 10 years ago and has questionable family history of colon cancer.

CASE 9

The patient is an 18-year-old woman who had unprotected sex with a "blind date" last night.

RESOLUTIONS

CASE 1

What methods of contraception would you discuss?

What are the major advantages, disadvantages, and effectiveness of each method?

TABLE 6.10.1. Methods and Advantages and Disadvantages of Each Method.

Method	Advantages	Disadvantages
Oral contraceptives	Convenient	Daily use (pill only)
		No protection from sexually transmitted infection
Patch	Easy to use	No protection from sexually transmitted infection
Ring	Rapidly reversible	Expensive
		Need prescription
		Side effects
		No protection from sexually transmitted infection
Diaphragm	Can insert up to 6 hours before sex	Increased risk of urinary tract infection
	Decreased STI risk	Risk of toxic shock syndrome
	Decreased risk of cervical cancer	Possible sensitivity to the jelly
		Must be fitted properly
Intrauterine device (IUD)	Absence of metabolic effects (depending on type)	Risk of uterine perforation
		Risk of spontaneous abortion
	Improves menorrhagia	Risk of ectopic pregnancy
	May help endometriosis	Risk of bleeding
	May help fibroids	Possible pain
	Reversible	
Cervical caps	Protection for 48 hours	Risk of toxic shock syndrome
Norplant	Highly effective	Disruption of menstrual pattern
	Avoids risks of giving estrogen	Difficult removal
Female condoms	Some STI protection	Difficult to place properly
Depo-Provera	Decreased menstrual flow	Unpredictable bleeding
	Easy to use	Changes in lipids may occur
	No estrogen	

What are the potential contraindications for each of the methods?

- *Oral contraceptives and other hormonal methods:*
  History of blood clots, pregnancy, thrombophlebitis, congestive heart failure, cerebrovascular disease (CVD), coronary artery disease. Breast/endometrial cancer, undiagnosed abnormal bleeding, jaundice, hepatic problems, Leiden factor V mutation, severe headaches when using oral contraceptives, diastolic BP ≥ 90 or hypertension, cardiac/renal dysfunction, impaired glucose tolerance, depression, varicose veins, smoker ≥ 35 years old, sickle cell disease, jaundice during pregnancy, hepatitis/or mononucleosis in past year, breast-feeding, asthma, primary relative with CVD, diabetes mellitus (under age 50), ulcerative colitis, use of drugs that interact with migraines (if migraines are not accompanied by focal neurological signs then the migraine is not a contraindication).
- *IUD:*
  Absolute contraindications are: pelvic inflammatory disease (PID) within last the 3 months; pregnancy. Relative contraindications are: Ectopic pregnancy, abnormal vaginal bleeding, history of endometriosis, infection after an abortion in the last 3 months, poor access to health care, impaired ability to check string, known or suspected bleeding disorder, valvular heart disease, anatomic variations (that might cause difficulty with insertion), severe dysmenorrhea, history of fainting or vasovagal episodes, allergy to copper (Paraguard IUD), history of impaired fertility, steroid use, small uterus, cervical stenosis, polyps, fibroids, HIV, multiple sex partners, high risk for STIs/PID.
- *Diaphragm/condom:* Allergy to latex (can have nonlatex condoms).
- *Sponge:* Allergy to sponge.

What workup should be done before prescribing oral contraceptives? Should a patient be given a prescription on the initial visit for this concern? What aspects need to be considered before making the decision?

- Obtain the patient's height, weight, blood pressure, and other vital signs. Take a thorough history including history of deep vein thrombosis, STI, and dysmenorrhea. Ask the patient when the last menstrual period occurred, the results of the last Pap smear, and the date of the test. Is the patient a smoker? Does she drink alcohol and how much? What was the age of menarche?
- Use lab studies to rule out an STI and pregnancy. Give the prescription for the contraceptive today if the patient is not pregnant by urine test in the office. Consider the patient's likelihood of compliance with a daily dose. Obtain a CBC, LFTs, and lipids.

The patient asks when she should start her pills and when she will be protected from pregnancy.
She needs a backup method during the first pack. She should start the pill the first day of the cycle or on the first Sunday after her period begins. If she starts on the day of menses, then she is protected. If she starts within 6 days of the first day of her period, then she will need protection for 21 days.

What issues regarding the use of a diaphragm or IUD should be addressed?
It is important to discuss the need for compliance with when using a diaphragm, the risk of pregnancy, and the need to use spermicide. Be sure to discuss a history of urinary tract infections, and check whether the patient is pregnant now.

CASE 2

What issues would you discuss at this office visit?
Discuss the possibility of pregnancy and how she would react if she were found to be pregnant during this visit. Discuss birth control options, the advantages and disadvantages of each method, and contraindications to each method.

Should the IUD have been suggested to her at the time she used it? Why or why not?
No, the IUD was contraindicated at that time in all nulliparas. However, at this time the IUD can be used in appropriately selected nulliparous women with no increase in the risk of tubal infertility.

What would be the treatment plan?
Rule out reasons for the missed period, do a pregnancy test, a physical exam, and a pelvic exam. Fit the patient for a diaphragm or send her to a gynecological nurse practitioner who is trained to do the fitting. Follow up with the patient after she has used the diaphragm to evaluate its effectiveness and her opinion of the method.

CASE 3

Consider a BCP. However, she may not be compliant and is a smoker, but she is under age 35 years. Alternatives: Nuva ring and a condom.

CASE 4

Consider a diaphragm with spermicide or a BCP. Monitor blood pressure. Alternatives: IUD or Depo-Provera.

CASE 5

Consider a diaphragm with spermicide or a cervical cap. These can be used for intermittent sexual activity. Alternatives: Condom with spermicide or a BCP.

CASE 6

A BCP and Norplant are contraindicated. Consider sterilization, as she would be a high-risk obstetrical patient. May give a low dose BCP, but must monitor her carefully. Alternatives: Diaphragm with spermicide or cervical cap.

CASE 7

Consider a low dose BCP and a condom.

CASE 8

Consider a diaphragm with spermicide or a cervical cap because of intermittent sexual activity. Alternative: Condoms with spermicide.

CASE 9

This patient needs emergency postcoital contraception.

REFERENCES AND RESOURCES

Hawkins, J. W., Roberto-Nichols, D. M., & Stanley-Haney, J. L. (2008). *Guidelines for nurse practitioners in gynecologic settings* (9th ed.). New York: Springer.

MacKay, H. T. (2010). Gynecologic disorders. In S. J. McPhee, & M. A. Papadakis (Eds.), *Current medical diagnosis & treatment* (pp. 674–704). New York: McGraw Hill, Lange.

Section 7

Men's Health Cases

Case 7.1 Fatigue

By Geraldine F. Marrocco, EdD, APRN, CNS, ANP-BC

SUBJECTIVE

Fred, a 62-year-old male, presents to the primary care clinic with the chief complaint of fatigue. Upon further questioning, he also reports some difficulty concentrating and a decreased sex drive.

Further review of symptoms reveals dry skin, left-knee weakness, occasional heartburn, polyuria, and wheezing on exertion. He denies chest pain or palpitations. He reports being on antidepressants in the past but did not take them as directed. He is easy to get along with, forthcoming in his complaints, and describes his fatigue as a little bit more pronounced in the last couple of months. He also complains of erectile dysfunction, which he has noticed is worse in the last few years, especially since his diabetes is out of control.

Past Medical and Surgical History: Significant for uncontrolled type 2 diabetes, insulin dependent. The patient reports a last hemoglobin A1c of 10.2. He also has hypertension, gout, obstructive sleep apnea (with refusal to wear CPAP), and hyperlipidemia. His past surgical history includes a deviated septum repair 20 years ago.

Family History: His mother died at the age of 81 of Parkinson disease; his father died at the age of 56 of Hodgkin disease; and he has one sister who is alive and well at the age of 58.

Screening: He had a negative colonoscopy in 2008. His most recent PSA value was 3.1 in 2007.

Social history: He reports drinking 2 drinks of hard liquor daily. He quit smoking 20 years ago and drinks 4 cups daily of coffee. He reports not adhering to his prescribed diabetic diet and has many financial and marital stressors at home. He is self-employed with some college education.

Medications:

Humalog, 75/25, 20 units in the morning and 20 units at night
Nexium, 40 mg daily
Crestor, 10 mg daily
Allopurinol, 300 mg daily
Trazadone, 150 mg at night
Lopid, 600 mg twice daily
Baby aspirin, 81 mg daily
Micardis, 40/12.5 daily
Actos, 30 mg daily

Allergies: He has no known drug, food, or environmental allergies; and his immunizations are up to date.

Clinical Case Studies for the Family Nurse Practitioner, First Edition. Edited by Leslie Neal-Boylan.
© 2011 John Wiley & Sons, Inc. Published 2011 by John Wiley & Sons, Inc.

OBJECTIVE

Vital Signs: T: 98; P: 72; RR: 20; B/P: 138/90. His weight is 312 lbs, and his height is 58 inches.

General: He has a very pleasant attitude. He is a morbidly obese male, calm, pleasant and in no acute distress.

Skin: His color is pale. His skin is clear. Small senile keratosis is noted on his left arm.

HEENT: Negative.

Neck: He appears to have short neck syndrome. He has no palpable nodes, no JVD.

Cardiovascular: Regular rate and rhythm. S1 and S2 are normal.

Respiratory: Chest is clear to auscultation.

Abdomen: Obese, nontender; and bowel sounds are present.

Musculoskeletal: Full range of motion.

Genital: He has normal genitalia. There is no evidence of swelling. His testicular exam is normal, and there is appropriate hair growth.

CRITICAL THINKING

Which diagnostic or imaging studies should be considered to assist with or confirm the diagnosis?
___CBC
___Comprehensive metabolic panel
___Lipid profile
___Urinalysis with microalbumin and microanalysis
___Serum testosterone

What is the most likely differential diagnosis and why?
___Hypogonadism
___Sexual dysfunction
___Depression
___Parkinson disease

What is your plan of treatment?

Are there any referrals needed/?

What would be relative and absolute contraindications to the treatment plan of testosterone therapy?

Are there standardized guidelines that would help in this case?

NOTE: The author would like to recognize Amanda La Manna, RN, ANP for her contribution to the editing of this case.

RESOLUTION

Diagnostic Testing: In order to get a better picture of Fred's status and the reason for his symptoms, it is appropriate to order a CBC, comprehensive metabolic panel, lipid profile, urinalysis with microalbumin and microanalysis, and serum testosterone levels. The CBC will rule out systemic illness and give a picture of general health. The comprehensive metabolic panel will show Fred's diabetes control, kidney and liver function, and fluid status. The lipid profile will evaluate the status of his hyperlipidemia, while the urine studies will evaluate several aspects of Fred's diabetes control. The serum testosterone will evaluate for hypogonadism.

Relevant test results for Fred include a free testosterone level of 128 ng/dL. Normal levels for a young adult male are 300–1000 ng/dL. In men older than 60 years with signs or symptoms of androgen deficiency, a total testosterone level below 200 ng/dL is almost always clinically significant.

What is the most likely differential diagnosis and why?
Secondary hypogonadism:
Given the objective report of clinically significant low testosterone, we can conclude that Fred has secondary hypogonadism. This explains his decreased sexual function, along with his lowered concentration and impaired mood.

However, looking further into the constellation of Fred's symptoms and conditions, it becomes evident that there is interplay of many factors. Fred's uncontrolled diabetes is a wildcard, as it can also contribute to his decline in sexual function. The problem is autonomic neuropathy that results from failure of the small vessels that lead to vasodilation. In addition, it is known that obesity leads to lower free and total testosterone levels. Adding in Fred's probable depressive syndrome completes the clinical picture that shows many overlaps in symptoms. However, an objective diagnosis of hypogonadism can be confidently made considering the laboratory results. Diagnosis is made via evaluation of serum testosterone levels.

It is known that blood concentrations of testosterone and prehormones are significantly lower in older men than younger men, as they begin a gradual decline at midlife. In aging men who have not always had symptoms, hypogonadism is referred to as secondary, since the problem is not a primary dysfunction of the testes. Signs and symptoms of secondary hypogonadism due to aging include decreased muscle mass and strength, decreased bone mass, decreased libido (desire), erectile dysfunction, impaired mood, and impaired sense of well-being.

The diagnosis of male sexual dysfunction can include any or all of the following categories: (1) decreased libido, (2) erectile dysfunction, (3) ejaculatory insufficiency, or (4) impaired orgasm. Fred reports both decreased libido and erectile dysfunction, which can have several different etiologies. Decreased libido can occur due to psychogenic factors, medications, androgen deficiency, substance use or abuse, or central nervous system disease. Erectile dysfunction can occur due to psychogenic factors, medications, endocrine disorders, aging, or systemic illness. Diagnosis is generally made on subjective reporting, and treatment is symptom based.

Fred reports being on antidepressants in the past, which alludes to a previous diagnosis of depressive disorder. Today, Fred's report of altered mood, fatigue, sexual dysfunction, poor concentration, substance use, and personal stressors all suggest the possibility of a depressive syndrome.

What is your plan of treatment?
As an initial approach to Fred's low testosterone, an appropriate treatment is testosterone therapy. There are several different administration modalities, including intramuscular (IM) injections, skin patches, and transdermal gel preparations. IM injection is widely used and is an appropriate choice for Fred. The recommended dose is 150–200 mg IM every 2–3 weeks. The testosterone transdermal patch delivers 5 mg of testosterone daily but has a high incidence of skin irritation. There are other patch preparations that are larger and cause less irritation, but they may have a tendency to fall off with activity. The transdermal testosterone gel is widely used and the dosage is 5–10 mg of 1% testosterone gel applied daily. It causes little skin irritation, though there is a possibility for transfer through direct skin contact. Since Fred has difficulty with daily medication compliance, bringing him to the clinic for routine injections is a wise choice.

In adjunct to testosterone therapy, Fred should be educated about medication compliance. Explaining to him the importance of diabetes control and the interplay of his numerous symptoms may be an effective approach.

Since Fred will be coming to the office for routine injections to start, there will be opportunities to reassess his symptoms. There will also be an opportunity to assess whether Fred or his spouse should be instructed in injection administration. Follow-up intervals should occur between every 4 and 6 months to evaluate progress, symptoms, and blood levels. Blood levels should be drawn periodically to evaluate whether his serum testosterone has returned to normal levels. Therapy could continue for as long as 3–4 years.

Are there any referrals needed?
Education about diet and exercise should be reinforced; and, if he is willing, he should be given a referral for nutritional counseling.

What would be relative and absolute contraindications to the treatment plan of testosterone therapy?
Testosterone therapy is absolutely contraindicated in those with carcinoma of the prostate or of the male breast, as these cancers require androgens for proliferation. Testosterone therapy should be used with caution in older men with enlarged prostates, with urinary symptoms, or elevated hematocrit.

Are there standardized guidelines that would help in this case?
The American Association of Clinical Endocrinologists Medical Guidelines for Clinical Practice for the Evaluation and Treatment of Hypogonadism in Adult Male Patients—2002 Update. (http://www.aace.com/pub/pdf/guidelines/hypogonadism.pdf)

REFERENCES AND RESOURCES

AACE Hypogonadism Task Force (2002). American association of clinical endocrinologists medical guidelines for clinical practice for the evaluation and treatment of hypogonadism in adult male patients—2002 update. *Endocrine Practice, 8,* 439–456.

Gibbs, R. S., et al. (2008). *Danforth's Obstetrics and Gynecology.* Philadelphia, PA: Lippincott Williams & Wilkins.

Goroll, A. H., & Mulley, A. G. (2009). *Primary care medicine: Office evaluation and management of the adult patient.* Philadelphia, PA: Lippincott Williams & Wilkins.

Case 7.2 Testicular Pain

By Geraldine F. Marrocco, EdD, APRN, CNS, ANP-BC

SUBJECTIVE

Richard is a 45-year-old male who is an established patient. He arrives at the primary care office with the chief complaint of "extremely painful" right testicular pain for 3 hours. He reports no history of trauma. He reports that the pain came on gradually over the last 3 hours and is associated with some mild dysuria, but no urethral discharge. Pain is described as a 9 on a 0–10 series. He denies fever, nausea, or vomiting. He reports a loss of appetite due to extreme pain.

Past Medical/Surgical History: Significant for COPD, GERD, hypertension, and chronic tendonitis in right elbow since fracture in 2007. He also reports a gastrointestinal infection that responded very well to Cipro. His past surgical history includes only a cervical laminectomy in 1996.

Family History: His mother is alive at the age of 87 and has diabetes mellitus type 2. His father died at the age of 79 from leukemia and prostate cancer. He has 4 sisters and 2 brothers who are all alive and well.

Social History: Works as a plumber and has been married for 20 years. He reports being in a monogamous sexual relationship with his wife. He lives in a single family home and has smoked 1 pack per day for the last 30 years. He denies alcohol or substance abuse and drinks tea daily.

Medications:

Nexium, 40 mg in a.m.
Advair Inhaler, 250/50 1 puffs twice daily
Atacand, 16/12.5 mg
Spiriva inhaler, 1 puff daily

Allergies: No known drug allergies, but has seasonal allergies and an allergy to peanuts.

OBJECTIVE

General: Visibly grimacing and teary eyed, not smiling. His skin is flushed.

Vital Signs: T: 98.2 F; P: 80; BP: 136/84; RR: 18.

Clinical Case Studies for the Family Nurse Practitioner, First Edition. Edited by Leslie Neal-Boylan.
© 2011 John Wiley & Sons, Inc. Published 2011 by John Wiley & Sons, Inc.

Respiratory: CTA bilaterally.

Cardiac: RRR: S1/S2; no murmurs, clicks, gallops, or rubs.

Genitourinary: Scrotal exam reveals obvious edema and redness of the right scrotal area. The area is very painful to touch or lift. There is no evidence of urethral discharge. The testes are tender to palpation, but the position of the testes is consistent and normal. When in the supine position, with elevation of the testes, Richard notes a slight decrease in pain, which is called Phren's sign. Transillumination of the testes is negative for masses. The rectal exam reveals some prostate tenderness.

CRITICAL THINKING

Which diagnostic or imaging studies should be considered to assist with or confirm the diagnosis?
__Doppler ultrasound
__Urinalysis
__Urine culture and sensitivity
__Gram stain

What is the most likely differential diagnosis and why?
__Sexually transmitted infection
__Testicular torsion
__Epididymitis
__Testicular tumor
__Trauma

What is your plan of treatment?

Are there any referrals needed?

NOTE: The author would like to recognize Amanda La Manna, RN, ANP for her contribution to the editing of this case.

RESOLUTION

Diagnostic Testing: To rule out the emergent condition of testicular torsion, it is appropriate to obtain a stat Doppler scrotal ultrasound. In addition, it is appropriate to order a urinalysis for routine analysis and a culture and sensitivity test to evaluate for infection of the urinary tract. If there was urethral discharge, a gram stain of the discharge would be appropriate, as well.

The results of the Doppler indicated that there was no testicular torsion. A pulse Doppler and a color Doppler were performed, revealing both testicles to be normal in size and to have a homogenous echotexture. The right testicle measured 4.4 × 2.2 × 2.4 cm, and the left testicle measured 2.98 × 2.0 cm. There was no intratesticular or extratesticular mass present. No abnormal fluid was noted in bilateral scrotal sacs, and there was no evidence of testicular torsion. Urinalysis was negative.

What is the most likely differential diagnosis and why?
Epididymitis
As testicular torsion and testicular mass were ruled out via ultrasound and there was no report of trauma, the differential can be narrowed down to STI or epididymitis. There was no urethral discharge on exam. Coupled with the patient's report of monogamy, this suggests that the cause of the pain is not a sexually transmitted infection. The acute pain and positive Phren's sign on exam point strongly toward epididymitis.

Epididymitis is a bacterial infection and inflammation of the epididymis, which is the tube connecting the testicle with the vas deferens. It is the most common cause of acute scrotal pain in all age groups, though it is most common among sexually active men younger than 35. In the younger age group, the infection is most often due to *Chlamydia trachomatis* or *Neisseria gonorrheae*. In men who have anal intercourse, epididymitis can be caused by *Escherichia coli*. In older men, the cause is often a urinary tract infection. On exam, the affected testis will transilluminate, and there will be a positive Phren's sign.

While some sexually transmitted infections can lead to epididymitis, it is possible for some infections to affect the ductus deferens and/or the testicles. Those included are chlamydial infection, gonorrheal infection, and syphilis infection.

Testicular torsion should be suspected whenever a man complains of scrotal pain, as it is an emergent condition that can, if left untreated, lead to ischemia of the affected testis. It presents acutely as a firm, tender mass, often associated with nausea and vomiting. Testicular torsion occurs more often in young men, and the incidence is 1 in 4000 in men younger than 25 years of age. No exam finding can completely rule out testicular torsion. Therefore, it must be ruled out via a Doppler study due to its emergent nature. A Doppler study will reveal decreased blood flow to the testis in a case of torsion.

Testicular malignancy is most prevalent in young men ages 15–35 years, where the incidence is 4 in 100,000. Symptoms include a hard, heavy, firm, nontender mass. There will often be scrotal swelling in the affected testis, and about 18%–46% of testicular tumors will cause discomfort or pain. Upon exam, the affected testis where the mass is located will not transilluminate.

Though uncommon, testicular trauma should be a consideration when presented with a case of scrotal pain. Usually the affected individual will identify a recent injury or trauma. Classifications of disorders due to trauma include blunt trauma, penetrating trauma, degloving trauma, and testicular rupture.

What is your plan of treatment?
Without knowing the offending bacterial organism, empiric treatment of the infection is appropriate at this stage. Fluoroquinolones and cephalosporins are suggested empiric treatments, as are sulfonamides. In this case the patient was treated with ciprofloxacin, 500 mg twice daily for 3 weeks.

To address the patient's acute pain, a relatively strong analgesic was indicated. In this case, the patient was appropriately prescribed Vicodin ES, 1 tab by mouth twice daily. It is also important to review supportive measures, such as sitz baths, rest, elevation of the testes, ice packs, and anti-inflammatory agents.

The patient being treated for epididymitis should be brought back in 2 weeks to evaluate the success of treatment. If treatment is successful in symptom reduction, the antibiotics should be completed. If symptoms still persist, the patient should be further evaluated by a specialist.

Are there any referrals needed?
In the cases of recurrent infection or failure to respond to treatment, it would be appropriate to consult with or refer the patient to a urologist.

REFERENCES AND RESOURCES

De Cassio Saito, O., de Barros, N., Chammas, M. C., Oliveira, I. R. S., & Cerri, G. G. (2004). Ultrasound of tropical and infectious diseases that affect the scrotum. *Ultrasound Quarterly, 20*(1), 12–18. Retrieved from http:// ovidsp.ovid.com/ovidweb.cgi?T=JS&NEWS=N&PAGE=fulltext&D=ovftg&AN=00013644-200403000-00003

Goldman, L., & Ausiello, D. (2008). *Cecil textbook of medicine* (23rd ed.). Philadelphia: Saunders.

Goroll, A. H., & Mulley, A. G. (2009). *Primary care medicine: Office evaluation and management of the adult patient.* Philadelphia, PA: Lippincott Williams & Wilkins.

Wampler, S. M., & Llanes, M. (2010). Common scrotal and testicular problems. *Primary Care: Clinics in Office Practice, 37*(3), 613–626. doi:10.1016/j.pop.2010.04.009

Case 7.3 Prostate Changes

By Meredith Wallace Kazer, PhD, APRN, A/GNP-BC

SUBJECTIVE

Roy presents to the primary care practice for his 6-month checkup. He has been seen here every 3–6 months over the past 6 years. Roy is a 75-year-old man who is generally healthy and who has well-managed hypertension and coronary artery disease. In addition to his semi-annual visits to the practice, he also sees a cardiologist annually.

During this visit, his review of systems is negative. He denies shortness of breath (SOB), dyspnea on exertion (DOE), chest pain, palpitations, headaches, dizziness, nausea, vomiting, or diarrhea. He complains of a little urinary hesitancy and difficulty starting his stream. This has been going on for "some time now" He says it doesn't bother him much and he's getting used to it. He denies pain and burning on urination. He denies a past history of urinary tract infection or problems with his prostate gland. His bowels are regular with an occasional need for prune juice or Metamucil. He is sexually active with his wife, and sexual function is adequate with the assistance of oral erectile agents.

Past Medical and Surgical History: Hypertension; erectile dysfunction; dyslipidemia.

Social History: Roy lives at home with his wife and works part-time at a local grocery store. He has a son and a daughter who are both married professionals who live close by. He has 4 grandchildren. He has an occasional social drink, but does not smoke. His income comes primarily from social security and a small pension from his previous career as a banker. He also supplements his income with his part-time job. He is very involved with his family and attends Catholic services weekly. He is in generally good health and visits his primary care provider every 6 months for followup of his chronic medical illnesses.

Family History: His family is healthy. Both parents are deceased. His father died in his fifties of a heart attack. His mother recently died at age 92.

Medications: HCTZ, 25 mg; Lisinopril, 20 mg; Lipitor, 20 mg every day (QD); Metamucil and Cialis, as needed

Allergies: NKDA.

OBJECTIVE

General: Awake, alert, and oriented. Erect posture. He appears clean and well kept. Clothes are appropriate.

Vital Signs: He is 5 ft 9 inches and weighs 180 lbs. BP: 164/92; P: 110. 02 sat 99%. He is afebrile with a temperature of 97.8.

Eyes: Clear sclera; PERRLA.

Ears: Mild wax buildup; clear and intact tympanic membranes bilaterally.

Mouth: Intact oral mucosa.

Respiratory: Lungs are clear with no adventitious sounds.

Cardiac: Regular heart rate, S1/S2; no abnormal heart sounds.

Abdomen: Soft, nontender; and bowel sounds are present in all 4 quadrants. He has no scars or lesions on his abdomen, and his umbilicus is midline.

Skin: Dry and intact.

Extremities: No pedal edema; positive pedal pulses.

Neuromuscular: 2+ deep tendon reflexes bilaterally and equal strength. Gait is normal with full range of motion of all extremities.

Rectal: Digital rectal examination (DRE) reveals no abnormalities.

CRITICAL THINKING

Which diagnostic or imaging studies should be considered to assist with or confirm the diagnosis?
__CBC
__Urinalysis
__Metabolic panel
__Prostate specific antigen (PSA) test
__Urine culture and sensitivity
__Transrectal ultrasound

What is the most likely differential diagnosis and why?
__Urinary tract infection (UTI)
__Benign prostatic hypertrophy (BPH)
__Prostate cancer
__Testicular cancer
__Pyelonephritis
__Sexually transmitted infection

What is your plan of treatment?

Does the patient's psychosocial history impact how you might treat this patient?

What if the patient also had kidney failure?

What are the best treatment options for this patient with each of the differentials listed?

Are there any standardized guidelines that you should use to assess or treat this case?

RESOLUTION

Diagnostic Testing: An important point to consider is whether or not this patient should have had a PSA test at all. Controversy exists as to whether the PSA test should be used to screen men for the presence of disease, as the goal of screening is to decrease mortality and improve quality of life. The U.S. Preventive Services Task Force (USPSTF) has recently recommended that men over 75 years of age forego PSA screening due to limited benefit and increased risk for physical and psychological harm (2008). During this routine visit, the patient agrees to have a complete metabolic panel drawn, complete blood count (CBC), and prostate specific antigen (PSA). Because of the urinary symptoms, a urinalysis and a culture and sensitivity test should be ordered. Diagnosis of prostate cancer is confirmed following biopsy guided by transrectal ultrasound. The ultrasound is used to direct the placement of the needle to extract the specimens. The urologist may opt for a transperineal or transrectal approach to perform the biopsy (ACS, 2009). Roy's CBC and metabolic panel are all within normal limits. Urinalysis is negative; PSA reading is 6.2 ng/dL. His readings over the past 4 years are revealed in the figure below (Figure 7.3.1):

> The USPSTF concludes that the current evidence is insufficient to assess the balance of benefits and harms of prostate cancer screening in men younger than age 75 years. Thus, The USPSTF recommends against screening for prostate cancer in men age 75 years or older. This recommendation is a level D. This means that the USPSTF recommends against it because there is moderate or high certainty that the screening has no net benefit or that the harms outweigh the benefits. (Accessed from http://www.ahrq.gov/clinic/USpstf/uspsprca.htm#summary.)

What is the most likely differential diagnosis and why?
Possible *prostate cancer:*
What is most curious in Roy's case is his rapidly rising PSA value over the past year. Normal PSA values are between 0 and 4.0 ng/mL; values greater than 4.0 may warrant additional followup dependent on a number of patient characteristics including, but not limited to, age, ethnicity, body mass index, height, and a family history of prostate cancer. The PSA levels revealed in the graph are very suspicious for prostate cancer. Most telling is the doubling of the PSA values over the past year. However, elevated PSA levels may also be the result of benign prostatic hypertrophy, older age, inflammation, or ejaculation within 2 days of testing (ACS, 2009). Values lower than 4.0 in African American men and those who are obese also call for additional followup by a healthcare provider as research has shown that these factors may result in high risk for prostate cancer. (Freedland et al., 2008; Sanchez-Ortiz et al., 2006).

Prostate cancer is the most commonly diagnosed cancer in U.S. men (American Cancer Society, 2008), and 64% of all prostate cancers are diagnosed in men older than 65 years (American Cancer Society, 2008). A tumor growing in the prostate gland will produce pressure on the urethra and manifest in the symptoms described.

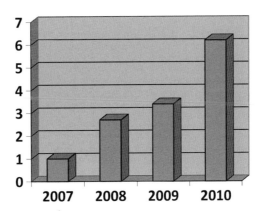

Figure 7.3.1. Roy's PSA values over past five years.

Urinary tract infection (UTI)

UTI is an obvious differential given the symptoms that Roy presented with. UTIs are relatively rare, in adult males, but increase dramatically after the age of 60 related to conditions of the prostate (Howes & Pillow, 2009). In Roy's case, a UTI could be confirmed or ruled out with a simple in-office normal urinalysis. In this case, Roy did not have a UTI. Had he had a urinary tract infection, the urinalysis would have revealed white blood cells. Had this been the case, culture and sensitivity testing of the urine sample would have revealed an antibiotic that would be appropriate to treat him.

The next differential is benign prostatic hyperplasia. Gerber (2009) states that BPH is a condition resulting from benign enlargement of the prostate gland. This is very common in adult males over the age of 50. Urinary symptoms result from increased pressure on the urethra from the surrounding enlarged prostate. An enlarged prostate can easily be determined through the use of a digital rectal examination (DRE) in the office or upon referral to a urologist. BPH may also be accompanied by an elevated PSA value. BPH is effectively treated with alpha-1-adrenergic antagonists to relax prostate and bladder muscle contractility—Tamsulosin (Flomax); terazosin (Hytrin). Men should be cautioned about the hypotensive effects of these medications. Alternative medications in the form of 5-alpha-reductase inhibitors to reduce the size of the prostate gland (Finasteride) (Proscar) or dutasteride (Avodart) may be prescribed but could have the side effect of erectile dysfunction. In Roy's case, a digital rectal exam revealed a normal-size prostate. However, he was referred to a urologist for further evaluation.

What is your plan of treatment?

In Roy's case, symptoms have been present for some time; and the PSA values for this patient have been gradually increasing over the past several years. However, the PSA has doubled over the last year, which is cause for concern and referral. The next steps for this patient would be referral to a urologist. The diagnostic testing would likely entail a digital rectal exam (DRE). DRE is helpful in finding abnormalities in the prostate; but the exam covers only the small, palpable portion of the gland. Thus, if a tumor is in an area of the prostate gland that is not palpable, it may not be detected. Transrectal ultrasound (TRUS) guided biopsy of the prostate gland would likely be the next step in the diagnosis of this patient. The biopsy results are categorized using a grading system, referred to as the Gleason Staging system. This system assigns a grade to each of the 2 largest areas of cancer in the biopsy samples. Grades range from 1 to 5, with 1 being the least aggressive and 5 being the most aggressive. The 2 grades are then added together to produce a Gleason score. A score of 2 to 4 is considered low grade; 5 through 7, intermediate grade; and 8 through 10, high grade. A high Gleason score indicates that the cancer is more likely to grow quickly (ACS, 2009). Roy had a positive biopsy for Gleason stage 6 prostate cancer.

Treatment options for Roy would include radical prostatectomy, external beam radiotherapy, brachytherapy, cryotherapy, or active surveillance. The treatment decision would be made by Roy with discussion with his family and health care provider. However, given his age and the modest survival benefits of treatment, as well as the fact that all available therapeutic modalities for localized prostate cancer result in significant risk of adverse effects such as sexual dysfunction, urethral strictures, urinary incontinence, and bowel problems, active surveillance may be a good option. Active surveillance (AS) is becoming a more accepted prostate cancer management option. For men like Roy, with early-stage prostate cancer, AS provides an alternative to surgery or radiation therapy. That is, men make the decision to actively monitor their disease with the knowledge that treatment remains an option.

Regardless of his treatment choice, Roy will continue followup with a urologist. However, Roy will continue to visit his primary care provider for followup of other medical problems. During these visits, he should be questioned to ensure visits with the urologist every 6 months at a minimum. PSA values can be drawn with annual blood work and sent to the urologist for followup. Of course, changes in PSAs should be reported to the patient and the urologist immediately, as rising PSAs after treatment are problematic in the prostate population. PSAs should still be monitored after treatment completion.

Does the patient's psychosocial history impact how you might treat this patient?

The fact that the patient is married underscores the need to determine the impact of treatment on his sexual relationship. Thus, the adverse effects of treatment should be discussed with this patient prior to decision-making. While his urologist or medical oncologist will discuss this, the patient may still have questions regarding the impact of treatment on urinary and sexual structures and their subsequent impact on quality of life. These must be considered carefully.

What if the patient also had kidney failure?
As kidney failure has a potential to shorten lifespan, and would prevent radical treatments, the presence of this disease would greatly impact treatment options. In conjunction with the patient's age, a chronic illness such as kidney failure may make this patient a good candidate for active surveillance above other treatment options.

Are there any standardized guidelines that you should use to assess or treat this case?
The American Urological Association has published guidelines on the treatment of localized prostate cancer. This is available at http://www.auanet.org/content/guidelines-and-quality-care/clinical-guidelines.cfm.

REFERENCES AND RESOURCES

American Cancer Society (2008). *American cancer society. Cancer facts & figures 2008*. Atlanta: American Cancer Society.

American Cancer Society (2009). *American cancer society. Cancer facts & figures 2009*. Atlanta: American Cancer Society.

American Cancer Society. Retrieved from http://www.cancer.org/docroot/lrn/lrn_0.asp

American Urological Association (2010). American urological association treatment guidelines and resources. Retrieved from http://www.auanet.org/content/guidelines-and-quality-care/clinical-guidelines.cfm

Freedland, S. J., Wen, J., Wuerstle, M., Shah, A., Lai, D., Moalej, B., . . . Aronson, W. J. (2008). Obesity is a significant risk factor for prostate cancer at the time of biopsy. *Urology, 72*(5), 1102–1105.

Gerber, G. (2009). Benign prostatic hyperplasia (BPH, enlarged prostate). Retrieved from http://www.medicinenet.com/benign_prostatic_hyperplasia/article.htm

Howes, D. S., & Pillow, M. T. (2009). Urinary tract infection. Male. EMedicine. Retrieved from http://emedicine.medscape.com/article/778578-overview

John Hopkins Prostate Health Alerts (2010). Retrieved from http://www.johnshopkinshealthalerts.com/alerts_index/prostate_disorders/25-1.html

National Cancer Institute (2010). Retrieved from http://www.cancer.gov/cancertopics/types/prostate

Sanchez-Ortiz, R. F., Troncoso, P., Babaian, R. J., Lloreta, J., Johnston, D. A., & Pettaway, C. A. (2006). African-American men with nonpalpable prostate cancer exhibit greater tumor volume than matched white men. *Cancer, 107*(1), 75–82.

U.S. Preventive Services Task Force (2008). Screening for prostate cancer: U.S. preventive services task force recommendation statement. *Annals of Internal Medicine, 149*(3), 185–191.

Us TOO. International Prostate Cancer Education and Support Network. www.ustoo.org

Section 8

General Adult Health

Case 8.1 Weight Gain and Fatigue

By Vanessa Jefferson, MSN, BC-ANP, CDE

SUBJECTIVE

Maxwell is a 40-year-old homosexual African-American male and corporate lawyer who first came to the health maintenance organization 3 years ago. At that time, he had not been to a primary care provider since graduating from law school. The patient admitted to a sedentary life style, a weight gain of 25 pounds within the past 2 years, and occasional fatigue and headache.

Past medical history: None significant.

Past surgical history: Significant for a tonsillectomy at the age of 7.

Family history: Significant for thyroid disease, hypertension, type 2 diabetes, hyperlipidemia, and obesity.

OBJECTIVE

VISIT THREE YEARS AGO

Vital signs: 220 pounds with a height of 6 ft 1 inch and a body mass index of 29. Blood pressure: 140/88; radial pulse: 78; temperature: 98.7; and respiratory rate: 16.

Physical examination: Significant for acanthosis nigricans and central adiposity.

Diagnostic test results: Fasting lipids revealed total cholesterol of 182, a low density lipoprotein level of 106, a high density lipoprotein level of 57, and a triglyceride level of 95. His fasting blood glucose was 95, and an A1c was 5.6. His thyroid stimulating hormone level was 0.24. A routine electrocardiogram documented normal sinus rhythm and rate.

Diagnoses: Stage 1 hypertension (due to the elevation of blood pressure) and hypothyroid disease (since the thyroid stimulating hormone level was abnormally low).

Plan: The patient was started on both hydrochlorothiazide 25 mg by mouth daily and levothyroxine 0.25 mcg by mouth daily. He was counseled regarding lifestyle modifications, inclusive of preparing

Clinical Case Studies for the Family Nurse Practitioner, First Edition. Edited by Leslie Neal-Boylan.
© 2011 John Wiley & Sons, Inc. Published 2011 by John Wiley & Sons, Inc.

and eating a low-sodium and low-fat diet. Maxwell was encouraged to start a routine exercise program of at least 30 minutes of modest aerobic activity such as walking as if to catch a bus. He was also encouraged to lose 5%–7% of his body weight. These lifestyle modifications have proven effective in diabetes prevention and maintenance, as well as in control of blood pressure and lipid levels. The patient was informed regarding the mechanism of action of both medications, duration of action, contraindications, and adverse effects. The patient was also instructed to take the levothyroxine on an empty stomach first thing in the morning.

THREE-MONTH FOLLOW-UP VISIT

Vital signs: Blood pressure of 128/76.

Diagnostic test results: Thyroid stimulating hormone level = 3.37. Basic metabolic panel: Blood urea nitrogen level of 14; creatinine level of 0.98; sodium level of 137; potassium level of 3.5; and a chloride level of 104.

Plan: The patient was given a list of potassium containing foods and reminded to eat 1 or 2 items daily due to a low potassium level. He was instructed to continue to take the hydrochlorothiazide.

TWO YEARS LATER

SUBJECTIVE

Maxwell has been very busy climbing the corporate ladder and has not been in for a physical examination or lab work for 2 years. Now he presents with complaints of extreme fatigue for the past 2 months and low libido. He states that he feels fatigued all the time, and sleep does not seem to relieve it. He is able to work, but has limited socialization and participation in outside activities due to fatigue. He reports sleeping for 8–10 hours a night, with his sleep being interrupted by a need to go to the bathroom at least twice. He awakens fatigued.

Sexually, he has a morning erection but not as strongly as in previous months. He has limited sexual desire. He is able to have an erection with intercourse, but it is less of an erection than previously. He states that he has been in a monogamous relationship for the past 2 years. He admits to a 15-pound weight gain over the past 2 years. He reports that he experiences occasional constipation and some cold intolerance. He denies fever, night sweats, and tobacco or drug use and reports socially drinking several glasses of red wine per week.

Past medical history: Remains significant for hypertension and hypothyroidism.

Past surgical history: Remains the same.

Family history: His father died recently from a heart attack.

Medications: Hydrochlorothiazide, 25 mg PO QD; levothyroxine, 0.50 mcg PO; multivitamin, 1 capsule PO QD; and fish oil capsules, 2000 mg PO QD. There are no known drug allergies or no known food allergies.

OBJECTIVE

Vital signs: Temperature: 98.6; radial pulse: 76; blood pressure: 134/80; oxygen saturation: 99%; height: 6 ft 1 inch; weight: 235 lb (15-lb weight gain); and body mass index: 31. Physical exam is unremarkable except for the following findings:

Skin: Poor skin turgor; acanthosis nigricans.

Mouth: Dry oral mucosa.

Abdomen: Central adiposity.

Lymph: No significant lymphadenopathy.

Rectal: Hemoccult negative for occult blood.

CRITICAL THINKING

Which diagnostic or imaging studies should be considered to assist with or confirm the diagnosis?
___Stool hemoccult
___Complete blood count
___Thiamine
___Iron studies
___Complete metabolic panel
___Rapid HIV test
___HIV viral load test
___HbA1c
___Thyroid stimulating hormone
___Testosterone
___Urine analysis
___Tuberculosis testing
___Urine microalbumin/creatinine ratio

What is the most likely differential diagnosis and why?
___HIV and/or AIDS
___Pernicious anemia
___Hypothyroidism uncontrolled
___Hypogonadism

What is the most likely differential diagnosis and why?

What is your plan of treatment?

Are any referrals needed?

Does the patient's psychosocial history impact how you might treat this patient?

What if this patient were female?

What if the patient were over age 65?

What if the patient was over the age of 80?

Are there standardized guidelines that should be used to assess and treat this patient?

RESOLUTION

Diagnostic testing: The basic metabolic panel reveals the following : Creatinine level: 0.89; blood urea nitrogen, 14; sodium: 137; potassium: 3.5; chloride: 104. Liver function tests are within normal limits. Rapid HIV test is negative. Complete blood count—white blood count: 5.7; hemoglobin: 14.3; hematocrit: 43.2; macrocytic corpuscle volume: 84; fasting blood glucose: 168; A1C: 8.5. Testosterone is within normal limits. Erythrocyte sedimentation rate is within normal limits. Urinalysis is positive for 2+ glucose; trace protein.

What is the most likely differential diagnosis and why?

Diabetes mellitus type 2:

Maxwell has had a gradual onset of fatigue over the past few months, which presents as a classic symptom of diabetes. Noted also is nocturia, which awakens him at least 2 times during the night. Polyuria and/or nocturia are also classic presenting symptoms, due to the glucose concentrated urine creating a diuretic effect. He also has had a 15-lb weight gain over the past 2 years. His body mass index has progressed from 29 (which is the overweight category) to 31 (the obese category). Obesity is a leading cause of insulin resistance. He reports a sedentary lifestyle which contributes to the obesity and the insulin resistance. Low libido may be related to a lack of energy in conjunction with some erectile dysfunction relevant to the hyperglycemia causing an autonomic neuropathy.

Fatigue is a major symptom reported with inadequately treated hypothyroidism, HIV, anemia and inadequate testosterone levels. The patient does have a history of hypothyroidism and therefore may require additional levothyroxine due to a thyroid hormone deficiency. Also the patient did report occasional constipation, some cold intolerance, and significant weight gain. Patients with hypothyroidism have a diminished red blood cell mass, which may present as a macrocytic anemia. A small percentage of patients with hypothyroidism have the occurrence of pernicious anemia. Therefore, anemia is a relevant differential diagnosis. The patient reports that he is in a monogamous homosexual relationship and denies fevers and night sweats and has had a positive weight gain; however it would be wise to rule out the diagnosis since he is in a high risk category. African Americans have the highest rates of HIV and AIDS in the United States. Maxwell exhibits high-risk behavior since he is a male who is sexually active with a male. Symptoms of HIV are often nonspecific but may include fatigue. The patient has numerous risk factors for diabetes due to family history, hypertension, increased body mass index, sedentary lifestyle, and being African American. Detection of hypogonadism in males with sexual dysfunction is warranted. Male hormone deficiency can be a cause of fatigue as well as sexual dysfunction.

What is your plan of treatment?

The patient has a moderate degree of hyperglycemia ranging from 151 to 250. Therefore, diet, exercise, and 1 oral agent is appropriate therapy with which to begin. The patient's creatinine and liver function studies are within normal limits. Metformin 500 mg daily in the evening is initially started. The patient is instructed to take 1 tablet daily with the first bite of food in the evening. He is informed regarding the mechanism of action, contraindications, adverse effects of the metformin, and the need to remain hydrated while taking the medication to prevent lactic acidosis.

If he is unable to drink oral solutions and/or hold liquids down, then he should stop the metformin and call the office. If the metformin is tolerated well without significant gastrointestinal affects, then the patient is told to increase the dose of metformin to twice a day following the week of initiation. Basic education is taught surrounding diabetes signs and symptoms and potential treatment. Lifestyle modifications are again stressed concerning consumption of a heart-healthy diet and routine modest aerobic exercise of 30 minutes, 5 days a week. The patient receives instruction in self–blood glucose monitoring and use of the glucose meter. Prescriptions are written for the metformin, a glucose meter, and supplies of strips and lancets. Additional and routine diabetes management lab work is ordered such as fasting lipids and a urine microalbumin/creatinine ratio.

The patient is instructed to call the office in 1 week for followup regarding the use of the glucose meter and blood glucose readings. At that time, it should be determined if the patient should receive another phone call or return to the clinic sooner than 1 month. Otherwise, the patient will be scheduled to return to the clinic to see this clinician in a month for followup of self–blood glucose monitoring results and possible adjustment of medications. Repeat the HbA1C in 3 months along with fasting lipids and a urine microalbumin/creatinine ratio if any of the previous levels are abnormal.

Are any referrals needed?

A referral to a dietitian is appropriate for a discussion related to meal planning, cooking methods, and portion control. An ophthalmology referral for a dilated eye exam in 3 months will allow time for improved glycemia and improved vision. A referral should be made to a certified diabetes educator for further diabetes education and co-management. Offer the patient the opportunity to attend a series of diabetes education classes. A podiatry referral for diabetic foot care and management should be considered. If the low libido persists following normoglycemia, then a referral to a urologist would be appropriate.

Does the patient's psychosocial history impact how you might treat this patient?
This patient's psychosocial history does not impact how this patient will be treated.

What if this patient were female?
If this were a female patient, more questioning would have occurred to assess her menstrual cycle, including the duration and the amount of flow of her menses. A ferritin level would have been included in the initial workup. Also a pregnancy test may be indicated. More attention would have been spent on an initial evaluation for depression. The Becks Depression Inventory would have been useful.

What if the patient was over age 65?
If the patient were 65 years or older, more emphasis would have been initially placed on determining if any cancer markers were present. The initial evaluation would have also included a chest x-ray.

What if the patient was over the age of 80?
Metformin may not be the first drug of choice since impaired renal function and the greater potential for dehydration exists in this age group. The possibility of lactic acidosis is higher in this age group, though it rarely occurs. Patients over the age of 80 should have a normal creatinine clearance documented prior to beginning therapy. All patients on metformin should have their liver function test and creatinine checked annually.

Are there standardized guidelines that should be used to assess and treat this patient?
Use Clinical Practice Guidelines provided by the American Diabetes Association 2010.

REFERENCES AND RESOURCES

American Diabetes Association (2010a). Diagnosis and classification of diabetes. *Diabetes Care, 33*(Suppl. 1), S62–S69. doi:10.2337/dc10-S062.

American Diabetes Association (2010b). Executive summary: Standards of medical care in Diabetes—2010. *Diabetes Care, 33*(Suppl. 1), S4–S10. doi:10.2337/dc10-S004.

American Diabetes Association (2010c). Standards of medical care in diabetes—2010. *Diabetes Care, 33*(Suppl. 1), S11–S61. doi:10.2337/dc10-S011.

Centers for Disease Control and Prevention (2010). HIV/AIDS and African-Americans. Retrieved July 7, 2010, from http://www.cdc.gov/hiv/topics/aa/index.htm

Diabetes Prevention Program Research Group (2002). Reduction in the incidence of type 2 diabetes with lifestyle intervention or metformin. *The New England Journal of Medicine, 346*(6), 393–403. doi:10.1056/NEJMoa012512.

Inzucchi, S. (2010). *Diabetes facts and guidelines* (13th ed.). North America: Takeda Pharmaceuticals North America, Inc.

Moneyham, L., Sowell, R., Seals, B., & Demi, A. (2000). Depressive symptoms among African-American women with HIV disease. *Scholarly Inquiries in Nursing Practice, 14*(1), 9–39.

Rosenthal, T. C., Majeroni, B. A., Pretorius, R., & Malik, K. (2008). Fatigue an overview. *American Family Physician, 78*(10), 1173–1179.

Steer, R. A., Cavalieri, T. A., Leonard, D. M., & Beck, A. T. (1999). Use of the beck depression inventory for primary care to screen for major depression disorders. *General Hospital Psychiatry, 21*(2), 106–111. doi: 10.1016/S0163-8343(98)00070-X.

Unger, J. (2007). *Diabetes management in primary care.* Philadelphia: Wolters Kluwer Health/Lippincott Williams & Wilkins.

Case 8.2 Fatigue

By Geraldine F. Marrocco, EdD, APRN, CNS, ANP-BC

SUBJECTIVE

Maryanne, a 78-year-old female widow, presents to the primary care clinic with the chief complaint of feeling very tired lately. She also complains of some nasal congestion. She arrives with her daughter, who provides some gaps in the medical history. The daughter notes that Maryanne's fatigue has been a complaint for about 16 months.

Further review of systems provided by the daughter reveals a concern that her mother seems to have slight confusion, increased fatigue, poor appetite, and a bitter taste sensation when eating. Maryanne eats 3 small meals daily, and she's had some unintentional weight loss over the past few months. She reports a marked decrease in energy level. She denies nausea, vomiting, or emotional lability. She does not eat red meat.

Past medical history: Significant for hypertension for many years; type 2 diabetes mellitus that is not well controlled on oral meds; high cholesterol for many years; lymphedema in lower extremities bilaterally since adolescence; benign lung densities per chest x-ray; and a report of "Mediterranean anemia." She had cataract removal surgery in 2009. She sees a podiatrist every 3 months and sees a retinopathist periodically. Her last visit was today, and her exam was negative.

Family history: Her mother died at age 81 with DM and hypertension. Her father died of lung cancer. She has two brothers ages 81 and 83, both with hypertension and one with prostate cancer.

Social history: Born in California and has four children; does not use tobacco currently; quit smoking over 20 years ago. She denies ETOH use or history of substance abuse. She does not drink coffee and does not exercise. Her typical day includes watching television and doing housework. She lives independently in an adult community in Alabama and has a homemaker 3 times weekly. She is a retired cook. She has one daughter who lives nearby.

Medications:

- Glucophage, 1000 milligrams BID
- Avandia, 4 mg daily
- Protonix, 40 mg daily
- Glucotrol, 10 mg daily
- Aricept, 10 mg daily at night
- Cardia, 240 mg daily in AM

Clinical Case Studies for the Family Nurse Practitioner, First Edition. Edited by Leslie Neal-Boylan.
© 2011 John Wiley & Sons, Inc. Published 2011 by John Wiley & Sons, Inc.

- Lisinopril, 10 mg daily
- Diovan, 160/12.5 BID
- Aspirin, 81 mg daily
- Crestor, 5 mg daily
- Zetia, 10 mg daily
- Coreg, 12.5 mg BID
- Lasix, 20 mg daily
- Potassium, 10 mEq daily
- Actonel, 35 mg weekly.
- Multivitamin, over the counter
- B12
- Tylenol, as needed for pain

Allergies: No known drug allergies and is up to date on her immunizations.

Additional ROS:

Skin: Complains of dry skin.

HEENT: Denies any dizziness or blurry vision. No headaches except for + right ear pain. Sometimes difficulty swallowing.

Cardiovascular: Denies chest pain or palpitations.

Respiratory: Occasional cough and has noticed more shortness of breath recently. Sleeps on 2 pillows.

Gastrointestinal: Denies abdominal pain or bloating. She does not have any regurgitation. No nausea or vomiting. She has a bowel movement daily which is normal, brown in color, and normal consistency. She does not report any blood in her stool.

Musculoskeletal: Reports joint pain in her knee, especially her left knee.

Psyche: Generally happy, social, but most recently not engaged due to fatigue and weakness.

OBJECTIVE

General: She is a 78-year-old female who is pleasant, slightly confused, and moderately anxious. Her daughter is present during the visit. The patient defers to her daughter for clarification of events and details. Daughter and mother have a positive working relationship with evidence of support and caring.

Vital Signs: T: 98.2; P: 86; RR: 28; SaO$_2$: 93; B/P: 140/70. Her weight is 191 pounds, and her height is 64 inches.

Skin: Clear, slightly grayish color.

HEENT: Hair thinning, gray at roots, silky texture. Sclera nonicteric, pupils dilated since she just came from the retinopathist (examination of her eyes deferred). Oral mucosa, pink moist intact.

Neck: Supple, no JVD, no bruits. Thyroid nonpalpable. No lymphadenopathy.

Cardiovascular: Heart regular rate and rhythm. PMI is at 5th intercostal space left sternal border; + systolic murmur II/VI. Pulses positive all extremities. There is bilateral lower leg edema; chronic lymphedema; no ulcerations; skin intact; no hair growth; no pitting.

Respiratory: Lungs clear to auscultation. Transverse/AP diameter 2/1.

Abdomen: BS+, obese, soft, nontender. No hepatomegaly; no splenomegaly; no hernia.

Neurological: CN I–XII grossly intact. Mental status 30/30 (Folstein Mini Mental Status Exam).

Geriatric depression screen: No evidence of depression.

Musculoskeletal: Walks with a cane; s/p right knee replacement 2007. Full ROM; no deformities; muscle strength appropriate for age.

CRITICAL THINKING

Which diagnostic or imaging studies should be considered to assist with or confirm the diagnosis?
___CBC
___FBS
___CMP
___HbA1c
___TSH
___Ultrasound
___Urea breath test
___Iron studies

What is the most likely differential diagnosis and why?
___Chronic kidney disease
___Anemia (type?)
___COPD
___Obstructive sleep apnea
___Dementia
___Depression
___Gastric ulcer

What is the plan of treatment?

What is the plan for follow-up care?

Are any referrals needed at this time?

Are there standardized guidelines that you should use to assess or treat this case?

NOTE: The author would like to recognize Amanda La Manna, RN, ANP for her contribution to the editing of this case.

RESOLUTION

Diagnostic tests: CBC: Hemoglobin and hematocrit were 10.1/29.5; FBS: 149; potassium 4.8; BUN: 42; creatinine 1.44 (estimated glomerular filtration rate [GFR] was 35)

What is the most likely differential diagnosis and why?
Chronic kidney disease (CKD) stage 3:
The GFR of 35 points directly to CKD, stage 3. The low hemoglobin clearly suggests anemia, though the specific etiology is unknown. There are several mainstays of CKD management, which include blood pressure control, volume management, anemia management, and sodium/potassium management. The JNC-7 lists 130/80 to be the target blood pressure of an individual with CKD and HTN. ACE-I and ARBs are pharmacotherapy options that have been proven to be renoprotective, so switching to one of these agents for blood pressure control is wise. In addition, thiazide and loop diuretics are excellent choices for hypertensive patients with CKD. Since individuals with CKD can be at risk

for hyperkalemia and hypernatremia, particularly if also diabetic, management of sodium and potassium levels is crucial. This can be done via dietary restriction of 2 g/day of each sodium and potassium (Goroll & Mulley, 2009).

Maryanne also has anemia secondary to CKD, stage 3. The BUN and creatinine lab values lead us to evaluate Maryanne's kidney function. The general health of an individual's kidney is determined by the glomerular filtration rate, 35 in this case. A decrease in GFR correlates with a change in histology secondary to kidney disease. The stages of chronic kidney disease (CKD), as defined by the National Kidney Foundation, are as follows:

CKD is defined as kidney damage or GFR $< 60\,\text{mL/min}/1.73\,\text{m}^2$ for at least 3 months. Kidney damage is defined is abnormal pathology, abnormal blood values, abnormal urine studies, or abnormal imaging.

- Stage 1: Kidney damage with normal GFR (≥ 90)
- Stage 2: Kidney damage with mild decrease in GFR (60–89)
- Stage 3: Moderate decrease in GFR (30–59)
- Stage 4: Severe decrease in GFR (15–29)
- Stage 5: Kidney failure (GFR < 15 or dialysis) (National Kidney Foundation [NKF], 2002).

The workup for anemia of CKD is initiated when the hemoglobin value is less than 12 g/dL in a postmenopausal female. Anemia of CKD can be most commonly attributed to decreased production in erythropoietin by the kidneys or to iron deficiency. Other causes of anemia of CKD include blood loss, hypothyroidism, acute and chronic inflammatory conditions, and hemoglobinopathies.

Maryanne also appears to have dementia, a condition that is characterized by a progressive decline in intellectual functioning. The functional decline tends to involve the memory, cognitive capacities, and adaptive behavior. Dementia does not involve alteration in consciousness. Dementia may start as mild cognitive impairment in its earliest stages, which refers to an isolated loss of memory without difficulty in other cognitive functions. Alzheimer's disease is the leading cause of dementia, though depression in the older adult can also present similarly. Other symptoms of depression in the older adult include hopelessness, anhedonia, and fatigue. Assessment of dementia is further evaluated with a mental status examination (Goroll & Mulley, 2009).

When evaluating chronic fatigue, malignancy must always be on the differential. The clinical picture often also includes severe involuntary weight loss, depression, and apathy. Laboratory studies (CBC) are paramount for ruling out a cancer.

OSA might be considered as a differential diagnosis. It occurs when the nasopharyngeal airway patency is compromised during sleep. Risk factors include obesity, increased neck circumference, deviated septum, nasal polyps, and enlarged tonsils. Presentation includes snoring, disturbed sleep, daytime sleepiness, chronic fatigue, and personality change. The easiest way to determine whether OSA is appropriately on the differential is to have the patient observed by another during sleep to evaluate for snoring (Goroll & Mulley, 2009).

COPD is known as irreversible and progressive decline in lung function due to obstruction of airflow, airway inflammation, and reduction in the expiratory flow rate. Individuals with COPD often have a history of smoking, asthma, or environmental/work exposure to irritants. COPD refers to chronic bronchitis or emphysema. Symptoms include shortness of breath, wheezing, and increased work of breathing. On examination, lung sounds can include fine or coarse crackles and wheezes. In emphysema, the AP diameter of the chest is increased, and lung sounds can be distant (Goroll & Mulley, 2009).

What is the plan of treatment?

To manage and further evaluate the anemia secondary to CKD, it is necessary to order further lab tests, particularly iron studies. In the meantime, it is appropriate to start treatment of erythropoietin. The iron studies to be ordered are CBC, indices, reticulocytes, serum iron, TIBC, and ferritin. If those studies reveal iron deficiency, treatment should be changed to iron replacement. If those values are normal, it means that the deficiency is in fact due to the damaged kidneys producing less than normal erythropoietin. Specific changes to Maryanne's medication regimen should be as follows:

- Discontinue Glucophage,
- Discontinue Avandia.
- Begin Actos, 30 mg daily (for glycemia control)
- Discontinue Lasix
- Begin HCTZ 25 mg daily (thiazide diuretic for hypertension)
- Begin Procrit, 2000 units subcutaneously 3 x week (erythropoietin for anemia)
- Continue Actonel 35 mg weekly

What would be your plan for follow-up care?

The following lab studies should be ordered at this time and discussed as soon as the results become available: Repeat CBC; TSH; LFTs; chemistry panel; BUN/creatinine; Hgb A1C; micro urinalysis; ferritin, serum iron, TIBC, reticulocytes; and R/O thalassemia.

Further diagnostic tests that are appropriate include a CT scan of the chest, abdomen, and pelvis with contrast (if not contraindicated), a mammogram, and a transvaginal US of the uterus.

Are any referrals needed at this time?

Referrals should be initiated to hematology and nephrology.

Are there standardized guidelines that you should use to assess or treat this case?

The National Kidney Foundation has published guidelines for the management of CKD and its common comorbid conditions. KDOQI Clinical Practice Guidelines for Chronic Kidney Disease: Evaluation, Classification, and Stratification (http://www.kidney.org/professionals/KDOQI/guidelines_ckd/toc.htm)

REFERENCES AND RESOURCES

Goroll, A. H., & Mulley, A. G. (2009). *Primary care medicine: Office evaluation and management of the adult patient.* Philadelphia, PA: Lippincott Williams & Wilkins.

National Kidney Foundation (2002). KDOQI clinical practice guidelines for chronic kidney disease: Evaluation, classification, and stratification. *The American Journal of Kidney Disease, 39*(2 Suppl. 1), S1–S266.

Case 8.3 Morning Headache

By Kathy J. Booker, PhD, RN

SUBJECTIVE

Andrew is a 42-year-old African American male who presents with BP 168/92 and morning headaches. Andrew reports headaches upon arising approximately 2 times per week. This morning prompted his coming to the office for evaluation, as he felt some lightheadedness and chest tightness that resolved following his shower. He has never been told that his blood pressure was high, but he has not been seen in the office for 6 years. His last visit was for bronchitis and treatment with antibiotics.

Past medical/surgical history: He has no surgical history.

Family history: His father is deceased at age 65 from an acute MI; one brother died at age 50 with acute MI, following abdominal aortic aneurysm surgery. He has 4 other siblings in good health.

Social history: He has been dealing with several life issues including the death of a child and a reduction in his work hours at a local manufacturing plant. He smokes 2 packs of cigarettes per day, leads a sedentary life outside of work, and is overweight at 6 ft 2 inches and 255 pounds (BMI = 33). He reports generally good health. His smoking history is 44 years. He is married and has 3 remaining children, aged 12, 15, and 17. His oldest son was killed in a car accident 2 months ago. He drinks moderately, generally 2–3 beers 4–5 times per week. He reports drinking more heavily on the weekends. He and his wife are active in their church. He is a high-school graduate and makes approximately $50K annually. His wife has a full-time position that supplements the family income to approximately $90K. For 3 months, his business has experienced a downturn; and there have been mandatory furlough days, which have required their family spending to be seriously curtailed, although they are able to meet their financial obligations at this time.

Medications: He is on no prescription medications at this time. Andrew takes a daily aspirin and a multivitamin, but no prescription medications.

Allergies: No known allergies. He reports being lactose intolerant.

Clinical Case Studies for the Family Nurse Practitioner, First Edition. Edited by Leslie Neal-Boylan.
© 2011 John Wiley & Sons, Inc. Published 2011 by John Wiley & Sons, Inc.

OBJECTIVE

General: Patient appears older than his stated age; frowning.

Vital signs: BP on arrival is 188/92. After 20 minutes, repeat BP is 180/90. P: 94; R: 20; T: 98.2 F.

HEENT: Cranial nerves intact. EENT exam negative.

Neck: No lymphadenopathy.

Skin: Skin warm and dry.

Respiratory: Lung sounds vesicular over peripheral fields; harsh, bronchial breath sounds in upper lobes bilaterally; moist cough audible; no adventitious breath sounds.

Cardiovascular: No jugular venous distention at 30 degree elevation. Heart sounds strong 3/4; grade 2/6 systolic murmur at left sternal border, 5th ICS. Abdominal and peripheral vascular assessments negative; pedal and post tibial pulses 2+/4+.

Abdomen: Tender over right upper quadrant. Tympany predominates. Liver border WNL, spleen and kidneys nonpalpable.

Neuromuscular: Romberg's sign negative; gait relaxed and symmetrical; no pronator drift. Full ROM all extremities.

CRITICAL THINKING

Which diagnostic or imaging studies should be considered to assist with or confirm the diagnosis?
___Electrocardiogram
___Troponin
___CBC
___Electrolytes
___Serum cholesterol panel

What is the most likely differential diagnosis and why?
___Obstructive sleep apnea
___Hypertension
___Dyslipidemia
___Cardiovascular disease
___Diabetes mellitus
___COPD

What is the plan of treatment?

What is the plan for follow-up care?

Are any referrals needed at this time?

What if this patient were female?

What if the patient were also diabetic?

Are there any standardized guidelines that you should use to assess or treat this case?

RESOLUTION

Diagnostic tests: ECG: The ECG shows nonspecific T wave changes; no evidence of acute ischemia. Troponin: <0.4. CBC: Slightly elevated RBCs, otherwise, WNL. Electrolytes: WNL. Total cholesterol: 240; HDL: 58; LDL: 166; Triglycerides: 196.

What is the most likely differential diagnosis and why?
Hypertension:
Morning headaches and the development of hypertension may also suggest obstructive sleep apnea. Daytime sleepiness and patterns of snoring should be explored. If either is present, he should be referred for a sleep study. With this patient's strong family history of early CHD, immediate treatment of his hypertension is indicated. Close monitoring of his altered cholesterol panel values is also indicated. If he is able to improve his exercise and diet and reduces weight subsequent to these changes, cholesterol levels may improve. Since he had nonspecific T wave changes, a repeat ECG in 6 months would be important. Teaching for signs and symptoms of acute coronary syndrome is extremely important.

What is the plan of treatment?

- Start the patient on antihypertensive therapy. Recent work (Feldman et al., 2009) suggests that a combination low-dose regimen is more effective than monotherapy. Potential combinations of diuretic with ACE inhibitors or combination diuretic with aldosterone receptor blocking drugs (ARB) are more effective and cause fewer side effects. Begin with lower dosages with increases of baseline dosages if BP targets less than 140/90 or less than 130/80 for diabetic patients are not reached.
- URGENT—stop smoking. Prescribe nicotine substitute patch and discuss plans for smoking cessation.
- Recommend low-fat, low-salt diet (DASH) high in fruits and vegetables; provide a referral to a dietitian and explain that lowering salt and eating fruits, vegetables and low-fat dairy products was found to be particularly effective in reducing blood pressure in minority patients (Moore et al., 1999)
- Encourage walking a minimum of 3–5 days per week. Schedule gradual increases in length and time after 2-week initiation.

What is the plan for follow-up care?

- Return for BP check in 1 week.
- Encourage patient to monitor BP at home twice daily and keep a log.
- Encourage a log of daily walking activity with BP.
- Recheck serum cholesterol in 3 months.

Are any referrals needed at this time?

- Referral for stress testing.
- Explore need for grief counselling.
- Refer to dietitian for dietary assistance.
- Refer to stop smoking clinic or web-guided smoking cessation program

What if this patient were female?
The initial treatments and counseling would be the same in females. In educating about the signs of acute coronary syndrome, women should be told about atypical symptoms including dyspnea, and pain radiating to jaw and back.

What if the patient were also diabetic?
Diabetes increases the risk of CAD, and additional teaching for glycemic control and risk factors associated with diabetes would be required. BP targets are set at a lower point (<130/80) in patients with DM to reduce CAD risk.

Are there any standardized guidelines that you should use to assess or treat this case?
The use of the DASH guidelines for dietary moderation, and the hypertension management guidelines (Chobanian et al., 2003) are useful. The American Heart Association has sponsored a campaign "Get with the Guidelines" that provides additional patient education material and research summaries for healthcare providers online at http://www.americanheart.org.

REFERENCES AND RESOURCES

Chobanian, A. V., Bakris, G. L., Black, H. R., Cushman, W. C., Green, L. A., Izzo, J. L. Jr., et al. and The National High Blood Pressure Education Program Coordinating Committee (2003). Seventh report of the Joint National Committee on prevention, detection, evaluation, and treatment of high blood pressure. *JAMA, 289,* 2560–2571.

Chobanian, A. V., & Hill, M. (2000). National Heart, Lung, and Blood Institute workshop on sodium and blood pressure: A critical review of current scientific evidence. *Hypertension, 35,* 858–863.

Feldman, R. D., Zou, G. Y., Vandervoort, M. K., Wong, C. J., Nelson, S. A. E., & Feagan, B. G. (2009). A simplified approach to the treatment of uncomplicated hypertension. A cluster randomized, controlled trial. *Hypertension, 53,* 646–653.

Moore, T. J., Vollmer, W. M., Appel, L. J., Sacks, F. M., Svetkey, L. P., Vogt, T. M., et al. (1999). Effect of dietary patterns on ambulatory blood pressure: Results from the dietary approaches to stop hypertension (DASH) trial. *Hypertension, 34,* 472–477.

Rathore, S. S., Ketcham, J. D., Alexander, G. C., & Epstein, A. J. (2009). Influence of patient race on physician prescribing decisions: A randomized on-line experiment. *Journal of General Internal Medicine, 24*(11), 1183–1191.

Rosendorff, C., Black, H. R., Cannon, C. P., Gersh, B. J., Gore, J., Izzo, J. L. Jr., et al. (2007). Treatment of hypertension in the prevention and management of ischemic heart disease. A scientific statement from the American Heart Association Council for High Blood Pressure Research and the Councils on Clinical Cardiology and Epidemiology and Prevention. *Circulation, 115,* 2761–2788.

Sacks, F. M., Obarzanek, E., Windhauser, M. M., Svetkey, L. P., Vollmer, W. W., McCullough, M., et al. (1995). Rationale and design of the Dietary Approaches to Stop Hypertension (DASH 2). *Annals of Epidemiology, 5,* 108–118.

SUBJECTIVE

Henry, a 32-year-old male, presents with a report of facial pain for 5 days. He reports that he has a headache, especially when he bends down, and that his teeth hurt sometimes. On further questioning, Henry states that he had a cold about 14 days ago. He had rhinorrhea with clear drainage, mild sore throat, ear pressure, and mild headache. The symptoms cleared up after 1 week, and he felt fine, but then some of the symptoms returned about 5 days ago. Now he describes facial pain, headache upon waking, dental discomfort, and blood streaked nasal drainage. He has a history of seasonal allergic rhinitis.

Past medical history: Chicken pox at age 5 years; testicular torsion at age 15 years (no complications).

Family history: His family is well, although his mother and sister have migraine headaches.

Social history: He is happily married with 2 children. Henry works as a supermarket manager, is a nonsmoker, and denies other substance use.

Medications: Advil sinus with no relief; MVI; baby aspirin.

Allergies: Seasonal hay fever.

OBJECTIVE

General: NAD.

Vital signs: Henry is 6 feet 1 inch tall and weighs 165 pounds. His oral temperature is 99.5 Fahrenheit. BP is 128/84. Pulse is 74 and regular. Respirations are 12 and regular.

HEENT: Sclera are clear; PERRLA; EOMs intact. Tympanic membranes are clear and intact; there is no fluid. There is tenderness to palpation of the frontal and maxillary sinuses. Nares are erythematous and swollen. There is no obvious discharge. There is cobblestoning in the throat, but no erythema. Tonsils are +2. There are no exudates.

Clinical Case Studies for the Family Nurse Practitioner, First Edition. Edited by Leslie Neal-Boylan.
© 2011 John Wiley & Sons, Inc. Published 2011 by John Wiley & Sons, Inc.

Neck: There is no lymphadenopathy, and the thyroid is nonpalpable.

Cardiac: RRR, S1/S2; no murmurs, clicks, gallops, or rubs.

Respiratory: Clear to auscultation.

CRITICAL THINKING

Which diagnostic or imaging studies should be considered to assist with or confirm the diagnosis?
___CT scan of sinuses
___X-ray of sinuses
___CT scan of brain
___CBC
___CMP

What is the most likely differential diagnosis and why?
___Viral upper respiratory infection (URI)
___Acute sinus infection
___Asthma
___Migraine
___Allergic rhinitis
___Nonallergic rhinitis
___Vasomotor rhinitis
___Rhinitis medicamentosa

What is the plan of treatment?

What is the plan for follow-up treatment?

Are any referrals needed?

Is the family history of migraines relevant?

RESOLUTION

Diagnostic tests: None are necessary at this time. However, repeated sinus infections or episodes of sinusitis may warrant a CT scan of the sinuses.

What is the most likely differential diagnosis and why?
Acute sinus infection:
The headache, sinus pain and pressure, and dental pain all support his diagnosis. It is not uncommon for patients to experience blood streaked rhinorrhea. A typical course toward the development of sinusitis includes a cold or upper respiratory infection followed by the patient feeling improved or well. However, symptoms return; and they tend to be worse and include sinus pressure and pain. A sinus infection needs time to develop and typically follows a cold, URI, or allergies, as mucus and drainage accumulates in the sinus allowing bacteria or viruses to grow and fester.

Henry may also have allergic rhinitis which is characterized by cobblestoning in the throat, pale boggy mucosa, clear drainage, scratchy throat, itchy eyes, and an initial presentation after age 8 years old. However, any evidence of Henry's allergies would be superseded by his sinusitis symptoms. Children may have an obvious crease in their noses called an allergic salute that is caused by constantly rubbing the nose. People with allergies may also have epistaxis and frequent throat clearing accompanied by a cough. Mouth breathing, snoring, and creases beneath the lower eyelids (Dennie lines) are sometimes also present. It is not unusual to also have sinus pressure, tenderness, and headache.

Vasomotor rhinitis is a type of nonallergic rhinitis. It is unrelated to an allergic hypersensitivity, infection, structural lesions, systemic disease, or drug use. One can also have atrophic sinusitis (from normal aging), rhinitis medicamentosa (overuse of some over-the-counter medication), or rhinitis related to the hormonal changes of pregnancy. Nonallergic rhinitis may also be caused by foreign bodies in the nose, nasal polyps, neoplasms, cocaine use, hypothyroidism, anatomic variations, and NARES (nonallergic rhinitis with eosinophilia syndrome). In NARES, there is eosinophilia in the nasal drainage, but skin and in vitro tests for allergens are negative.

TABLE 8.4.1. Plan of Treatment.

Illness	Patho	S/Sx	Treatment
Common cold :URI	Antigen, inflammatory response: edema, WBCs, congestion. Airborne, direct contact. Rhinovirus, coronavirus, parainfluenza virus, coxsackie, RSV. Incubation 1–5 days, virus shedding up to 3 weeks.	Mild fever possible, chills, body aches, rhinorrhea (possibly purulent), and ear congestion, HA. ≤7–10 days, peak 5 days.	Rest, fluids, analgesic, antipyretic. Atrovent nasal spray (anticholinergics), nasal spray. Afrin (watch for rebound): vasoconstriction. Dextromethorphan: Cough suppressant, may cause serotonin syndrome.
Allergic rhinitis	IgE mediated: Allergen specific IgE after T cell release. RXN is from subsequent exposure to allergen. Early phase: Prompt, lasts 1 hour. Late: Begins in 3–6 hours, gone in 12–24 hours. Early mediated by histamine. Late mediated by chemokines, cytokines, eosinophils, basophils. Eosinophils release leukotrienes.	Sneezing, pruritus, congestion, drainage, sometimes conjunctivitis. Pale, boggy nasal mucosa, allergic shiners, nasal salute, watery eyes, cobblestoning throat and nose.	Avoidance, antihistamines (Zyrtec, Allegra, Claritin), decongestants: oral or topical (watch for rhinitis medicamentosa), intranasal steroids, antileukotrienes (Singulair), intranasal cromolyn (prevention), allergy shots (prevention).
Sinusitis	Cause is usually viral URI. Sinus inflammation should resolve in <14 days. If symptoms worsen after 3–5 days or last >10 days, then probably bacterial infection. Nasal mucosa produces drainage, then congestion and swelling into sinus cavity. Hypoxia and mucus retention promote bacterial growth. *Streptococcus pneumoniae, Haemophilus influenzae, M. catarahallis.* Chronic: *Staphylococcus aureus* and anaerobic bacteria. Can also have fungal sinusitis.	>7 days of congestion, purulent rhinorrhea, PND, facial pain, pressure, ear/teeth pain, maybe cough, fever, nausea, fatigue, halitosis, impaired smell, taste. Chronic: Congestion, cough & PND, worse at night. PE: Mucosal edema (nasal), purulent nasal secretions, sinus TTP (not specific or sensitive). Nose: Deviated septum, polyps, epistaxis, foreign bodies, tumors.	Amoxicillin (875 mg bid) or Augmentin (XR bid × 2 weeks) Ceftin, Bactrim, Biaxin, Zithromax. Chronic: ABX 4–6 weeks and intranasal steroid: Flonase, Nasonex, Rhinocort AQ, Nasacort AQ; decongestant (Sudafed) mucolytic: guaifenesin, saline spray or irrigation.

What is the plan of treatment?

Treat patient for sinusitis and allergic rhinitis.

What is the plan for follow-up treatment?

There is no need for a scheduled followup unless the patient reports that symptoms have persisted beyond treatment or have worsened.

Are any referrals needed?

No referrals are needed at this time. However, a referral to an EENT may be warranted for repeated episodes. An allergist might be worth a visit if it is deduced that allergies are the inciting causes of each episode of sinusitis.

Is the family history of migraines relevant?

Migraine headaches often appear in families. They tend to be more common in women than in men. The symptoms of migraine and sinusitis are often mistaken for each other, and each condition may be misdiagnosed as the other.

REFERENCES AND RESOURCES

Bhattacharyya, N. (2009). Approach to the patient with chronic nasal congestion and discharge. In A. H. Goroll, & A. G. Mulley (Eds.), *Primary care medicine* (pp. 1415–1422). Philadelphia: Lippincott.

Kormos, W. A. (2009). Approach to the patient with sinusitis. In A. H. Goroll, & A. G. Mulley (Eds.), *Primary care medicine* (pp. 1402–1407). Philadelphia: Lippincott.

Lustig, L. R., & Schindler, J. (2010). Ear, nose, & throat disorders. In S. J. McPhee, & M. A. Papadakis (Eds.), *Current medical diagnosis & treatment* (pp. 179–214). New York: McGraw Hill, Lange.

Case 8.5 Burning Epigastric Pain after Meals

By Leslie Neal-Boylan, PhD, CRRN, APRN-BC, FNP

SUBJECTIVE

Meredith is a 63-year-old female who presents with worsening epigastric pain. She describes it as burning pain that starts over the sternum and radiates upward to her neck. The pain occurs approximately 30–45 minutes after every meal and continues for about 4.5 hours thereafter. Heavy meals, coffee, and spicy foods make the discomfort worse; and she is most uncomfortable when she lies down at night. She has to prop herself on 3 pillows every night to decrease the pain, so she refrains from eating close to bedtime. Meredith also describes a sour taste in her mouth when she lies down and has awakened occasionally with coughing and regurgitation. The pain has been worsening over the past 3 months and occurs daily. The discomfort interferes with her quality of life. She has had some mild relief with Maalox and Tums. Meredith also reports an intermittent nonproductive cough and feeling hoarse when she talks. She denies any fevers, chills, dysphagia, odynophagia, weight loss, fatigue, shortness of breath, abdominal pain, nausea, changes in bowel habits, blood in the stool, or urinary symptoms.

Past medical history: Hyperlipidemia.

Family history: Noncontributory.

Social history: Meredith has smoked ½ ppd for 30 years; drinks a bottle of wine by herself each Friday and Saturday night. She has a history of marijuana use when in college but none currently. She is widowed and works as an elementary school teacher.

Medications: HCTZ, 12.5 mg PO daily; Lipitor: 10 mg.

Allergies: Penicillin.

OBJECTIVE

General: Meredith is well appearing, in no apparent distress, and is moderately obese.

Vital signs: She is afebrile. BP is 160/100. HR is 86 and regular. Respirations are 14 and regular, and oxygen saturation is 96% on room air.

Clinical Case Studies for the Family Nurse Practitioner, First Edition. Edited by Leslie Neal-Boylan.
© 2011 John Wiley & Sons, Inc. Published 2011 by John Wiley & Sons, Inc.

HEENT: Unremarkable except for some moderate erythema in the posterior pharynx and some dental erosion. Her teeth are stained, as well. There are no abscesses.

Neck: There is no cervical lymphadenopathy, and the thyroid is nonpalpable. Carotids are +2 without bruits.

Cardiac: Regular rate and rhythm without murmurs, clicks, gallops, or rubs.

Respiratory: Lungs are clear bilaterally.

Abdomen: Is soft and obese without bruits but with positive bowels sounds. There is mild epigastric tenderness on palpation but without rebound guarding. There is no organomegaly.

Rectal: Brown stool with a trace of positive on guaiac testing.

Skin: Is without rashes, lesions, or ulcers.

CRITICAL THINKING

Which diagnostic or imaging studies should be considered to assist with or confirm the diagnosis?
___CBC with differential
___Metabolic panel
___Liver function tests
___Urinalysis
___ECG
___Chest x-ray
___*H. pylori* testing
___Endoscopy
___Colonoscopy
___Fecal occult blood test
___Esophageal manometry and pH monitoring

What is the most likely differential diagnosis and why?
___Angina
___Myocardial infarction
___Gastroesophageal reflux disease (GERD)
___Gastric ulcer
___Duodenal ulcer
___Cholecystitis
___Gastrointestinal bleed

What is the plan of treatment?

Are any referrals needed at this time?

What are the patient's risk factors for this condition?

What are the possible complications of this condition?

RESOLUTION

Diagnostic tests: In this case, all of the diagnostic tests listed in the case presentation should be done. The clinician must rule out a cardiac condition (despite the mild success with antacid medication), pulmonary problem, ulcer, hepatitis, and infection. Since the guaiac was positive, a follow-up FOBT and/or colonoscopy should be done, especially if the patient has not had a colonoscopy done recently. If the FOBT is positive, then a colonoscopy must be done regardless of how long it has been since the last one. However, the gastroenterologist should be consulted about this and will need, in most places, to arrange the colonoscopy. The patient also will need an endoscopy, as her symptoms are severe. Possible complications of GERD and ulcers will need to be ruled in or out by an endoscopy. For a patient whose symptoms are not severe, the endoscopy can usually wait while the patient is monitored under conservative treatment with medication and diet changes.

What is the most likely differential diagnosis and why?
Gastroesophageal reflux disease:
This diagnosis is supported by the patient's symptoms of retrosternal burning pain that occurs after meals and is exacerbated by certain foods and heavy meals. The sour taste, coughing, and regurgitation are also relevant symptoms. The fact that Meredith has achieved some relief with Maalox and Tums helps the clinician to validate that the condition is probably related to reflux. A cardiac condition or an ulcer is unlikely to result in relief from an antacid.

What is the plan of treatment?
The first line treatment for GERD includes antacids, H2 blockers or proton pump inhibitors (PPI). (See Table 8.5.1). Meredith has already tried antacids but they are only providing minimal relief. At this point, Meredith should be started on a PPI once each day (with possibility of increase to twice each day if once a day is insufficient to control symptoms) for 4–8 weeks to see if that helps her symptoms to resolve. If her symptoms continue or if she develops dysphagia, weight loss, anemia, or odynophagia, she should be sent for an upper endoscopy. If these findings are normal but the patient continues to have symptoms, then the manometry and pH monitoring might be explored (small number of patients). If the endoscopy reveals abnormal results, such as Barrett's esophagus, the patient should be referred to a gastroenterologist.

Lifestyle modification (diet, weight loss, sitting up after meals and in bed at night) might be sufficient for patients with mild cases of GERD. Most people can come off of the PPI after 8–12 weeks or just change to an as needed basis. (See Table 8.5.2). However, Meredith has some troublesome symptoms that are affecting her quality of life. These modifications should still be recommended, but she should use the PPI therapy for 8–12 weeks. If she continues to have symptoms and requires twice-daily treatment after 12 weeks, she should be placed on the lowest dose possible with awareness of the possible adverse effects of long-term use (increased risk of *Clostridium difficile* and hip fractures).

TABLE 8.5.1. Medications Used to Treat GERD.

Antacids: Quick Onset, Short Duration	H2 blockers: OTC Dose Is ½ Prescription Dose. Longer Onset, Longer Duration	Proton Pump Inhibitors: Take 30 Minutes before Breakfast
Tums	Cimetidine	Omeprazole (also available with sodium bicarbonate)
Baking soda	Ranitidine	Rabeprazole
Maalox	Famotidine	Lansoprazole
		Pantoprazole

TABLE 8.5.2. Management of GERD.

Stage I: Lifestyle modification.
Stage II: OTC medications prn.
Stage III: Scheduled medications for 8–12 weeks: H2 blockers or PPIs (or can try H2 blockers for 8–12 weeks, THEN PPIs for 8–12 weeks).
Stage IV: Maintenance therapy with lowest possible dose.
Stage V: Surgery: Fundoplication.

Are any referrals needed at this time?

Most patients are treated based on a clinical diagnosis but some may need to be referred to a gastroenterologist for further testing and treatment. She should see the gastroenterologist if 12 weeks of a PPI is insufficient to resolve her symptoms. Intractable disease may require surgical treatment via fundoplication.

What are the patient's risk factors for this condition?

The risk factors that Meredith has include obesity and smoking.

What are the possible complications of this condition?

Possible complications of GERD include adenocarcinoma, Barrett's esophagus, aspiration pneumonia, severe esophagitis that results in odynophagia and dysphagia, esophageal hemorrhage, laryngitis, reflux induced asthma, unexplained wheezing, chronic cough, dental erosions, and a feeling of a lump in the throat.

REFERENCES AND RESOURCES

McPhee, S. J., & Papadakis, M. A. (2010). *Current medical diagnosis & treatment*. New York: McGraw-Hill Lange.

Case 8.6 Burning Chest Pain

By Kathy J. Booker, PhD, RN

SUBJECTIVE

Patricia is a 62-year-old female who calls the office at 10:00 a.m. for an appointment. She tells the receptionist that she is having mild chest pain and burning in the center of her chest. She has a history of GERD and the receptionist works her in for an 11:00 a.m. appointment. The history reveals that Patricia ate a very spicy meal, including 2 glasses of wine, at a local Mexican restaurant the evening prior to this visit. She reports a diet high in fat and salt. Last night, she took Tums and an additional omeprazole, with slight relief, but experienced significant dyspepsia from 7 p.m. to midnight, after which time she slept fitfully. This morning at 6:00 a.m., she awoke with epigastric burning and mild chest pain (rated at +4/10). She had no radiation of the pain, no nausea, no diaphoresis, and no associated symptoms. Her pain lasted until 10:00 a.m. and has dissipated in the past hour. She states that this is very similar to the symptoms she experienced when diagnosed 3 years ago with GERD.

Past medical/surgical history: GERD, depression, osteoarthritis, and glaucoma.

Family history: Mother died of myocardial infarction age 65 years. Otherwise, unremarkable.

Social history: Widowed with a supportive family. Nonsmoker.

Medications: Fluoxetine hydrochloride, 20 mg daily; omeprazole, 20 mg daily; ibuprofen, 300 mg as needed; and betaxolol hydrochloride, 2 gtts ou, bid.

Allergies: Penicillin and sulfa for seasonal allergies.

OBJECTIVE

General: She appears her stated age. She is rubbing her epigastric region gently and sitting upright.

Vital signs: BP: 144/86; P: 76; R: 22; T; 97.4. She is 5 ft 8 inches and weighs 186 lb.

HEENT: Negative.

Neck: No lymphadenopathy.

Respiratory: Lung sounds vesicular over peripheral fields bilaterally, with no adventitious sounds.

Clinical Case Studies for the Family Nurse Practitioner, First Edition. Edited by Leslie Neal-Boylan.
© 2011 John Wiley & Sons, Inc. Published 2011 by John Wiley & Sons, Inc.

Cardiovascular: Heart sounds strong. PMI at 5ᵗʰ ICS, left of sternum. No murmurs, rubs, or gallops. Peripheral vascular assessment negative. Pedal and post tibial pulses 2+/4+.

Abdomen: Tender over both upper quadrants and epigastrium. Percussion tympanic. Bowel sounds hyperactive. No liver enlargement noted. Spleen and kidneys nonpalpable. No aortic bruits.

Skin: Warm and dry.

CRITICAL THINKING

Which diagnostic or imaging studies should be considered to assist with or confirm the diagnosis?
___ECG
___Lipid panel
___CBC
___CMP
___Troponin
___ESR

What are the most likely differential diagnoses and why?
___GERD
___Dyslipidemia (type?)
___Myocardial infarction
___Cholecystitis
___Diverticulitis

What is your plan of treatment and follow-up care?

Are any referrals needed?

Does the patient's psychosocial history impact how you might treat this patient?

What if the patient were over age 65 or under age 13?

What if the patient were also diabetic?

Are there any standardized guidelines that you should use to assess or treat this case?

RESOLUTION

Diagnostic tests: ECG negative. Lipid panel: Total cholesterol: 308; LDL: 102; triglycerides: 440; HDL: 40.

What are the most likely differential diagnoses and why?
Exacerbation of GERD; hyperlipidemia:
While the chest pain could possibly be associated with coronary atherosclerosis, it was associated with a spicy meal and has elements consistent with GERD.

What is your plan of treatment and follow-up care?
Treatment should include the addition of lipid-lowering medication such as a statin. Initiation of simvastatin, 20 mg daily in the evening, is appropriate. Education on reducing saturated fats and replacing dietary trans fats is recommended (Kelly, 2010). Also, increasing exercise and fat reduction may lower lipids. Recheck LDL cholesterol in 4 weeks to adjust simvastatin, if necessary. Discuss dietary, activity levels, and cardiac risk reduction strategies in light of her postmenopausal status. Probe her current activities and determine whether hobbies should include physical activities to work toward the goal of walking or other physical activities 30 minutes daily.

Are any referrals needed?

Dietitian referral for dietary planning is recommended.

Does the patient's psychosocial history impact how you might treat this patient?

Evaluation of symptom management for the patient's depression may be warranted. Depression and lifestyle changes are often linked. As with many patients who need to introduce a number of lifestyle changes, working on a plan to deal with one issue at a time may be more manageable. Increasing physical activity may improve her depression, especially if social support networks are incorporated into her exercise changes.

What if the patient were over age 65 or under age 13?

Although Patricia is not at age 65, her postmenopausal status and her risk factors mirror those of an aging female. Her risk factors include age, sedentary lifestyle, being overweight, diet high in fats and salt, and elevated lipids. Children under age 13 with hyperlipidemia should be followed closely, first employing dietary modifications and adding statins, if necessary. In addition, birth control medications may increase blood lipids.

What if the patient were also diabetic?

Diabetes is now considered risk-equivalent with a prior coronary heart disease diagnosis in terms of risk for subsequent coronary events. Given the multiple risk factors promoting atherogenesis, more frequent monitoring of serum cholesterol, blood pressure monitoring, and active lifestyle changes would be even more pressing.

Are there any standardized guidelines that you should use to assess or treat this case?

The reference list includes National Clearinghouse Guidelines (2007) Evidence-Based Guidelines for Cardiovascular Disease Prevention in Women (Mosca et al., 2007).

REFERENCES AND RESOURCES

Kelly, R. B. (2010). Diet and exercise in the management of hyperlipidemia. *American Family Physician, 81*(9), 1097–1102.

Mosca, L., Banka, C. L., Benjamin, E. J., Berra, K., Bushnell, C., Dolor, R. J., . . . , Wenger, N.K., Expert Panel/ Writing Group, American Heart Association, American Academy of Family Physicians, American College of Obstetricians and Gynecologists, American College of Cardiology Foundation, Society of Thoracic Surgeons, American Medical Women's Association, Centers for Disease Control and Prevention, Office of Research on Women's Health, Association of Black Cardiologists, American College of Physicians, World Heart Federation, National Heart, Lung, and Blood Institute, American College of Nurse Practitioners (2007). Evidence-based guidelines for cardiovascular disease prevention in women: 2007 update. *Circulation, 115*(11), 1481–1501.

By Kathy J. Booker, PhD, RN

SUBJECTIVE

Oliver, a 48-year-old male, presents to the office with mild-to-moderate chest pressure with radiation to his back. Oliver reports that he was awakened from sleep at 7:00 a.m. with chest pressure, initially described as soreness across his anterior chest and through to his back. He rates his pain +6/10. He felt as though, if he could just belch, he would feel better. His wife drove him to the office to be here when it opened at 9:00 a.m. She tried to convince Oliver to go to the emergency room; but he emphatically refused, insisting on going to the office first. Upon arrival to the office, you take Oliver back to an examination room and instruct the receptionist to call 911.

Past medical/surgical history: Diabetes mellitus type 2.

Family history: He has a family history of premature coronary artery disease. His father died of acute myocardial infarction (AMI) at age 45. One brother died of AMI at age 49.

Social history: He has smoked for 25 years but has reduced his smoking to 1 pack per day since his brother's death 2 years ago. He has put on 25 pounds in the past 2 years and is generally sedentary.

Medications: Oliver was diagnosed with type 2 diabetes last year. He has been fairly well controlled with diet and Metformin, 500 mg daily. His last hemoglobin A1c 2 months ago was 7.4.

Allergies: Latex.

OBJECTIVE

General: He is anxious and shows Levine's sign as you enter the office room. He is slightly diaphoretic. He took an oral aspirin on the way to the office.

Vital signs: BP: 192/96; P: 102; R: 22; T: 97.8. His SpO2 is 90%.

ECG: His stat ECG shows ST segment depression and T wave inversion in leads II and III.

Cardiovascular: His heart tones are muffled with an S3 gallop. His hands and feet are cool to touch. Radial pulses are 2+. Pedal and posterior tibial pulses are 1+. He has neck vein distention of 5 cm

---

Clinical Case Studies for the Family Nurse Practitioner, First Edition. Edited by Leslie Neal-Boylan.
© 2011 John Wiley & Sons, Inc. Published 2011 by John Wiley & Sons, Inc.

with head of bed at 90 degrees. He has no carotid bruits, heaves, or thrusts. His PMI is at the 5th ICS, left mid-clavicular line.

Respiratory: He has harsh rhonchi in the upper lobes bilaterally and a nonproductive cough.

CRITICAL THINKING

Which diagnostic or imaging studies should be considered to assist with or confirm the diagnosis?
___Electrocardiogram
___Troponin
___Hemoglobin and hematocrit
___Electrolytes
___BUN and creatinine
___Transfer to emergency services with urgent cardiac catheterization.

What is the most likely differential diagnosis and why?
___Acute coronary syndrome
___Pulmonary embolism (PE)
___Gastric reflux

What is your plan of treatment?

Are any referrals needed?

Does the patient's family history impact how you might treat this patient?

What are the primary health education issues?

What if this patient were female?

What if the patient lived in a rural, isolated setting?

Are there any standardized guidelines that you should use to assess/treat this case?

RESOLUTION

Diagnostic tests (within 2 hours of Arrival to Care): ECG: Inferior wall myocardial ischemia; troponin: 6 ng/dL; chem panel: Na, K, Cl WNL; BUN: 20; creatinine: 0.8; serum glucose: 189. (Figure 8.7.1)

What is the most likely differential diagnosis and why?
Acute coronary syndrome (ACS): probable non-ST elevation myocardial infarction (NSTEMI):
The patient has positive family history, history of diabetes mellitus, and a long smoking history—all risk factors for ACS. The symptoms are consistent with ACS and the ECG changes are reflective of myocardial ischemia in the inferior (II, III, and aVF) lateral (V5 and V6) leads.
The sudden onset of chest pain is a hallmark sign of PE. Oliver also demonstrates tachypnea, hypertension, and neck vein distention, all of which may be seen with PE. Pulmonary embolism is generally associated with more dyspnea and seldom presents with epigastric distress.
Oliver reports feeling a need to belch. Gastric reflux can often cause symptoms of chest pain or pressure. A positive smoking history and being overweight are risk factors for gastric reflux.
However, the presence of ischemia on the ECG makes a diagnosis of GERD unlikely.

What is your plan of treatment?
Urgent transport by the EMS system to nearest interventional cardiology service is required. The ECG demonstrates myocardial ischemia and, coupled with the serious symptoms, is a medical emer-

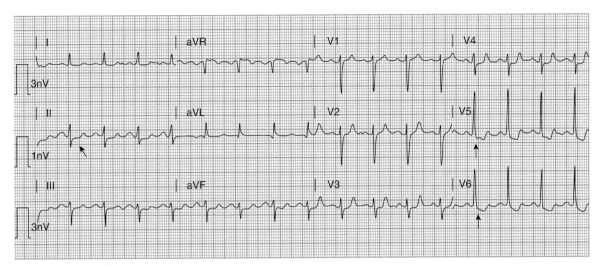

Figure 8.7.1. Oliver's ECG.

gency. Since Oliver is tachypneic and has chest discomfort, pulmonary embolism is likely the top differential diagnosis. However, the preponderance of history and symptoms point to acute MI. Pain onset in early morning hours is common with AMI symptoms; Oliver's pain began at 7:00 a.m. He did not report pain consistent with PE, which often is accompanied by deep vein thrombosis. In addition, PE is generally associated with more severe dyspnea and oxygen desaturation. Coronary artery catheterization will dictate the terminal intervention, with possible angioplasty and stent placement. Calling the hospital and faxing the office ECG would allow for more rapid definitive care for this patient.

Oliver will need a number of lifestyle changes in light of his diagnosis. Management of his multiple risk factors will be attempted with the addition of medications to prevent recurrence; but major lifestyle changes are warranted, including the addition of exercise, smoking cessation, dietary changes, and preventative measures to improve his risk profile. Despite his family history, Oliver has continued a number of risky behaviors that will be very difficult to change all at once. Supportive education and reinforcement of small gains will be needed as he seeks to implement changes in his lifestyle. He and his wife need education about activating the emergency medical system, and he needs to be advised against driving independently to the office or hospital in the event of future chest pain episodes.

Are any referrals needed?
Oliver will be followed by a cardiologist. He will undergo cardiac catheterization, which will allow for assessment of his coronary artery perfusion, interventions such as angioplasty and stent placement, and ventriculography, which will allow for ejection fraction estimation. If acute MI is confirmed, the most definitive treatment will be completed. If stents are possible to stabilize the coronary lesions, this will be done; if coronary artery bypass is required, he will be hospitalized for approximately 4–5 days. If CAD is confirmed, he will be discharged on additional medications, including a beta blocker, ACE inhibitor, IIb/IIIa inhibitor, and daily aspirin. He will be referred to cardiac rehabilitation post intervention so that he may be monitored during recovery as he increases his exercise capacity.

Does the patient's family history impact how you might treat this patient?
Oliver will be placed on similar treatments as any patient following an AMI. However, his family history requires a more aggressive approach to management of lipids, hypertension, and diabetes.

What are the primary health education issues?
Smoking cessation is the top priority. Smoking is a primary risk factor. A full cholesterol panel should also be ordered and a healthy diet begun. Exercise and risk factor reduction are also key elements in the educational process. Educational efforts with diabetes management should also be reinforced.

What if this patient were female?

Women often present with symptoms that differ from men. Common symptoms in women include chest discomfort with radiation to the jaw. Radiation of pain to the back, similar to one of Oliver's symptoms, is also a primary presenting symptom in women. Women may also present with dyspnea more often than men.

What if the patient lived in a rural, isolated setting?

Anticipatory education would be strongly recommended for anyone with the family history presented in this scenario. Since Oliver had both a father and a brother who died early with cardiovascular disease—and particularly if he lived in a rural area—he should be counseled to become familiar with the emergency medical services in his area, taught to keep chewable aspirin on hand, taught to take one immediately with the onset of chest pressure or pain that might resemble cardiac symptoms and be given detailed steps to take for recognition and early intervention to prevent a heart attack.

Are there any standardized guidelines that you should use to assess/treat this case?

The American Heart Association has published standards for care in both NSTEMI and STEMI; nurse practitioners should be familiar with these standards.

REFERENCES AND RESOURCES

Anderson, J. L., Adams, C. D., Antman, E. M., et al. (2007). ACC/AHA 2007 guidelines for the management of patients with unstable angina/non-ST-elevation myocardial infarction: A report of the American College of Cardiology/American Heart Association Task Force on Practice Guidelines (Writing Committee to Revise the 2002 Guidelines for the Management of Patients With Unstable Angina/Non-ST-Elevation Myocardial Infarction) developed in collaboration with the American College of Emergency Physicians, the Society for Cardiovascular Angiography and Interventions, and the Society of Thoracic Surgeons, endorsed by the American Association of Cardiovascular and Pulmonary Rehabilitation and the Society for Academic Emergency Medicine. *Journal of the American College of Cardiology, 50*, 1–157.

Krumholz, H. M., Anderson, J. L., Bachelder, B. L., Fesmire, F. M., Fihn, S. D., Foody, J. M., . . . Nallamothu, B. K. (2008). ACC/AHA 2008 performance measures for adults with ST-elevation and non-ST elevation myocardial infarction: A report of the American College of Cardiology/American Heart Association task force on performance measures. *Circulation, 118*, 2596–2648.

Lieberman, K. (2008). Interpreting 12-lead ECGs: A piece by piece analysis. *Nurse Practitioner, 33*(10), 28–35.

Wasylyshyn, S. M., & El-Masri, M. M. (2009). Alternative coping strategies and decision delay in seeking care for acute myocardial infarction. *Journal of CV Nursing, 24*, 151–155.

Case 8.8 Chest Pain and Dyspnea without Radiation

By Kathy J. Booker, PhD, RN

SUBJECTIVE

A 60-year-old man, Zachary, presents with sharp chest pain relieved by leaning forward. Zachary reports that he has had increasing chest pain over the past 3 days. His pain is rated at +5/10 and is accompanied by dyspnea, especially when walking. His pain is lessened by sitting upright and leaning forward. He has no radiation of the pain to his jaw, back, or arms. With the development of the dyspnea, he became worried and sought treatment.

Past medical history: He has been well for the past 2 years aside from a recent upper respiratory infection (2 weeks ago) and a history of gout.

Family history: His father died at age 58 of an MI. His mother had COPD and died at age 75.

Social history: He works as a commodities broker. He commutes to the city daily from out of state and is married and has 3 children, ages 16–25.

Medications: Zachary is on allopurinol, 300 mg daily, for gout and takes ibuprofen regularly for joint stiffness and pain in his right elbow and both knees. He also takes a daily Ecotrin and supplemental glucosamine.

Allergies: No allergies.

OBJECTIVE

General: Zachary is dyspneic at rest. He is completely upright and sitting forward on the exam table. His color is ashen.

Vital signs: BP: 142/94; P: 92; R: 28; T: 100.8. Height is 6 ft 4 inches. Weight is 247 lb.

Skin: Cool and dry.

HEENT: Negative.

Clinical Case Studies for the Family Nurse Practitioner, First Edition. Edited by Leslie Neal-Boylan.
© 2011 John Wiley & Sons, Inc. Published 2011 by John Wiley & Sons, Inc.

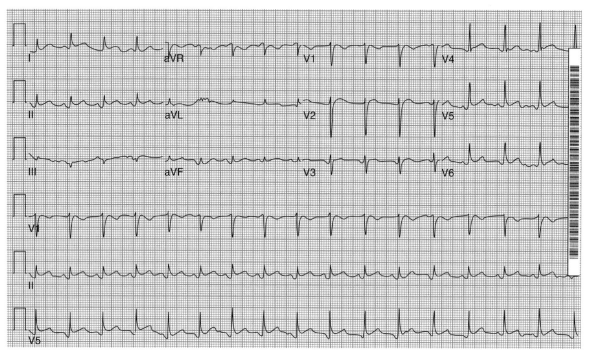

Figure 8.8.1. Zachary's ECG.

Cardiovascular: He has 6-cm jugular venous distention at 90 degrees. Heart tones: S1/S2 strong, with audible pericardial friction rub; no murmurs. He has trace ankle edema. Pedal and posterior tibial pulses are 1+/4.

Respiratory: CTA bilaterally.
   You get an ECG.

CRITICAL THINKING

Which diagnostic or imaging studies should be considered to assist with or confirm the diagnosis?
___Measure blood pressure for pulsus paradoxus
___Repeat ECG
___Echocardiogram
___CBC
___Electrolytes
___Sedimentation rate
___Serial troponins (stat, 12 and 24 hours).

What is the most likely differential diagnosis and why?
___Acute myocardial infarction
___Pericarditis
___Infectious cardiomyopathy

What is your plan of treatment?

What is your plan for follow-up care?

Are any referrals needed?

What if this patient had recently sustained an acute myocardial infarction?

Are there any standardized guidelines that you should use to assess/treat this case?

RESOLUTION

Diagnostic tests: Measure blood pressure for pulsus paradoxus. This is done by initially taking the BP and then retesting systolic BP during inspiration to see if it is lower with inspiratory effort. With pericardial tamponade, cardiac compression caused lowering of the systolic BP as the inspiratory mechanics increase venous return, increasing ventricular preload, placing strain on the left ventricular capacity to pump. Repeat the ECG. Arrange for the following tests: Echocardiogram, CBC, electrolytes, and sedimentation rate, serial troponins (stat, 12 and 24 hours).

What is the most likely differential diagnosis and why?
Pericarditis:
The most likely diagnosis is acute pericarditis. The chest pain, ECG findings and pattern of symptoms, including elevated temperature, point to this diagnosis. Due to the complaints of chest pain over several days, an acute MI must be ruled out. Although the pattern of pain does not point to MI, especially since there is relief with leaning forward, this condition must still be ruled out especially given this patient's age and highly stressful job. While troponin I elevations are common in pericarditis (Brandt, Filzmaier, & Hanrath, 2001), the combination of serial ECG changes and echocardiographic findings will generally allow diagnostic specificity. Infectious cardiomyopathy can be ruled out with the echocardiogram. Zachary's recent history of prior URI and his pattern of dyspnea bring this condition into the realm of possibility. Generally, the onset is abrupt; and progressive heart failure, including all chamber enlargement, jugular venous distention, and severe dyspnea ensue. These symptoms are similar to those seen with severe pericardial effusion/tamponade.

What is your plan of treatment?
Once myocardial infarction is ruled out, Zachary should be started on an anti-inflammatory drug such as Indocin. Echocardiography will quantify the degree of pericardial effusion and guide further therapy. If the pericardial effusion is small, observation is indicated. If the pericardial effusion is moderate to large, pericardiocentesis or a pericardial window will be considered based on patient's condition progression and symptoms.

What is your plan for follow-up care?
Following hospitalization, the patient should be seen in 2 weeks. A repeat echocardiograph is indicated to ensure resolution of the effusion. A careful review of Zachary's lifestyle management of gout is also indicated, and serum urate levels should be checked (goal 5–6 mg/dL).

Are any referrals needed?
Yes, the patient needs a cardiology consultation for definitive diagnosis and treatment. Admit the patient to the hospital, order a cardiology consult, and order the following upon admission: troponin, CBC, electrolytes, and sed rate.

What if this patient had recently sustained an acute myocardial infarction?
Dressler's syndrome, or post-MI pericarditis, would be the suspected diagnosis if the patient had recently sustained an acute myocardial infarction. Generally, the pericardial sac has approximately 15–30 mL of fluid between the pericardial layer and the epicardial layer to allow for smooth filling and contraction. When inflammation develops, the fluid in this layer may increase considerably, compressing the ventricular muscle and preventing filling, reducing cardiac output and raising central venous pressure. Symptoms of dyspnea and discomfort are common. If the onset of fluid accumulation occurs rapidly, severe symptoms may develop and emergent treatment by pericardiocentesis may be required.

Are there any standardized guidelines that you should use to assess/treat this case?
The Imazio, Spodick, Brucato, Trinchero, and Adler (2010) article offers excellent summaries of medical therapy for pericarditis, including a strong overview of anti-inflammatory drugs, tapering

regimens if prednisone is used, and an overview of treatment patterns, incorporating the latest published standards. In addition, Choi (2010) provides a wonderful summary of lifestyle changes that help reduce the incidence of gout. These are helpful in reducing overall cardiac risk factors as well.

REFERENCES AND RESOURCES

Brandt, R. R., Filzmaier, K., & Hanrath, P. (2001). Circulating cardiac troponin I in acute pericarditis. *American Journal of Cardiology, 87,* 1326–1328.

Choi, H. K. (2010). A prescription for lifestyle change in patients with hyperuricemia and gout. *Current Opinion in Rheumatology, 22,* 165–172.

Hilaire, M. L., & Wozniak, J. R. (2010). Gout: Overview and newer therapeutic developments. *Formulary, 45,* 84–90.

Imazio, M., Spodick, D. H., Brucato, A., Trinchero, R., & Adler, Y. (2010). Controversial issues in the management of pericardial diseases. *Circulation, 121,* 916–928.

Imazio, M., Spodick, D. H., Brucato, A., Trinchero, R., Markel, G., & Adler, Y. (2010). Diagnostic issues in the clinical management of pericarditis. *The International Journal of Clinical Practice, 10,* 1–9.

Khandaker, M. H., Espinosa, R. E., Nishimura, R. A., Sinak, L. J., Hayes, S. N., Meiduni, R. M., & Oh, J. K. (2010). Pericardial disease: Diagnosis and management. *Mayo Clinic Proceedings, 85,* 572–593.

Punja, M., Mark, D. G., McCoy, J. V., Javan, R., Pines, J. M., & Brady, W. (2010). Electrocardiographic manifestations of cardiac infectious-inflammatory disorders. *American Journal of Emergency Medicine, 28,* 364–377.

Case 8.9 Persistent Cough and Joint Tenderness

By Kathy J. Booker, PhD, RN

SUBJECTIVE

Alice, a 42-year-old female, presents with a persistent dry cough and joint tenderness. She was treated for an upper respiratory infection 1 month ago with only slight improvement in upper respiratory symptoms. At the time of onset of symptoms, she also had flu-like symptoms, including vomiting and chills, which have resolved. The cough persisted and the joint tenderness has worsened over the past week. She is mildly febrile and notes that both elbows are painful with any arm movement. She reports night sweats for 1 weeks' duration. She has been taking ibuprofen, alternated with acetaminophen every 4 hours. She has also noted gradual dyspnea with activities.

Past medical history: She has a history of breast cancer and GERD.

Family history: Noncontributory.

Social history: She lives in a rural farming community in the Southeast.

Medications: Prilosec, ibuprofen, and acetaminophen.

Allergies: Alice has no allergies.

OBJECTIVE

General: Coughing.

Vital signs: BP: 122/64; P: 92; R: 26; T: 100.8.

Skin: Warm and dry.

HEENT: Negative.

Neck: No JVD.

Cardiovascular Heart tones bounding; no thrills, rubs, or murmurs. No peripheral edema. All pulses 3+/4.

Clinical Case Studies for the Family Nurse Practitioner, First Edition. Edited by Leslie Neal-Boylan.
© 2011 John Wiley & Sons, Inc. Published 2011 by John Wiley & Sons, Inc.

Respiratory: Bronchovesicular breath sounds audible over anterior chest; posterior breath sounds diminished. Course crackles audible in posterior bases. Harsh, nonproductive cough is evident during lung assessment.

Abdomen: Soft, with active bowel sounds.

Neuromuscular: Range of motion of elbow and wrist restricted due to pain. Deep tendon reflexes slightly hyperactive in lower extremities.

CRITICAL THINKING

Which diagnostic or imaging studies should be considered to assist with or confirm the diagnosis?
___Chest x-ray
___CBC
___ABGs
___X-ray
___MRI
___CT of chest

What is the most likely differential diagnosis and why?
___Pneumonia
___Bronchitis
___Tuberculosis
___Blastomycoses dermatitidis (BD)
___Osteomyelitis

What is the most likely differential diagnosis and why?

What is your plan for follow-up care?

What further diagnostic tests are needed?

What is your plan for follow-up care?

Are any referrals needed?

Are there any standardized guidelines that you should use to assess/treat this case?

RESOLUTION

Diagnostic tests: The chest x-ray showed a right upper lobe mass and diffuse right infiltrates. CBC results: Marked elevations in WBC, eosinophils, and segmented neutrophils. ABGs: pH: 7.34; PaO2: 55; PCO2: 48; HCO3: 26; SaO2: 89.

What is the most likely differential diagnosis and why?
Blastomycoses dermatitidis (BD):
BD is a fungal infection identified in the yeast form from sputum or tissue culture. It may present as a pulmonary mass or a head/neck mass. BD may mimic histoplasmosis or tuberculosis. The spores are generally inhaled and transmitted through the lymphatic system. Presenting symptoms are often similar to influenza, accompanied by a dry, hacking cough. Diagnosis requires microscopic visualization of spores from a tissue or sputum sample. In this patient, the combination of dry cough, hypoxemia, and CBC changes point to the potential for BD.

What is your plan for follow-up care?
Alice is admitted to the hospital for further workup and treatment of her tachypnea and hypoxemia. A pulmonary consult is ordered. Given her history, an urgent bronchoscopy is scheduled. She is started on supplemental oxygen by venti-mask at 40%.

BD infections are generally treated with amphotericin, followed by oral antifungal therapy. When fulminant fungal infections develop in the lungs, a restrictive pattern of respiratory failure is the general trajectory. As the infection spreads, inflammation and injury to alveolar tissue results in ventilation, and perfusion mismatching and true shunting develop, with resultant hypoxemia. At the peak of the infection, respiratory failure may require continuous positive airway pressure or total ventilator support. Pulmonary neoplasm is a distinct possibility, especially given her history of breast cancer. However, the prodromal and admitting symptoms do not align with a malignancy. Untreated, BD manifests in joint pain which explains Alice's joint pain.

What further diagnostic tests are needed?
Bronchoscopy will allow for direct evaluation of the mass and cytology analysis of tissue or sputum sample.

What is your plan for follow-up care?
Completion of the full therapy is essential to prevent recurrence of BD. Supplemental oxygen may be necessary. Pulmonary function testing will be required to follow resumption of function. Unlike obstructive disorders associated with air trapping, restrictive pattern pulmonary disorders generally cause severe restrictions in total lung capacity, reduced tidal volumes and potentially severe hypoxemia. Amphotericin B (AmB) is toxic to the liver and is difficult to tolerate, causing a number of side effects. Baseline liver function tests should be measured prior to starting therapy. During therapy with AmB, electrolytes should be measured every 48–72 hours and liver enzymes measured once weekly during therapy.

Are any referrals needed?
Alice should be followed by pulmonary medicine for at least 1 year.

Are there any standardized guidelines that you should use to assess/treat this case?
The Infectious Diseases Society of America issued a clinical practice update in 2008 (Chapman et al., 2008). This published guideline makes recommendations for treatment based on age, clinical status, and severity of symptoms. Drug therapy guidelines for pulmonary and extrapulmonary treatment include intravenous amphotericin for those with severe infections, followed by oral itraconazole. The practice guidelines also review monitoring parameters.

REFERENCES AND RESOURCES

Chapman, S. W., Dismukes, W. E., Proia, L. A., Bradsher, R. W., Pappas, P. G., Threlkeld, M. G., & Kauffman, C. A. (2008). Clinical practice guidelines for the management of blastomycosis: 2008 update by the Infectious Diseases Society of America. *Clinical Infectious Diseases*, 46(12), 1801–1812.

Kauffman, C. A. (2007). Clinical practice guidelines for the management of patients with histoplasmosis: 2007 update by the Infectious Diseases Society of America. *Clinical Infectious Diseases*, 45, 807–825.

Saccente, M., & Woods, G. L. (2010). Clinical and laboratory update on blastomycosis. *Clinical Microbiology Reviews*, 23(2), 367–381.

Wheat, L. J., Freifeld, A. G., Kleiman, M. B., Baddley, J. W., McKinsey, D. S., Loyd, J. E., & Kauffman, C. A. (2007). Clinical practice guidelines for the management of patients with histoplasmosis: 2007 update by the Infectious Diseases Society of America. *Clinical Infectious Diseases*, 45, 807–825.

Case 8.10 Nonhealing Skin Lesion

By Geraldine F. Marrocco, EdD, APRN, CNS, ANP-BC

SUBJECTIVE

John, a 36-year-old Caucasian male, presents to the primary care clinic for a routine followup for the treatment and management of hypertension. During the visit, he mentions that he has several lesions on his lower left leg and abdomen that are not healing. He has tried over-the-counter antibiotic ointments, and these areas are not getting better. The areas are not painful, and he has had no fever. He has also noticed similar lesions on the arms and legs of his 2 children, ages 6 and 8 years. He attributes this spread to a possible spider bite or tick bite. He wants to be tested for Lyme disease since he is active outdoors with his children. He denies joint pain, and the rest of his review of systems is negative.

Past medical history: Hypertension.

Past surgical history: None.

Family history: Noncontributory.

Social history: Lives at home with his wife and 2 children. Works as fundraising representative for a nonprofit organization. Is very active outdoors with his family. His hobbies include camping, biking, and Nordic skiing.

Medications: HCTZ, 25 mg daily; lisinopril, 10 mg daily.

Allergies: No known drug or food allergies.

OBJECTIVE

General appearance: 36-year-old male, pleasant, in no acute distress; good eye contact.

Vital signs: T: 98.2; P: 86; RR: 18; SO2: 99; B/P: 128/70. His weight is 190 lbs, and his height is 71 inches.

HEENT: Negative.

Neck: Thyroid nonpalpable. No lymphadenopathy.

Cardiac: Regular rate and rhythm. No murmur, rub, gallop, or click.

Clinical Case Studies for the Family Nurse Practitioner, First Edition. Edited by Leslie Neal-Boylan.
© 2011 John Wiley & Sons, Inc. Published 2011 by John Wiley & Sons, Inc.

Respiratory: Lungs clear to auscultation. No wheeze; no crackles.

Abdomen: BS+; nondistended; nontender, soft. No organomegaly appreciated.

Neurological: A&O x 4, CN II–XII grossly intact. Patient Health Questionnaire (PHQ) depression scale 0/2.

Musculoskeletal: Full ROM. No deformities. Muscle strength 5/5.

Skin: Lesions of left lower leg are round, erythematous, nonhealing with scant exudates. No lymphadenopathy. No rash or erythema migrans noted.

CRITICAL THINKING

Which diagnostic or imaging studies should be considered to assist with or confirm the diagnosis?
___Skin cultures
___CBC with differential
___Urinalysis
___Metabolic panel
___HBA1c

What is the most likely differential diagnosis and why?
___Spider bite
___Cellulitis
___Community acquired Methicillin-resistant *Staphylococcus aureus* (CA-MRSA)
___Lyme disease
___Contact dermatitis

What is your plan of treatment?

Are there any referrals needed?

Are there standardized guidelines or resources that would help in this case?

NOTE: The author would like to recognize Amanda La Manna, RN, ANP for her contribution to the editing of this case.

RESOLUTION

Diagnostic testing: A culture is the most definitive diagnostic test for a nonhealing skin lesion. The Centers for Disease Control (CDC) recommends that MRSA be considered in the differential for all skin and soft tissue infections, especially those that are purulent or consistent with a complaint of spider bite. The culture is done via a small biopsy or drainage from the site of the lesion. Cultures were taken of John's lesions and they grew CA-MRSA and many positive gram-positive cocci.

What is the most likely differential diagnosis and why?
CA-MRSA:
CA-MRSA is an infection of staphylococcus bacteria that is resistant to the beta-lactam group of antibiotics. Most infections of community acquired MRSA are of the skin, as opposed to hospital acquired MRSA, which can occur in many sites (Centers for Disease Control and Prevention [CDC], 2010). Those people with CA-MRSA usually are without typical MRSA risk factors, which include recent hospitalization, surgery, or other invasive or habitual medical scenarios.

The disease presentation of CA-MRSA tends to be similar to that of methicillin-susceptible *Staphylococcus aureus* (MSSA), which refers to a purulent infection of the skin and soft tissue. MRSA skin lesions are very often confused with spider bites by both the patient and the clinician (Gorwitz,

Jernigan, Powers, & Jernigan, 2006). Specific symptoms include pustules or boils that are red, swollen, and painful, often with exudates or ulceration. The lesions often happen at sites of visible skin trauma (cuts, abrasions) and areas covered by hair. Transmission of CA-MRSA occurs via close or skin-to-skin contact. The infection can also live on surfaces, thus making households or day care centers prime locations for transmission.

It is important to note that spider bites are rare medical events, and most spider bites result in benign, self-limiting, local reactions that resolve spontaneously within 1 week (Vetter & Swanson, 2010). Recluse spiders can sometimes cause a bite that is necrotic, though this is an uncommon complication with a distinct clinical picture.

When a skin infection is without a head, without a distinct center, or without exudates, it could be a possible cellulitis without abscess, which itself is still a bacterial infection. Regardless, it is important to culture any suspected skin lesion to determine the offending organism in order to tailor therapy (Centers for Disease Control and Prevention [CDC], 2007).

What is your plan of treatment?

The primary treatment recommendation for management of a CA-MRSA skin infection is incision and drainage of the lesion (Gorwitz et al., 2006). Often, this may be the only treatment, particularly if the case and the patient are both uncomplicated. Clinicians should use their clinical judgment as to whether or not to involve treatment with antibiotics. Antibiotic therapy should be guided by the susceptibility profile of the organism. Commonly chosen antibiotics for CA-MRSA skin infections include doxycycline and minocycline, which are contraindicated in patients younger than 8 years old. Clindamycin is also effective, but should be used with caution because of a side effect profile of causing *C. difficile*. The organism appears to be gaining some resistance to clindamycin, as well. A third effective option is trimethoprim-sulfamethoxazole (Stevens et al., 2005).

More serious infections can develop from uncomplicated CA-MRSA skin infections; therefore, patients should be given precautions if conditions worsen or do not improve within 48 hours of treatment initiation. MRSA is reportable in some states, so it is important to check with one's state health department with confirmed cases of MRSA and other infectious diseases (Centers for Disease Control and Prevention [CDC], 2010).

John should have an incision and drainage of his skin lesions; and since he has young children who are likely also infected, it would be appropriate to treat him with adjuvant antibiotics. He should also be instructed about proper wound care and given anticipatory guidance about skin lesions in the future. Any of the previously discussed antibiotic therapies would be appropriate in this case. John should be encouraged to disinfect his home and to seek care for his children, as it is likely that they are also infected.

Are there any referrals needed?

It would be appropriate, but not necessary, to involve an infectious disease specialist in John's care if one is available. He should also be encouraged to have his children seen by their primary care provider, disclosing that there is an identified case of CA-MRSA in the household. It is within the scope of the family practice clinician to perform the incision and drainage and treat with antibiotics, though it is appropriate to refer if the case becomes more complicated.

Are there standardized guidelines or resources that would help in this case?

The CDC has a valuable web resource for both healthcare professionals and consumers, which includes information in CA-MRSA & HA-MRSA. http://www.cdc.gov/mrsa/index.html.

In addition, the Infectious Diseases Society of America (ISDA) has published practice guidelines for the diagnosis and management of skin and soft-tissue infections (Stevens et al., 2005).

REFERENCES AND RESOURCES

Centers for Disease Control and Prevention (2007). Outpatient management of skin and soft tissue infections in the era of community-associated MRSA. Available at http://www.cdc.gov/mrsa/treatment/outpatient-management.html

Centers for Disease Control and Prevention (2010). MRSA infections. Available at http://www.cdc.gov/mrsa/index.html

Gorwitz, R. J., Jernigan, D. B., Powers, J. H., Jernigan, J. A., & Participants in the CDC Convened Experts' Meeting on Management of MRSA in the Community (2006). Strategies for clinical management of MRSA in the community: Summary of an experts' meeting convened by the Centers for Disease Control and Prevention. Available at http://www.cdc.gov/ncidod/dhqp/ar_mrsa_ca.html

Stevens, D. L., Bisno, A. L., Chambers, H. F., Everett, E. D., Dellinger, P., Goldstein, E. J. C., & Wade, J. C. (2005). Practice guidelines for the diagnosis and management of skin and soft-tissue infections. *Clinical Infectious Diseases*, *41*, 1373–1406.

Vetter, R. S., & Swanson, D. L. (2010). Approach to the patient with a suspected spider bite: An overview. In D. S. Basow (Ed.). Retrieved from http://www.uptodate.com/home/index.html

Case 8.11 Aching in Legs

By Leslie Neal-Boylan, PhD, CRRN, APRN-BC, FNP

SUBJECTIVE

John is a 67-year-old male who reports increasing fatigue and aching in his legs for the last 3 months. He also has pain when walking long distances, but the pain is relieved when he stops walking and especially when he elevates his legs. He denies pain at night when his legs are elevated and states that, while he has noticed lower extremity swelling during the day, this is never present upon waking in the morning. He also reports a painless lesion on his ankle.

John denies trauma, chest pain, and shortness of breath or palpitations. He experiences occasional impotence but has not taken any medication for it, as he rarely engages in sexual activity. He describes the aching in his legs as "heaviness." He denies any cardiac history or current problems, renal dysfunction, lymphedema, or exposure to pelvic radiation.

Past medical history: Hypertension; dyslipidemia; diabetes mellitus.

Family history: Father: hypertension; mother: diabetes and dyslipidemia.

Social history: He drinks 1 beer 3 nights each week. He hasn't smoked for 20 years and denies current or past use of recreational drugs. Mr. Jones, although a retired engineer, works 3 days a week at a local hardware store "for fun" and is on his feet all day when he works. He lives happily and comfortably with his wife of 40 years in a single family home. They travel often to see their children and grandchildren who live across the United States.

Medications: Bystolic, 20 mg daily; Lipitor, 20 mg daily; Metformin, 1000 mg twice each day. He rarely takes NSAIDs.

Allergies: NKDA.

OBJECTIVE

General: The patient is afebrile, in no apparent distress. Obese, pleasant, and cooperative.

Vital signs: BP: 130/85. HR is 72 and regular. RR is 14 and regular. Pulse oximetry is 98%.

Clinical Case Studies for the Family Nurse Practitioner, First Edition. Edited by Leslie Neal-Boylan.
© 2011 John Wiley & Sons, Inc. Published 2011 by John Wiley & Sons, Inc.

Skin: Without pallor, and there is no clubbing. There is an ulcer with ragged edges measuring 0.5 cm x 0.5 cm on the left ankle above the medial malleolus.

HEENT: Head is normocephalic and nontender. There is no temporal artery dilatation. Eyes: PERRLA; EOMs are intact. There is no AV nicking or papilledema.

Neck: Carotids are +2 and without bruits.

Cardiovascular: RRR: S1/S2; without murmurs, clicks, gallops, or rubs. Upper and lower extremity pulses are +2 and regular. Capillary refill is <3 seconds.

Abdomen: No bruits. Bowel sounds are present throughout. There is no AAA, no organomegaly, and no inguinal lymphadenopathy.

Extremities: Lower extremities reveal a reddish brown pigment of the calves with skin that is thick and warm. There are visible and palpable varicosities throughout both legs. However, the saphenous veins are not visible or palpable. Ankle edema is present and pitting +2.

CRITICAL THINKING

Which diagnostic or imaging studies should be considered to assist with or confirm the diagnosis?
___Chest x-ray
___Duplex Doppler ultrasound
___Ankle brachial index
___MRI of left lower extremity
___CMP

Which differential diagnoses should be considered at this point?
___Peripheral arterial disease (PAD)
___Chronic venous insufficiency (CVI)
___Deep vein thrombosis (DVT)
___Venous stasis ulcer
___Arterial ulcer
___Post-phlebitis syndrome
___Lymphedema
___Neuropathic ulcer
___Infection
___Vasculitis
___Trauma

What is the plan of treatment?

Are any referrals appropriate?

What are the differences between venous disease and arterial disease?

How should the clinician differentiate between venous ulcers and arterial ulcers?

RESOLUTION

Diagnostic tests: A chest x-ray would be helpful, as would a CT of the chest if a pulmonary embolism was suspected. Measuring ABI is helpful to assess arterial disease. An MRI of the left lower extremity would not be helpful in this case.

What is the most likely differential diagnosis and why?
Chronic venous insufficiency that has resulted in a venous stasis ulcer:
The following risk factors and findings support the diagnosis: Obesity, intermittent claudication, prolonged standing, lower extremity edema, and an ulcer located near the medial malleolus that has an irregular border and is painless. The frequency of travel, in addition to these factors, puts John at risk for a deep vein thrombosis (DVT).

The reddish brown pigment (called hemosiderin) and the thickened warm skin are characteristic of venous insufficiency. Patients often have varicosities that may become superficially inflamed (phlebitis). Patients with CVI are at increased risk of DVT, which tends to be painful rather than achy but should be ruled out by Duplex Doppler ultrasound.

Lymphedema is typically painless. This patient could certainly have a neuropathic ulcer given his history of diabetes, but neuropathic ulcers typically present on the feet. Neuropathy is often characterized by a tingling, burning feeling in the lower extremity. There is decreased sensation and the ulcer often forms from a callous that the patient does not feel. Mr. Jones' history of diabetes, hypertension, and smoking are not risk factors for CVI, although they are risk factors for peripheral artery disease (PAD).

What is the plan of treatment?
John should lose weight to take pressure off of his blood vessels. Walking should be encouraged with elevation of the legs at rest. He should avoid prolonged standing, but wearing compression stockings (20–0 mm Hg) can help enhance venous blood flow.

Are any referrals appropriate?
As John is a diabetic, his healing process will undoubtedly be delayed, and every precaution should be taken to avoid expansion and progression of the ulcer. He should be referred to a vascular surgeon for evaluation. Following this visit, his wound care can be managed in the nurse practitioner's office or by a wound, ostomy, continence nurse (WOCN) working in home health care. Both the primary care practitioner and the vascular surgeon should evaluate the ulcer regularly on followup. However, if the patient receives home care, the providers will often rely on the home health nurses for reports regarding the patient's condition.

What is/are the difference(s) between venous disease and arterial disease? (See Table 8.11.1.)

TABLE 8.11.1. Differences Between Venous Disease and Arterial Disease.

Venous Disease Risk Factors	Treatment	Arterial Disease Risk Factors	Treatment
Prolonged standing	Do not rub or massage legs.	Smoking	Smoking cessation
Increased body weight	Weight loss	Lack of exercise	Exercise
Failed muscle pump function	Exercise	Increased fat, cholesterol, and sodium in the diet	Improve diet
Trauma	Start with compression stockings (must rule out arterial disease first).	Hypertension	Control blood pressure ($\leq$120/80)
Pregnancy	For venous ulcers:	Dyslipidemia	Maintain LDL <100 mg/ dL (<70 mg/dL for diabetic)
Genetic predisposition	Multilayered inelastic dressings (Unna boot) or sequential pump therapy		Antiplatelet therapy (Plavix)
	Surgical treatment if no improvement		Angiography with or without stenting
	Possible biopsy of ulcer, especially if not healing or is atypical		Atherectomy
			Endarterectomy
			Arterial bypass

How should the clinician differentiate between venous ulcers and arterial ulcers? (See Table 8.11.2.)

TABLE 8.11.2. Differences Between Venous Ulcers and Arterial Ulcers.

Venous Ulcers	Arterial Ulcers
Irregular borders	Regular borders
Shallow wound bed	Base of yellow material or eschar
No eschar	Scant or absent granulation tissue
No underlying structures are seen.	More likely to see underlying structures
Positive palpable pulses	Absent or decreased palpable pulses
Painless	Painful
Ankle, lower leg, above medial malleolus	Hair loss
	Waxy skin
	Cool

REFERENCES AND RESOURCES

Buczkowski, G., Munschauer, C., & Vasquez, M. A. (2009). Chronic venous insufficiency. *Clinician Reviews, 19*(3), 18–24.

Legendre, C., Debure, C., Meaume, S., et al. (2008). Impact of protein deficiency on venous ulcer healing. *Journal of Vascular Surgery, 48*(3), 688–693.

Robertson, L., Evans, C., & Fowkes, F. G. (2008). Epidemiology of chronic venous disease. *Phlebology, 23*(3), 103–111.

Case 8.12 Difficulty Breathing

By Kathy J. Booker, PhD, RN

Janis, a 59-year-old female, presents with tachypnea, dyspnea on exertion, and mild chest discomfort. She was diagnosed with emphysema 4 years ago and was placed on bronchodilator therapy. She has an 80 pack year history of smoking. "I feel short of breath when I walk, and my chest is sore." She describes her chest soreness as mild pressure, rated as 2 on a 1–10 scale. The pain is over the anterior thorax, more pronounced in the ribs, which she believes has developed from coughing hard. She states that she has had a nonproductive cough for 4 days and feels more fatigued than usual.

Past medical history: She has osteoarthritis in the hands and knees. She has a surgical history of appendectomy and cholecystectomy. In the past year, she has had 2 exacerbations of her COPD and has attempted to stop smoking, using nicotine gum replacement unsuccessfully.

Family history: Noncontributory.

Social history: She lives with her husband who also smokes 2 packs of cigarettes per day and cares for her elderly mother, who lives with them and is frail but ambulatory.

Medications: Albuterol MDI, 90 mcg/inhalation, 2 puffs as needed every 4–6 hours; ipratropium bromide MDI, 18 mcg/inhalation, 2 puffs 4 times/day; ibuprofen as needed for arthritic pain.

Allergies: Janis is allergic to Keflex and penicillin.

OBJECTIVE

General: Janis is dyspneic at rest, sitting. Use of accessory muscles evident. Pursed lip breathing noted.

Vital signs: BP: 122/64; P: 92; R: 26; T: 100.2; SpO2: 88. AP to transverse ratio is 1:1.

Skin: Warm and dry.

HEENT: Negative.

Cardiovascular: RRR: S1/S2; no murmurs, clips, rubs, or gallops. No evidence of peripheral edema. Posterior tibial and dorsalis pedis pulses 2+/4+.

Respiratory: Lungs have diffused wheezing and crackles in the right upper lobe. Tenderness to palpation along intercostal spaces on right and left anterior and lateral thorax from 2nd to 5th intercostal spaces. PFT conducted 2 months prior to visit showed obstructive flow patterns and reduced FEV1/FVC.

Abdomen: Soft, with bowel sounds; tympanic to percussion.

Neurologic: Negative.

CRITICAL THINKING

Which diagnostic or imaging studies should be considered to assist with or confirm the diagnosis?
___Spirometry
___CXR
___CBC
___ABGs
___ECG
___Echocardiogram
___CT of the chest

What is the most likely differential diagnosis and why?
___COPD exacerbation
___Pneumonia
___Asthma
___Pulmonary neoplasm

What is your plan of treatment?

What is your plan for follow-up care?

Are any referrals needed?

What additional risk factors are evident for this patient?

Are there any standardized guidelines that you should use to treat this patient?

RESOLUTION

Diagnostic tests:

- Spirometry: FEV1/FVC <.70; FEV1 50% predicted.
- Chest X-Ray: Overdistention of lungs; flattened diaphragm; mild cardiomegaly.
- CBC: WNL except slight elevation of RBCs.
- ABGs: pH: 7.36; PCO$_2$ 55; PO$_2$: 60; HCO$_3$: 29; SaO2: 89.
- ECG: Sinus tachycardia; frequent PVCs; no ischemia; right axis deviation.

What is the most likely differential diagnosis and why?
COPD:
Many community-acquired pneumonias manifest in the right lung due to the right mainstem bronchus angulation. However, given the absence of infiltrates (evidence for pneumonia) or suspicious lesions on CXR (pulmonary neoplasm), the most likely diagnosis is exacerbation of COPD. The ECG is not suspicious for coronary ischemia although it identifies changes commonly found with pulmo-

nary hypertension, including right axis deviations, often seen with right ventricular enlargement secondary to pulmonary hypertension. The decline in ABGs is concerning. Janis is very close to acute respiratory failure and would require hospitalization if PaO_2 and SaO_2 were much below their current values. Since Janis is able to perform her metered dose inhaler therapies competently and she has noticeable improvement in her dyspnea with the administration of a nebulizer bronchodilator treatment, with adjustments in her medications, she will likely show improvement. Janis should revisit smoking cessation treatments. She is approaching the point at which home oxygen is needed (paO_2 less than 55 mmHg; SaO_2 less than or equal to 88) (Brashers, 2010).

What is your plan of treatment?

Add beclomethasone dipropionate, 42 mcg/inhalation MDI, 2 puffs 3–4 times per day, and change Janis's inhaled bronchodilator therapy to a long-acting form: salmeterol 12 mcg (range 4.5–12). Oral glucocorticoid therapy may also improve her recovery. Serious discussion about smoking cessation and the addition of pulmonary rehabilitation should occur at the time of the visit. She should be seen again in 2–3 days for repeat spirometry and clinical assessment of her lungs.

What is your plan for follow-up care?

Janis may improve with pulmonary rehabilitation. Prescription or over-the-counter smoking cessation medication should be recommended. She should be instructed to call in the case of increased temperature, dyspnea, or chest pain. Plan to review risk factors with Janis at the next visit, and invite her husband to attend. Working with Janis to improve overall health is essential. Smoking cessation and pulmonary rehabilitation are top evidence-based treatments for COPD (Rabe et al., 2007). Her current trajectory places her at grave risk for continued decline and early mortality.

Are any referrals needed?

Annual evaluation by a pulmonologist is recommended. Once her condition has improved, she should also be referred to a cardiologist for further workup to rule out coronary artery disease (CAD). In light of this risk, an assessment of her lipids and an evaluation of her diet are recommended to examine other lifestyle modifications that might slow the development of CAD. With ECG evidence of right axis deviation, it is likely that her right ventricle may be enlarged secondary to pulmonary hypertension. This places her at risk for progression to heart failure (cor pulmonale). These serious affects of her condition require careful discussion so that she is fully informed of her risks and can make informed decisions about her future. Her husband should be invited to meet with the medical team to discuss his risks and how his continued smoking may be contributing to Janis's condition.

What additional risk factors are evident for this patient?

Janis is at great risk for coronary artery disease and lung cancer. She should also have an annual influenza vaccine, given her progression of disease. A pneumococcal vaccine is also advisable.

Are there any standardized guidelines that you should use to treat this patient?

Careful review of the progression and treatment recommendations (Rabe et al., 2007) provide evidence-based guidelines for stages of COPD. These highlight the 4 components of management, including assessment and monitoring of the disease and its progression, reduction of risk factors, management of stable disease, and exacerbations. In addition, the Agency for Healthcare Research and Quality (2008) provides guidance for acute respiratory conditions that serve as helpful targets for acute or chronic condition management.

REFERENCES AND RESOURCES

Agency for Healthcare Research and Quality (2008). ACR Appropriateness criteria acute respiratory illness. National Guideline Clearinghouse. Available: http://www.guideline.gov/summary/summary.aspx?doc_id=13678

Brashers, V. L. (2010). Alterations of pulmonary function. In K. L. McCance, S. E. Huether, V. L. Brashers, & N. S. Rote (Eds.), *Pathophysiology: The biologic bases for disease in adults and children* (6th ed., pp. 1266–1309). Chapter 33. Maryland Heights, MO: Mosby Elsevier.

Falk, J. A., Kadiev, S., Criner, G. J., Scharf, S. M., Minai, O. A., & Diaz, P. (2008). Cardiac disease in chronic obstructive pulmonary disease. *Proceedings of the American Thoracic Society, 5,* 543–548.

Kuzma, A. M., Meli, Y., Meldrum, C., Jellen, P., Butler-Lebair, M., Koczen-Doyle, D., . . . Brogan, F. (2008). Multidisciplinary care of the patient with chronic obstructive pulmonary disease. *Proceedings of the American Thoracic Society, 5,* 567–571.

Rabe, K. F., Hurd, S., Anqueto, A., Barnes, P. J., Buist, S. A., Calverley, P., . . . Zielinski, J. (2007). Global strategy for the diagnosis, management, and prevention of chronic obstructive pulmonary disease: GOLD executive summary. *American Journal of Respiratory Critical Care Medicine, 176*(6), 532–555. Available http://ajrccm.atsjournals.org/cgi/reprint/176/6/532

Sarna, L., Cooley, M. E., Brown, J. K., Chernecky, C., Elashoff, D., & Kotlerman, J. (2008). Symptom severity 1 to 4 months after thoracotomy for lung cancer. *American Journal of Critical Care, 17,* 455–467.

Case 8.13 Wrist Pain and Swelling

By Leslie Neal-Boylan, PhD, CRRN, APRN-BC, FNP

SUBJECTIVE

Rosa, a 29-year-old Latina woman, presents for evaluation of wrist pain and swelling. She developed symptoms about 3 months ago and has noted progressive worsening since that time. In addition, she has tenderness across the balls of her feet with any weight bearing. The pain is worse when she is inactive and improves with activity. The symptoms have significantly impacted her ability to perform her job as a receptionist in a busy office. She denies any recent trauma to her hands or feet or other joint pain.

She notes stiffness in the feet and ankles as well as 4 hours of overall morning stiffness that improves only marginally for the rest of the day. She has noted increased fatigue and weakness in the last few months. She often naps when she gets home from work and has curtailed her social activities significantly. Rosa denies fever, chills or other systemic symptoms. Rosa denies dry eyes or dry mouth, changes in her vision, neck or shoulder stiffness, chest pain or difficulty breathing. She denies ever having previous episodes of these symptoms. Rosa denies any rashes, lesions or ulcers, any changes in her hair, skin or nails, any polyuria, polydipsia, or polyphagia. She does not recall being bitten by any insects recently and spends most of her time indoors. Rosa denies any weight loss, history of pregnancy or any memory changes. She is not aware of having any recent infection, nor has she experienced any problems with her bowel or bladder function. She denies numbness or tingling in any part of her body.

Past medical history: None.

Family history: No family history of any inflammatory or autoimmune disease, except for a cousin with systemic lupus erythematosus.

Social history: Rosa is single, but several family members live nearby. She barely supports herself without assistance, but her parents occasionally give her money for extras. She denies a history of smoking, or drug use. She does drink with friends on the weekends, consuming 1–2 mixed drinks or beers on Friday and Saturday evenings. She states that she is generally happy but would like to settle down with someone in a monogamous relationship. She verbalizes her fear of having a serious disease during the visit today.

Medications: Rosa takes only birth control pills and a multivitamin daily.

Clinical Case Studies for the Family Nurse Practitioner, First Edition. Edited by Leslie Neal-Boylan.
© 2011 John Wiley & Sons, Inc. Published 2011 by John Wiley & Sons, Inc.

OBJECTIVE

General: Rosa appears to be in no apparent distress.

Vital signs: Rosa weighs 110 lbs, and her height is 63 inches. She has an oral temperature of 100 degrees Fahrenheit. BP is 120/70. HR is 64 and regular. Respiratory rate is 12 and regular.

HEENT: Her head is normocephalic and nontender. There are no scalp lesions or apparent alopecia. PERRLA, with EOMs intact. Sclerae are clear without visible scleritis. There is no malar rash or any lesions or ulcers on her face or buccal mucosa.

Neck: There is no cervical or other lymphadenopathy. Her thyroid is nonpalpable. CNs II–XII are grossly intact.

Cardiac: The cardiac exam reveals RRR S1/S2 with no murmurs, clicks, gallops, or rubs.

Respiratory: Lungs are clear bilaterally.

Skin: The skin is clear.

Abdomen: Soft without organomegaly, tenderness, or bruits.

Neuromuscular: There is moderate synovitis (swelling) of the MCP and PIP joints bilaterally and of the MTP joints bilaterally. The patient has limited ROM of the UE and LE digits due to pain. There are no nodules noted on any extremity. The Phalen's, Finkelstein's, and Tinel's tests are negative. There is no warmth or redness of any joint. DTRs are +2 throughout.

CRITICAL THINKING

Which diagnostic or imaging studies should be considered to assist with or confirm the diagnosis?
___Rheumatoid factor
___ESR
___CRP
___CCP
___ANA, C3 and C4
___Anti-DS DNA
___CMP
___CBC
___HLA-B27
___SS-B
___SS-A
___Imaging studies

Which differential diagnoses should be considered at this point?
___Osteoarthritis
___Rheumatoid arthritis
___Systemic lupus erythematosus
___Carpal tunnel syndrome
___Sjögren's syndrome

What is the plan of treatment?

Are any referrals needed at this time?

Would the primary diagnosis be different if the patient were 55 years old?

Would there be treatment considerations if the patient had a history of tuberculosis?

RESOLUTION

Diagnostic tests and differential diagnoses:

Rheumatoid arthritis (RA):

The patient most likely has rheumatoid arthritis (RA). There are several findings that support this diagnosis: Wrist and foot pain and swelling, more than 1 hour of morning stiffness, fatigue, and weakness. According to the American College of Rheumatology 1987 criteria for a diagnosis of rheumatoid arthritis, the patient must have 4 of the following 7 criteria for at least 6 weeks:

1. Morning stiffness lasting more than one hour.
2. Arthritis pain in 3 or more joints.
3. Swelling in the hand joints.
4. Symmetrical joint swelling.
5. Erosions or decalcifications on x-rays of the hands.
6. Rheumatoid nodules.
7. Abnormal rheumatoid factor

Rosa has had the symptoms mentioned in the first 4 criteria for 3 months. Her diagnostic workup will include a rheumatoid factor and x-rays of the hands and feet.

Rosa is an unlikely candidate for OA because of her youth. She may have SLE as it is present in her family and the symptoms of SLE are similar to those in RA and also occur most often in young women. Her diagnostics should include tests for SLE, which include at this time: ANA (antinuclear antibody), C3, C4, and DS DNA (double stranded DNA). Sjögren's disease can also be ruled out—although the patient denies dry eyes or dry mouth—by testing her SS-A and SS-B levels. A rheumatoid factor, CRP (c-reactive protein), ESR, or CCP should be done to confirm inflammatory disease. In addition, a CBC can rule out anemia that often accompanies RA, and a CMP should be done to check the status of blood sugar, electrolytes, and liver function. Several treatments for RA require normal liver function. Carpal tunnel syndrome (CTS) often accompanies or follows a diagnosis of RA. In addition, the patient does perform repetitive movements in her job. The hand and wrist x-rays will be helpful in assessing whether there are erosions in the wrists, but a nerve conduction test might be done in the future on each wrist to evaluate for the loss of nerve function. This is not urgent at this point because tests during the physical exam were negative for CTS.

What is the plan of treatment?
The lab work and imaging studies described above should be performed, and the results should be evaluated and discussed with the patient at the follow-up visit. Treatment in the meantime should consist of NSAIDs such as ibuprofen or naproxen sodium. The patient can be provided with wrist splints and be encouraged to alternate ice and heat to the painful joints.

Are any referrals needed at this time?
A referral to a rheumatologist is appropriate at this time. However, if an appointment is not possible for several months, it is important to consult with the rheumatologist by phone regarding starting the patient on methotrexate. It is no longer considered advisable to wait more than 3 months before moving on to the next level of treatment after failing with one pharmaceutical remedy. Further, it may be advisable to give the patient a short course of prednisone during this time if symptoms flare, but this should be done in consultation with the rheumatologist.

Would the primary diagnosis be different if the patient were 55 years old?
If the patient were 55 years old, the diagnosis of RA would still be the most likely diagnosis, given the same history and presentation.

Would there be treatment considerations if the patient had a history of tuberculosis?

If the patient had a history of tuberculosis, the treatment might differ in that the rheumatologist would be likely to steer away from the use of TNF alpha inhibitors, which are often used to treat RA if methotrexate does not work sufficiently to control symptoms.

REFERENCES AND RESOURCES

Imboden, J., Hellman, D., & Stone, J. (2007). *Current diagnosis and treatment: Rheumatology* (2nd ed.). New York: McGraw-Hill Lange.

Case 8.14 Hand Numbness

By Michelle Wolfe Mayer, MSN, ANP-BC

SUBJECTIVE

Timothy is a right-hand dominant, 45-year-old Caucasian male. He presents with a complaint of intermittent "right hand numbness." He first noticed the numbness about 8 months ago, but it was so slight that he thought nothing of it. Some mornings he wakes up with tingling in his right arm. He then shakes his hand, and the tingling goes away. He now complains of sharp, shooting pains going up his right arm over the last month; and last week, he dropped his hammer a few times while working. He denies any redness, swelling, weakness, or recent trauma to his right hand. He denies symptoms in his left hand.

Past medical history: He dislocated his right shoulder playing basketball in high school. He occasionally has lower back pain and knee pain from all the sports he did in high school. He denies history of arthritis or fractures to the hands, arms, or neck.

Family history: His mother is 67 years old and has a history of hypothyroidism and osteoarthritis. She was diagnosed with hypothyroidism at age 45 and is being treated with levothyroxine on a daily basis. His father is 70 years old and had a stroke at age 50. After extensive rehabilitation, his father exhibits few deficits. His sister is 48 years old and obese with diabetes mellitus type 2. He denies family history of rheumatoid arthritis, osteoarthritis, gout, or carpal tunnel syndrome.

Social history: Timothy is a carpenter by trade. He owns a furniture repair business. He is right-hand dominant. He is married to a school teacher and lives in a house that he built in the country. He states he makes a decent living and is very concerned with his right hand as this will impact his livelihood. He has smoked about ½ to 1 pack of cigarettes per day for the past 15 years. He has tried to quit many times but has been unsuccessful. He drinks about a six pack of beer on the weekends.

Medications: He takes ibuprofen, 200 mg, 2–3 tablets, every few days for knee and back pain. Otherwise, he denies use of any prescription, supplemental, or herbal medications.

Allergies: He reports he gets a non-itchy rash when he takes amoxicillin. He can take penicillin without any problems. He denies any known allergies to food, latex, or the environment.

Clinical Case Studies for the Family Nurse Practitioner, First Edition. Edited by Leslie Neal-Boylan.
© 2011 John Wiley & Sons, Inc. Published 2011 by John Wiley & Sons, Inc.

OBJECTIVE

General: Timothy is a slightly overweight male, sitting comfortably, in no apparent distress.

Vital signs: Blood pressure: 135/80; pulse: 64 and regular; respirations: 14; temperature: 98.6 degrees Fahrenheit; height: 5 ft 10 inches; weight: 180 lb; BMI: 25.

Skin: Pale pink without rashes, lesions, or ulcers.

Respiratory: Clear without wheezes or crackles.

Cardiac: S1/S2 intact without murmurs, rubs, or gallops.

Peripheral vascular: Skin pink, warm, and dry without edema, lesions, or ulcers. Brachial, radial, and ulnar pulses 2+ equal and strong bilaterally. Nail beds pink with capillary refill <2 seconds bilaterally.

Musculoskeletal: Neck with full range of motion (FROM) without pain. Vertebral column in "S" shape without deformity or tenderness to palpation or percussion. No pain, tingling, or numbness with compression of the head onto the cervical neck. Shoulders and elbows aligned with full range of motion (FROM) bilaterally, without erythema, swelling, bruising, deformity, crepitus, or pain. Muscle strength 5/5. Forearms, wrist, and hands symmetrical without erythema, swelling, bruising, or deformity bilaterally. Palms without thenar wasting with FROM intact bilaterally. Hand grip strength 5/5 bilaterally. Right thumb abduction strength 4/5; left 5/5.

Neurological: Wrist and hands: Right wrist with pain first and second digit with direct compression of right median nerve; positive Phalen's test with pain and numbness. Negative Tinel's test. Sensation to light touch and 2-point discrimination intact in forearm and fingers equal bilaterally. Deep tendon reflexes: triceps, biceps, brachioradialis, patella, Achilles 2+ bilaterally.

CRITICAL THINKING

Which diagnostic or imaging studies should be considered to assist with or confirm the diagnosis?
___CBC
___Metabolic panel
___FBG
___TSH
___X-ray of wrists
___Nerve conduction velocity studies (NCV)
___Electromyography (EMG)
___MRI of neck
___X-ray of elbows
___X-ray of neck

What are your most likely differential diagnoses and why?
___Amyotrophic lateral sclerosis
___Multiple sclerosis
___Carpal tunnel syndrome
___CVA
___Pronator syndrome
___Osteoarthritis

What is the plan of treatment?

Are any referrals needed at this time?

What specific activities do you want to ask about?

What other important history questions must you ask so as not to miss an important differential diagnosis?

Why do you inspect for thenar atrophy?

Would your diagnosis change if Timothy complained of acute onset of paresthesias of the upper arm?

Why would you be concerned if Timothy's pain were past his elbows?

What significance does thumb strength have?

When would you consider referring Timothy?

What would you do if this patient were female and pregnant?

Are there any standardized guidelines available for you to use to assess or treat this case?

RESOLUTION

Diagnostic tests:

TABLE 8.14.1. Diagnostic Testing.

Complete blood count	Not necessary for diagnosis.
Chemistry profile	Not necessary for diagnosis.
Fasting plasma glucose	Yes, because of the family history and to rule out as a differential diagnosis. There is some controversy whether to obtain this lab test without suspicion of diabetes mellitus.
TSH	Yes, because of the family history and to rule out as a differential diagnosis. There is some controversy whether to obtain this lab test without suspicion of hypothyroidism.
X-ray of wrists	No. Conditions that you would obtain X-ray: History of trauma or suspicion of a tumor or bone spurs (Walker, 2010); history of a fracture or dislocation of carpal bone or distal radius and concern about malunion, wrist arthritis or mass (Shrivastava & Szabo, 2008).
Electrodiagnostic studies: Nerve conduction velocity studies (NCV) Electromyography (EMG)	Diagnosis is usually based on history and physical exam. May treat conservatively first prior to obtaining (Neal & Fields, 2010; Shrivastava & Szabo, 2008; Walker, 2010). Neal & Fields (2010) recommend obtaining NCV studies if no improvement occurs after 6 weeks after initiating conservative treatment. You would not be faulted for obtaining these studies at the time of diagnosis, especially with the presentation of muscle weakness. They can confirm the diagnosis and quantify the severity of the disease (Shrivastava & Szabo, 2008).
MRI	Not ordered unless the following are present: No relief from conservative treatment (Scanlon & Maffei, 2009) suspicion of tumors, ganglions, or lipomas of the forearm (Shrivastava & Szabo, 2008) or cervical radiculopathy.
X-ray of elbows	No, not necessary unless a history of trauma.
X-ray of neck	No, not necessary unless there is a history of trauma.

What are your most likely differential diagnoses and why?

Carpal tunnel syndrome:

Carpal tunnel syndrome (CTS) is the most likely diagnosis. Though it is more common in females than males, males may be afflicted with the condition, especially with a history of repetitive motion. In 50% of the cases, it will affect both wrists (Scanlon & Maffei, 2009). The gradual onset of numbness, pain, and even burning are typical. Symptoms can worsen at night because individuals may sleep with a flexed wrist. It is typical for patients to describe that shaking their hand helps to relieve the numbness (Scanlon & Maffei, 2009; Shrivastava & Szabo, 2008). This is known as the flick sign (Scalon & Maffei, 2009). The median nerve is a mixed nerve and transmits both sensory and motor neurons. The median nerve supplies sensation to the ventral aspect of the thumb, first 2 fingers, and half of the third and to the tips of the fingers on the dorsal aspect of the same digits (Walker, 2010). Since it is a mixed nerve, it also supplies motor movement to the muscles of the thenar eminence, which abducts, flexes, adducts, and medially rotates the thumb (Walker, 2010). It first affects sensation and then motor movement. The dropping of his hammer can represent the beginning of motor weakness.

Pronator syndrome:

Occurs with entrapment of the median nerve at the elbow. Pronator syndrome can mimic symptoms of CTS (Neal & Fields, 2010) and pain often occurs with repetitive motion of the forearm . It affects only sensation but not motor. Therefore, you would not see weakness or thenar atrophy. With pronator syndrome, the Tinel's and Phalen's tests are negative.

Cervical radiculopathy:

When dealing with nerve symptoms, you must always eliminate the possibility of circulation problems and determine whether the origin is from an upper motor neuron or lower motor neuron. When dealing with upper motor neuron entrapment syndromes, pain typically is not limited to the hand. According to Scanlon & Maffei (2009), if pain is located in the shoulder, upper arm, or neck, a cervical problem is suspected. With cervical radiculopathy, there may be point tenderness on vertebral palpation or percussion or pain with neck movement. Pain, weakness, or numbness or paresthesias when C 6/7 nerve root is compressed is indicative of a spinal cord problem (Walker, 2010). Cervical problems usually present bilaterally or shift from right to left. If spinal cord injury is suspected, this mandates immobilization, radiologic evaluation, and repeated neurological exams as motor symptoms may occur hours to days later (Neal & Fields, 2010).

What is the plan of treatment?

Prescribe a wrist splint for Timothy to wear at night. Advise careful use of topical and/or oral NSAIDS for pain relief. Advise avoidance of repetitive activities. Suggest a break, if possible, from his work. Consider a corticosteroid injection at this visit or in the future for pain relief.

Are any referrals needed at this time?

Refer for surgical evaluation in the following situations: Severe disease, such as symptoms lasting more than 1 year; muscle weakness or atrophy or abnormal electrodiagnostic studies (Scanlon & Maffei, 2009; Shrivastava & Szabo, 2008); or failure of conservative treatment to alleviate symptoms (Scanlon & Maffei, 2009).

What specific activities do you want to ask about?

Peripheral nerve injuries commonly occur in individuals who participate in recreational sports or specific occupational activities. Ask about repetitive motion activities, use of keyboard, hammering, knitting, piano playing which constantly flex the wrist.

What other important history questions must you ask so as not to miss an important differential diagnosis?

When deciding on a cause for median nerve compression, think about internal causes from decrease in tunnel space or external causes from edema or inflammation. This will narrow down whether the nerve compression is from repetitive motion; trauma; congenital malformations; medications that can increase edema; or metabolic, infectious, or inflammatory diseases/conditions such as rheumatoid arthritis, systemic lupus erythematosus, gout (Scanlon & Maffei, 2009), or obesity (Rettig, 2009).

Since rheumatoid arthritis, systemic lupus erythematosus, and gout can mimic CTS, asking about pain, swelling and erythema in other joints is important. Pain and swelling may indicate osteoarthritis. Other conditions that can cause swelling include hypothyroidism, heart failure, pregnancy, and any use of steroids. Also conditions that can cause neuropathy, such as diabetes mellitus, should be ruled out.

Why do you inspect for thenar atrophy?

The motor aspect of the thumb is innervated by the median nerve. The abductor pollicus brevis is only innervated by the median nerve and is responsible for abduction of the thumb. The opponeus pollicus flexes, adducts, and medially rotates the thumb. With a lower motor neuron entrapment injury, the nerve innervating the muscle is compromised causing decreased movement, resulting in muscular atrophy.

Would your diagnosis change if Timothy complained of acute onset of paresthesias of the upper arm?

Yes. Acute CTS is uncommon; and, if it does occur, is typically caused by a radial fracture or carpal injury (Pai, Pai, & Muir, 2009). Other considerations for nontraumatic acute CTS can develop secondarily from infective tenosynovitis, coagulopathies, false aneurysm, gout, or rheumatoid disorders (Pai, Pai, & Muir, 2009).

Why would you be concerned if Timothy's pain were past his elbows?

CTS pain may present as shooting pains radiating up to the elbow. If pain radiates past the elbow toward the shoulder or neck, consider a cervical cord problem (Scanlon & Maffei, 2009).

What significance does thumb strength have?

The motor aspect of the thumb is only innervated by the median nerve. Muscle weakness of the thumb is a strong indicator of median nerve entrapment.

What would you do if this patient were female and pregnant?

Pregnancy or any condition that increases estrogen may cause fluid retention, causing increasing pressure on the median nerve. Avoiding noxious stimuli, wrist splinting, ergonomic modification, and ultrasound treatment are the courses of treatment for pregnancy.

Are there any standardized guidelines available for you to use to assess or treat this case?

The National Guideline Clearing House published the American Academy of Orthopedic Surgeons evidenced-based practice guidelines for the diagnosis and treatment of carpal tunnel syndrome.

REFERENCES AND RESOURCES

American Academy of Orthopaedic Surgeons (2007). Clinical practice guideline on the diagnosis of carpal tunnel syndrome.

American Academy of Orthopaedic Surgeons (2008). Clinical practice guideline on the treatment of carpal tunnel syndrome.

Makepeace, A., Davis, W. A., Bruce, D. G., & Davis, T. M. (2008). Incidence and determinants of carpal tunnel decompression surgery in type 2 diabetes. *Diabetes Care, 31*, 498–500.

Neal, S. L., & Fields, K. B. (2010). Peripheral nerve entrapment and injury in the upper extremity. *American Family Physician, 81*, 147–155.

Pai, V., Pai, V., & Muir, R. (2009). Periarticular calcification causing acute carpal tunnel syndrome: A case report. *Journal of Orthopaedic Surgery, 17*, 234–237.

Rettig, A. C. (2009). Tests and treatment of overuse syndromes: 20 clinical pearls. *The Journal of Musculoskeletal Medicine, 26*, 263–271.

Scanlon, A., & Maffei, J. (2009). Carpal tunnel syndrome. *Journal of Neuroscience Nursing, 41*, 140–147.

Shrivastava, N., & Szabo, R. M. (2008). Decision making in upper extremity entrapment neuropathies. *The Journal of Musculoskeletal Medicine, 25*, 278–289.

Smith, C., O'Neil, J., Parasu, N., & Finlay, K. (2009). The role of ultrasonography in the assessment of carpal tunnel syndrome. *Canadian Association of Radiologists Journal, 60*, 279–280.

Walker, J. A. (2010). Management of patients with carpal tunnel syndrome. *Nursing Standard, 24*, 44–48.

Case 8.15 Depression

By Joanne DeSanto Iennaco, PhD, PMHCNS-BC, APRN

SUBJECTIVE

Steve is a 65-year-old married man who reports feeling down and worthless, is irritable, and has poor sleep. He feels guilty that he is no longer working and covering the household expenses. He reports difficulty falling asleep due to thoughts and worries that he cannot stop from running through his mind. He often wakes up at night and cannot get back to sleep. He states that sometimes he thinks everyone would be better off if he were dead. Steve reports pain from old shoulder and neck injuries. He describes himself as feeling tense all the time. Steve is a Vietnam War veteran, who worked as a fireman and emergency medical technician during his career. Steve took advantage of an early retirement package offered by his employer in the fall, as he was concerned he might end up laid off if he continued in his job and feared he could lose his retirement benefits. Steve has hypertension. Steve's wife has "had it with him hanging around, not doing anything but worrying all day." She reports he is not taking care of things around the house and has been forgetting to pay the bills. He reports he has few interests anymore and just can't get going to do things around the house. He rarely sees his friends from work anymore and has lost contact with old friends. He reports drinking more in the past few months, "probably at least two a day." He has gained 20 lb since his retirement.

Past medical history: Steve was diagnosed with hypertension at age 50. He experienced several job related injuries in his role as a fireman and EMT, including a neck and back injury when the fire engine he was riding in was hit and rolled over. He has chronic neck and lower-back pain. He has never had surgery.

Family medical history: Hypertension and colon cancer.

Social history: He lives with his wife in a house in a suburb, and attends church regularly. Finances are tight since Steve's retirement. Steve was a 1-pack-per-day smoker, but he quit when he was diagnosed with hypertension. He reports a history of alcohol use of >2 drinks per day and going out with friends for a drink in early adulthood. He decreased use to only 1 or 2 drinks per week once he was diagnosed with hypertension.

Medications: Hydrochlorothiazide, 25 mg PO QD; tramadol, 50 mg PO twice a day.

Allergies: No known allergies.

Clinical Case Studies for the Family Nurse Practitioner, First Edition. Edited by Leslie Neal-Boylan.
© 2011 John Wiley & Sons, Inc. Published 2011 by John Wiley & Sons, Inc.

OBJECTIVE

General: Cooperative, NAD.

Vital signs: BP: 136/80; P: 72; R: 16; T: 98.6; height: 6 ft 1 inch; weight: 224 lb; BMI: 30.

Cardiovascular: Carotids +2; pulses without bruits. Regular rate and rhythm, S1 and S2.

Respiratory: Lungs clear to auscultation bilaterally.

Musculoskeletal: Limited range of motion of the neck with lateral bending and flexion. Has full ROM of trunk and negative straight-leg raise.

CRITICAL THINKING

Which diagnostic or imaging studies should be considered to assist with or confirm the diagnosis?
___Metabolic panel
___Fasting lipid profile
___CBC
___CT of head

What is the most likely differential diagnosis and why?
___Major depressive disorder
___Generalized anxiety disorder
___Posttraumatic stress disorder (PTSD)
___Alcohol abuse or dependence:

What is your plan for treatment?

What is your plan for follow-up care?

Are any referrals needed?

Does the patient's psychosocial history impact how you might treat this patient?

What if the patient lived in a rural, isolated setting?

Are there any standardized guidelines that you should use to assess or treat this case?

RESOLUTION

TABLE 8.15.1. Diagnostic Tests.

Metabolic Panel	Fasting Lipid Profile
Na: 142 mL/dL	Cholesterol: 240
K: 4.3 mEq/L	LDL: 90 mg/dL
Glucose: 76 mmol/L	HDL: 42 mg/dL
Ca: 9.4 mg/dL	Triglycerides: 80 mg/dL
Cl: 98 mEq/L	
CO2: 24 mEq/L	
BUN: 78 mL	
Creatinine: 0.8 mg/dL	

What is the most likely differential diagnosis and why?
__Major depressive disorder:__
This diagnosis is supported by the number of symptoms that fit this disorder as well as Steve's recent attempt to cope with his changing role. Steve must be carefully assessed for suicidal ideation and intent. His statement that others would be better off if he were dead is indicative at least of passive suicidal ideation (thought). The clinician needs to understand whether Steve also has suicidal intent (plans to end his life).

To assess suicide risk, you would ask Steve if he has ever had specific thoughts about what he might do to act on his suicidal thoughts. Based on his response we would also ask if he has the means to carry out the plan he identifies (having a specific plan and the means greatly increase the risk of suicide). In addition you should be concerned about the lethality of the means he identifies. If Steve had any evidence of psychotic thinking, command hallucinations, impulsivity, or severe anxiety, his risk would be heightened. Other factors that increase risk include substance abuse history, a history of prior suicide attempts, or a family history of suicide death. Differential diagnoses would include:

1. *Major depressive disorder:* Steve reports several symptoms indicative of depression: "feeling down" or depressed, lack of interest (anhedonia), suicidal thoughts, worthlessness, guilt and worrying, sleep disturbance, weight gain, and decreased activity (r/o psychomotor retardation). Further history needs to be obtained to determine whether the depressed mood or anhedonia (and other symptoms) have been present nearly every day for at least 2 weeks. A comprehensive assessment of whether Steve is suicidal must be a priority of further discussion and followup.

2. *Generalized anxiety disorder:* Steve describes many worries that interfere with his sleep. He feels tense most of the time, is irritable, and has been having difficulty sleeping. Further information must be obtained about the worries he has to determine whether they are more than would be expected for a particular event or situation. In addition, it is not yet clear whether Steve is having difficulty controlling the worry or being able to relax or cope with anxiety. Finally, we would need to obtain a history of duration of symptoms, as the symptoms must be present for most days over the past 6 months for this condition to be diagnosed.

3. *Posttraumatic stress disorder:* Steve has several symptoms that may be a part of PTSD: Sleep disturbance, diminished interest, isolation from others, and irritability. Given Steve's work history as a fireman and EMT, as well as his being a Vietnam veteran, it is worthwhile to consider whether he might have PTSD that has not been diagnosed. To be diagnosed with PTSD, individuals must have been exposed to an event where there was some threat to their physical integrity or to someone else's and where they experienced fear and helplessness as a result. In addition, there must be symptoms of re-experiencing (distressing memories or dreams of event, flashbacks, or physical or psychological distress with cues related to the event), avoidance (of thoughts, feelings, activities, people involved with the trauma; feeling detached, diminished interest, or diminished participation), and increased arousal (sleep disturbance, irritability, hypervigilance, difficulty concentrating). Symptoms of this disorder must be present for more than 1 month to be diagnosed as PTSD.

4. *Alcohol abuse or dependence:* Steve reports increasing his use of alcohol recently. In addition he is not fulfilling his role obligations in his household. It is important to obtain a full history of use of alcohol and recent use. Information on whether use is interfering in any way with role performance is important. Alcohol is a central nervous system depressant; and if abuse is present, it precludes a clear diagnosis of other mental disorders.

What is your plan for treatment?
Treatment should include starting Steve on a SSRI to treat the depression. Given what appear to be anxiety related symptoms, an agent with properties to also treat anxiety would be beneficial. Citalopram, 10 mg PO QD, to start may be helpful with both the depression and Steve's anxiety symptoms. Education related to treatment with an SSRI is important so that he understands that it may take from 2 to 4 weeks for him to have a full effect from the medication, and that if he experiences anxiety, agitation, or worsening suicidal ideation he should contact you or seek assessment and treatment. He should be told that once he starts to feel better he needs to stay on the medication and may require treatment for 6–9 months to prevent return of symptoms; therefore, it is wise to teach

him that, when it is time to go off this medication, it is best to see you for instructions on slow tapering of the medication and for monitoring him for any change in status.

Sleep hygiene, increasing physical activity, coping skills, and encouragement to engage with support systems and in activities he has previously enjoyed would also be helpful. Referral to a mental health clinician is suggested, as psychotherapeutic approaches have been found to be as useful as medications and they may help Steve to change how he copes with difficulties in his life.

Steve should also be counseled related to weight loss; and he requires monitoring for changes in blood pressure and treatment of his hypertension.

What is your plan for follow-up care?

Steve should return within 2 weeks of starting on an antidepressant to be certain that he is not feeling more agitated or anxious as a result of starting treatment. In addition Steve should have his suicidal ideation re-evaluated at the follow-up visit to be certain that his condition is improving. Steve should be instructed to call if he experiences increased anxiety or suicidal thoughts or plans with the addition of the SSRI.

Are any referrals needed?

Referral to a mental health clinician would be beneficial, particularly given the high rates of recurrence of both depression and anxiety related disorders. Evidence suggests that the combination of psychotherapy and pharmacologic management of depression has better outcomes. If Steve has used a 12-step program like AA in the past, a referral now may be useful.

Does the patient's psychosocial history impact how you might treat this patient?

The patient's prior work and military history suggest a need to carefully assess for history of trauma that was not earlier identified and treated.

What if the patient lived in a rural, isolated setting?

Steve would have similar follow-up even if he lived in a rural area, although referral to a mental health clinician may be more difficult and he may have to travel a distance to a clinic.

Are there any standardized guidelines that you should use to assess or treat this case?

HEDIS guidelines suggest revisit/follow-up standards for those with depression.

The American Psychiatric Association has guidelines for the treatment of depression and for assessment of suicide on their website: http://www.psych.org/MainMenu/PsychiatricPractice/PracticeGuidelines_1.aspx.

REFERENCES AND RESOURCES

American Psychiatric Association (2000). *Diagnostic and statistical manual of mental disorders, fourth edition, text revision*. Washington, DC: American Psychiatric Association.

Culpepper, L. (2008). Treating depression and anxiety in primary care. *Primary Care Companion to the Journal of Clinical Psychiatry*, 10(2), 145–152.

Davidson, J. R. (2010). Major depressive disorder treatment guidelines in America and Europe. *The Journal of Clinical Psychiatry*, 71(Suppl. E1), e04.

Davis, B. (2004). Assessing adults with mental disorders in primary care. *The Nurse Practitioner*, 29(50), 19–27.

Kessler, D., Bennewith, O., Lewis, G., & Sharp, D. (2002). Detection of depression and anxiety in primary care: Follow up study. *BMJ*, 325, 1016–1017.

Sadock, B. J., Sadock, V. A., & Ruiz, P. (2009). *Kaplan & Sadock's comprehensive textbook of psychiatry* (9th ed.). Philadelphia: Lippincott, Williams & Wilkins.

Case 8.16 Anxiety

By Joanne DeSanto Iennaco, PhD, PMHCNS-BC, APRN

SUBJECTIVE

Sally is a 33-year-old married Caucasian female who works for a local newspaper and presents to your office with complaints of problems sleeping, fatigue, and difficulty "getting going." She reports intermittent awakening and usually having a lot of trouble waking up in the morning. She states she lies in bed in the morning and can't get up. She reports difficulty concentrating during the day and that she often loses her thoughts and has difficulty at work due to this. Recently it takes her longer to complete her work. She fears that if she doesn't start sleeping soon she will lose her job because she is not performing at her usual level; in addition, she is tired and irritable and is not getting along as well as normal with colleagues or family members. She said she feels tense all the time and has difficulty getting her job fears out of her mind. These symptoms have been increasingly difficult in the past 2 months, but present to a lesser degree over the past 8 months since she changed jobs. It is typical for her to wake up more than once during the night now; however, she never struggled to get back to sleep previously.

Past medical history: She reports having similar sleep problems after her college graduation when she wasn't sure what to do with her life. The sleep problems and anxiety resolved after she found a part-time job and then was hired by the company full-time. She denies prior history of psychiatric disorder or treatment. She has a history of gastroesophageal reflux disease (GERD). She has no other prior history of medical problems. She had a 30-lb weight gain after her first pregnancy, which she has been unable to lose. She has never had surgery.

Family history: She has a family history of ischemic heart disease in her father and uncles, and breast cancer in a maternal aunt.

Social history: She denies smoking, but drinks 1–2 glasses of wine with dinner. She is married and has 2 children ages 4 and 7. She has been more irritable with her family recently. They live in a large suburban town in a condominium complex. Her husband works at a local factory on the evening shift; she works days at a local newspaper. She has a few friends at work and a few friends from college who are not local. She sees friends less since having children. Her social life surrounds the activities of her children and husband. She has a degree in graphic arts, likes music, and likes reading.

Medications: Pantoprazole, 40 mg PO QD.

Allergies: None.

Clinical Case Studies for the Family Nurse Practitioner, First Edition. Edited by Leslie Neal-Boylan.
© 2011 John Wiley & Sons, Inc. Published 2011 by John Wiley & Sons, Inc.

OBJECTIVE

General: Sally appears restless and has dark circles under her eyes.

Vital signs: BP 118/72; pulse: 94; RR: 20; temperature: 98.6; height: 5 ft 4 inches; weight: 169 lb; BMI: 29.

CRITICAL THINKING

Which diagnostic or imaging studies should be considered to assist with or confirm the diagnosis?
___CBC
___TSH
___CMP
___Lipid panel
___LFTs

What are your next steps in assessment and determining a diagnosis?

What is the most likely differential diagnosis and why?
___Generalized anxiety disorder (GAD)
___ Major depressive disorder (MDD)
___Hyperthyroidism

What is the plan of treatment?

What is the plan for follow-up care?

Are any referrals needed at this time?

Does the patient's psychosocial history impact how you might treat this patient?

What if the patient were over age 65 or under age 13?

What if the patient lived in a rural, isolated setting?

RESOLUTION

TABLE 8.16.1. Diagnostic Tests.

Thyroid Panel	CBC & Differential	Metabolic Panel
TSH: 1.8 miU	WBC: $5.8 \times 10^3/mm^3$	Na: 139 mL/dL
T3:120 ng/mL	RBC: $5.1 \times 10^6/mm^3$	K: 4.2 mEq/L
T4: 6 ug/mL	Hgb:14.2 g/dL	Glucose: 88 mmol/L
	Hct: 38%	Ca: 10.1 mg/dL
	MCV: 88	Cl: 102 mEq/L
	MCH: 30	CO2: 27 mEq/L
	MCHC: 33	BUN: 87 mL
	Neutrophils: 60%	Creatinine: 0.9 mg/dL
	Lymphocytes: 30%	
	Monocytes: 6%	
	Eosinophils: 3%	
	Basophils: 0.8%	
	Thrombocytes: $225,000 \times 10^3/mm^3$	

What are your next steps in assessment and determining a diagnosis?

Sleep problems can be symptoms of a variety of psychiatric disorders. It is important to not only obtain more information about sleep patterns, but to also seek to identify or rule out the most common psychiatric disorders of having sleep abnormalities, anxiety disorders, and depression.

You ask her to tell you more about the sleep problem. She identifies that by the time it is 9 p.m., she is exhausted from the day; and she usually brings her laptop into her room and either catches up on her email or finishes some of the work she left at the office. She often falls asleep during this activity. She awakens frequently during the night often, because her children cry out in sleep or get up to use the bathroom. It is then difficult to go back to sleep. Eventually she might doze off, only to be awakened again later. In the morning she is exhausted when the alarm goes off, and she often feels unable to face the day.

When you inquire about how she feels unable to face the day, she tells you she initially just feels really tired. Once she starts to wake up, she feels like all the problems start to come into her mind and they overwhelm her. She often ends up feeling like she just wants to hide under the covers all day because she feels there is no way out and she feels she can't even see what she could do to change anything.

What is the most likely differential diagnosis and why?
Generalized anxiety disorder:

The patient presents with symptoms that are congruent with anxiety related problems versus mood oriented problems. There were no reports of depressed mood or sadness to suggest depression.

With diagnosis of any mental disorder, the Diagnostic and Statistical Manual of Mental Disorders (DSM-IV-TR) requires the clinician to determine that the distress experienced due to symptoms of a disorder must be clinically significant and that the symptoms must interfere with daily life or occupational function. There are 3 possible differential diagnoses in this case:

1. *Generalized Anxiety Disorder (GAD):* Presenting symptoms of feeling tense, fatigue, concentration problems, and difficulty sleeping are all symptoms that must be present for this diagnosis. She also expresses her worry about work, and difficulty getting the worry out of her mind. To diagnose GAD, there must be greater than expected anxiety or worry about events and situations and the person has difficulty controlling anxiety and worries.
2. *Major Depressive Disorder (MDD):* While she does not present reporting 1 of the 2 criteria that must be found to diagnose depression (depressed mood or lack of interest or pleasure in activities), she does have symptoms that occur in depression including insomnia, fatigue, and difficulty thinking and concentrating.
3. *Hyperthyroidism:* She presents with insomnia, fatigue, irritability, and nervousness, which are symptoms that may be present in individuals with hyperthyroidism. She also has a fast heart rate, which may be a physical sign of hyperthyroidism.

What is the plan of treatment?

Treatment should include prescription of an SSRI to manage the anxiety symptoms. Escitalopram, 10 mg QD, might be a good choice to start with, since it has some anxiolytic properties. Sleep hygiene interventions would be beneficial. Discussion of major stressors and potential coping mechanisms may help in the short term. Referral for psychotherapy, particularly cognitive behavioral therapy may help to have a stronger impact on how she handles stressors and events in her life.

What is your plan for follow-up care?

With prescription of an SSRI, particularly in a person with anxiety, it is wise to have a follow-up within the first 2 weeks of treatment to evaluate the effect of the medication, and to be sure that further anxiety or agitation are not being experienced with the SSRI treatment. There is a black box warning for SSRIs about the need to assess for response to medications and the potential for anxiety, agitation, and worsening of suicidal ideation or intent.

Are any referrals needed at this time?

In a patient who presents with mental health needs, it is always helpful to suggest referral to a mental health clinician for further evaluation and treatment and explain that talking with someone about their current difficulties may help to reduce the difficulties in coping with stressors and to prevent recurrence of the disorder. Evidence suggests that treatment with both psychotherapy and medication is more effective than either alone.

Does the patient's psychosocial history impact how you might treat this patient?
The fact that this patient has been largely well and not struggling in her adult years suggests that intervention might be successful in managing problems without complications. If the patient had a stronger history of anxiety symptoms since childhood, or had comorbid depression, these would suggest a need for careful followup and referral.

What if the patient were over age 65 or under age 13?
In an elderly patient, difficulties thinking or concentrating may relate to a change in cognition; and further assessment of mental status should be performed to rule out dementia. In a child under age 13, assessment and differential diagnosis might include attention deficit hyperactivity disorder (ADHD).

What if the patient lived in a rural, isolated setting?
For a patient in a rural or isolated setting it would be important to consider available community supports, particularly if referral is required for psychotherapy. Many rural areas may not have an abundance of mental health providers, and travel may be extensive to reach a provider.

REFERENCES AND RESOURCES

American Psychiatric Association (2000). *Diagnostic and statistical manual of mental disorders, fourth edition, text revision*. Washington, DC: American Psychiatric Association.

Kroenke, K., Spitzer, R. L., Williams, J. B. W., Monahan, P. O., & Lowe, B. (2007). Anxiety disorders in primary care: Prevalence, impairment, comorbidity, and detection. *Annals of Internal Medicine, 146*(5), 317–325.

Sadock, B. J., Sadock, V. A., & Ruiz, P. (2009). *Kaplan & Sadock's comprehensive textbook of psychiatry* (9th ed.). Philadelphia: Lippincott, Williams & Wilkins.

Stein, M. B. (2003). Attending to anxiety disorders in primary care. *Journal of Clinical Psychiatry, 64*(Suppl. 15), 35–39.

Case 8.17 Abdominal Bloating and Diarrhea

By Geraldine F. Marrocco, EdD, APRN, CNS, ANP-BC

SUBJECTIVE

Amelia, a 25-year-old Caucasian female, presents to the primary care clinic with the chief complaint of abdominal bloating and diarrhea, worsening over the past 2–3 months. This patient is generally healthy. Occasionally she comes to the clinic for acute illnesses. Her last visit was almost a year ago with flu-like symptoms. She goes to her gynecologist annually and considers this her routine health maintenance; her last visit was 6 months ago with no significant findings. She has a self-described long history of nonspecific gastrointestinal malaise. She bloats, feels nauseous, and has inconsistent voiding patterns with a tendency toward loose stools. Over the past 2 months, however, more than 60% of her stools have been loose, double the usual. She is voiding ~2 times per day, which feels frequent to her, although her elimination pattern has never been consistent. Generalized abdominal bloating has been increasing in frequency and intensity, now occurring 4–5 times per week, generally 1 hour after eating. There is associated generalized cramping and pain that she rates as a 6/10, though she is in no pain right now. She has vomited 3 times in as many weeks without resolution of symptoms. The patient denies making herself vomit. She reports that she had to leave work numerous times because of the pain and discomfort. Lying down and applying heat make her symptoms more tolerable; but this is an unsustainable management technique; and she is worried and frustrated. She has not done any recent traveling.

Past medical and surgical history: Allergic rhinitis.

Family history: Mother and father are alive and well, both with hypertension. Brother, 20, is alive and well with type 1 DM, which he manages well.

Social history: She is a college graduate currently working 50 hours per week for a community development nonprofit organization. She loves her job and sleeps well—though admittedly not enough—usually 6 or 7 hours per night. She goes to the gym for an hour 3–4 times per week, has an active social life, is applying to graduate school, and is generally pleased with her life. If she could change anything, "I'd add a couple hours to the day so I could slow down a little and still get things done. I'm pretty type A, which is why this stomach thing is bothering me so much." She drinks 2–3 cups of coffee a day; skips breakfast; eats a bagel, yogurt, and fruit for lunch; and usually goes out or eats "healthy" takeout for dinner. She drinks socially ~1 time per week, but denies tobacco or other drug use.

Medications: Yaz, daily (birth control); multivitamin daily; OTC Claritin, 1 tab PRN for allergy symptoms; OTC Mucinex, PRN for cold symptoms.

Allergies: Seasonal. No known drug or food allergies.

Screening: Routine blood work last year WNL, but showed borderline iron deficient anemia. Negative Pap test last year.

OBJECTIVE

General: Well-developed and well-nourished, 25-year-old female who looks her stated age. She is in no acute distress.

Skin: Clear.

HEENT: Unremarkable.

Neck: No lymphadenopathy.

Respiratory: Chest, clear to auscultation.

Cardiac: Regular sinus rhythm. No ectopy.

Abdominal: Symmetrical, nondistended, positive BS; nontender; no organomegaly.

CRITICAL THINKING

Which diagnostic or imaging studies should be considered to assist with or confirm the diagnosis?
___CBC
___Comprehensive metabolic panel
___TSH
___Tissue transglutimase antibodies, IgA
___Duodenal biopsy

What is the most likely differential diagnosis and why?
___Irritable bowel syndrome (IBS)
___Celiac Disease
___Inflammatory bowel disease (IBD)

What is your plan of treatment?

Are there any referrals needed?

Are there standardized guidelines or resources that would help in this case?

NOTE: The author would like to recognize Amanda La Manna, RN, ANP for her contribution to the editing of this case.

RESOLUTION

Diagnostic testing: In order to get a better idea of Amelia's gastrointestinal troubles, it is appropriate to order blood work, including a CBC, comprehensive metabolic panel, TSH, IgA antiendomysial antibody (EMA), and IgA antitissue transglutimase antibody (anti-tTG). It would not be appropriate to order a duodenal biopsy at this time, though it may be part of a diagnostic workup after the results of the current screening lab work are received. The CBC will show whether Amelia does, in fact, suffer from iron deficiency anemia, as this would be a crucial part of the clinical picture. It will also rule out systemic illness and give a picture of general health. The CMP will show Amelia's kidney and liver function, as well as her fluid status. The TSH will show thyroid function, and the IgA studies are part of the autoimmune workup for celiac disease.

The lab results are as follows: Hemoglobin: 11.7; HCT: 32; MCV: 80; Ferritin: 100; LFTs: normal; TSH: 2.08. The IgA antitissue transglutimase (anti-tTG) antibody was positive. The IgA antibody was positive.

What is the most likely differential diagnosis and why?
Celiac disease:
Amelia's abdominal bloating and diarrhea, along with her borderline iron deficiency anemia, points to a diagnosis of celiac disease. Celiac disease is an inflammatory condition of the small bowel that manifests due to an allergy or sensitivity to foods containing gluten. Foods that contain gluten include wheat, barley, and rye. Other classic symptoms of typical celiac disease include steatorrhea and weight loss. Celiac disease affects approximately 1% of the Caucasian population and is often under-diagnosed due to similar symptom presentation to other conditions, such as IBS and IBD. Atypical celiac disease presents without gastrointestinal symptoms, but with anemia, reduced bone mineral density, and abnormal liver function tests (Leeds, Hopper, & Sanders, 2008).

Screening for celiac disease should be done whenever an individual presents with chronic symptoms of abdominal pain and bloating, diarrhea, and weight loss. Initial screening can be done via blood work, and the IgA antiendomysial antibody and IgA antitissue transglutimase antibody tests are over 95% sensitive and specific when done together (Leeds et al., 2008).

There is inconclusive discussion in recent literature as to whether duodenal biopsy is necessary for diagnosis of celiac disease. Some sources state its necessity, while others suggest a trial of a gluten-free diet before instituting invasive (and expensive) diagnostic tests (van der Windt, Jellema, Mulder, Kneepkens, & van der Horst, 2010).

Celiac disease is difficult to diagnose due to its similar presentation to other gastrointestinal disorders. Irritable bowel syndrome, a functional and highly prevalent disorder, is characterized by severe disturbance in bowel functions. It affects as many as 1 in 6 Americans, and the prevalence is greater in white women, often with onset by the third or fourth decade of life (Goldman & Ausiello, 2008, 990). The Rome III diagnostic criteria describe IBS as "recurrent abdominal pain or discomfort at least 3 days per month in the last 3 months associated with 2 or more of the following: (1) improvement with defecation, (2) onset associated with a change in frequency of stool, and (3) onset associated with a change in form of stool (Rome, 2006)." It can be noted that Amelia's symptoms fall into the criteria of IBS. However, since approximately 10% of those diagnosed with IBS have celiac disease, the 2 conditions are not mutually exclusive and must both be considered in a workup (Goldman & Ausiello, 2008, 1032).

Another diagnosis to consider with individuals presenting with chronic loose stools is inflammatory bowel disease, which includes ulcerative colitis and Crohn disease. IBD hallmarks include bloody diarrhea, urgency, steatorrhea, fever, abdominal pain, and weight loss (Goldman & Ausiello, 2008, 1045). Both disease processes of IBD must be diagnosed via endoscopy. While Amelia's symptoms do not fit perfectly into this pattern, it is a differential to be considered if our initial diagnosis proves to be incorrect.

What is your plan of treatment?
Treatment for celiac disease is a lifelong commitment to a gluten-free diet (Goldman & Ausiello, 2008, 1034). Foods that contain wheat, barley, or rye must be omitted. In most individuals with gluten sensitivity, oats are well tolerated. Such a diet can be a challenge, as many foods today contain gluten derivatives. There are, however, many support networks, grocery stores, and restaurants that make a gluten-free life much easier.

In order to act conservatively and not to subject Amelia to invasive endoscopy immediately to confirm the diagnosis of celiac disease, it is appropriate to begin treatment with a trial of a gluten-free diet. After 1 month, Amelia should return to the clinic for reevaluation. Improvement of her symptoms would be sufficient to confirm celiac disease, following which she would be counseled further about the lifelong commitment. If Amelia's symptoms do not improve, it would be appropriate to send her for endoscopy or colonoscopy for further evaluation.

Are there any referrals needed?

A diagnosis of celiac disease involves lifelong management of one's diet, which is why routine meetings with a dietician should be strongly encouraged. If Amelia's symptoms were not alleviated by a gluten-free diet, it would also be appropriate to consider referral to a GI specialist.

Are there standardized guidelines or resources that would help in this case?

The Celiac Disease Foundation is an excellent resource for both the healthcare professional and the consumer. Information can be found about gluten-free support networks, as well as emerging research findings. http://www.celiac.org.

The American Gastroenterological Association has published guidelines and position statements for many GI diseases and syndromes at http://www.gastro.org.

The Rome foundation criteria for IBS can be found at http://www.romecriteria.org.

REFERENCES AND RESOURCES

Goldman, L., & Ausiello, D. (Eds.) (2008). *Cecil textbook of medicine* (23rd ed.). Philadelphia: Saunders.

Goroll, A. H., & Mulley, A. G. (2009). *Primary care medicine: Office evaluation and management of the adult patient.* Philadelphia, PA: Lippincott Williams & Wilkins.

Leeds, J. S., Hopper, A. D., & Sanders, D. S. (2008). Coeliac disease. *British Medical Bulletin, 88*(1), 157–170. Retrieved from Ovid (MEDLINE).

Rome, F. (2006). Guidelines—Rome III diagnostic criteria for functional gastrointestinal disorders. *Journal of Gastrointestinal & Liver Diseases, 15*(3), 307–312. Retrieved from Ovid (MEDLINE).

van der Windt, D. A., Jellema, P., Mulder, C. J., Kneepkens, C. M., & van der Horst, H. E. (2010). Diagnostic testing for celiac disease among patients with abdominal symptoms: A systematic review. *JAMA, 303*(17), 1738–1746. Retrieved from Ovid (MEDLINE).

Case 8.18 Elevated LFTs

By Geraldine F. Marrocco, EdD, APRN, CNS, ANP-BC

SUBJECTIVE

Jane, a 48-year-old Caucasian female, presents to the primary care clinic to establish care. She states that in 1980 she received a blood transfusion after sustaining injuries associated with a motor vehicle accident. She had tested positive for hepatitis C virus (HCV) in the past, but ignored any advice regarding treatment options. She brings a previous lab result with her today that shows an alanine aminotransferase (ALT) level of 55 IU/mL (range 8–35 IU/mL). The lab form also states, "HCV antibody is positive by enzyme immunoassay—confirmation is suggested." She states that she feels fine, but thought it best to get checked out. Her review of systems is negative.

Past medical history: Hypertension, dyslipidemia, hepatitis C.

Past surgical history: Ectopic pregnancy, age 26.

Family history: Noncontributory.

Social history: She works as a sales representative and is married with 3 children. Denies use of illegal drugs, denies alcohol abuse, and has no tattoos.

Medications: HCTZ, 25 mg daily; Crestor, 20 mg daily.

Allergies: No known drug or food allergies.

OBJECTIVE

General appearance: 48-year-old female; pleasant, in no acute distress; good eye contact.

Vital signs: T: 98.2; P: 86; RR: 28; SaO$_2$: 93; BP: 128/70. Her weight is 164 lb, and her height is 65 inches.

HEENT: Negative.

Neck: Thyroid nonpalpable. No lymphadenopathy.

Cardiovascular: Regular rate and rhythm. PMI is at 5th intercostal space, left sternal border. Pulses +2 all extremities.

Respiratory: Lungs clear to auscultation. AP/transverse diameter 1:2. No wheezes; no crackles.

Abdomen: Mild tenderness in right upper quadrant. BS+, no bruits. Nondistended, soft. No organomegaly. No ascites.

Neurological: A&O × 4, CN II–XII grossly intact. Depression scale: negative.

Musculoskeletal: Full ROM. No deformities. Muscle strength is 5/5.

CRITICAL THINKING

Which diagnostic or imaging studies should be considered to assist with or confirm the diagnosis?
___ALT/AST
___HCV RNA measurement (qualitative)
___Reflexive HCV RNA genotype, if positive

What is the most likely differential diagnosis and why?
___Acute hepatitis C viral infection
___Chronic hepatitis C viral infection
___False positive; resolved HCV infection

What is your plan of treatment?

Are there any referrals needed?

Are there standardized guidelines or resources that would help in this case?

NOTE: The author would like to recognize Amanda La Manna, RN, ANP for her contribution to the editing of this case.

RESOLUTION

Diagnostic testing: A positive HCV antibody test cannot differentiate acute, chronic, or resolved infection, since the result will remain unchanged after the initial infection rather than reflecting the current disease state. Further serological testing is needed to investigate the status of Jane's current disease. Liver enzymes should be repeated, as a 15-fold increase of AST/ALT can be indicative of acute infection. In addition, the HCV RNA qualitative test will determine the presence of the virus in the blood (viremia). A positive HCV RNA test will confirm that the infection is active and not resolved. The HCV RNA genotype is crucial for determining treatment regimen and prognosis. There are 4 known genotypes, 1–4.

Jane's subsequent lab results show her liver tests were significant for aspartate aminotransferase (AST) of 56 U/L, indicating mild elevation and alanine aminotransferase (ALT) of 76 U/L. The qualitative HCV RNA was positive, indicating the presence of hepatitis C (HCV), type 1b genotype.

What is the most likely differential diagnosis and why?
Chronic HCV:
Since Jane's liver enzymes were elevated but not extremely so, and since her qualitative HCV RNA test was positive, we can deduce that she has a chronic hepatitis C viral infection. HCV is the most common chronic blood-borne infection in the United States and is a leading cause of chronic liver disease. The majority of those infected with HCV will develop chronic hepatitis, as opposed to those infected with other strands of hepatitis, whose diseases tend to be self limiting (Alter et al., 1999). In addition, 20% of those with HCV will go on to develop cirrhosis within 10–20 years of initial infection (Goroll & Mulley, 2009, 556).

Risk factors for HCV include a history of intravenous drug use or cocaine use, along with an early age of sexual debut and greater than 10 sexual partners. The presence of herpes simplex virus type 2 is a risk factor, as is co-infection with hepatitis B (HBV). Associated factors include elevated liver enzymes, alcohol dependence, tattoos, body piercings, and history of a blood transfusion before 1997. Things that are not risk factors include working in a health profession, increased dental visits, or a history of surgery that *may* have included a blood transfusion (Alter et al., 1999). The strongest predicting risk factors of HCV infection are illegal drug use and high-risk sexual behavior. However, given Jane's history, it is likely that she initially contracted HCV from her blood transfusion 30 years ago.

Jane presented to the clinic with an already-known previous positive test for HCV, but for the unknown individual, it is important to consider HCV antibody testing for those with risk factors or otherwise unexplained liver enzyme tests.

It was possible that Jane had an acute HCV infection, though unlikely given her history of blood transfusion, her previous positive assay, and liver enzymes that were elevated, but not drastically so. If her AST/ALT had been closer to 15 times the normal values or if she had signs or symptoms, acute infection would have more likely been the cause.

It was also possible that Jane had previously suffered an acute infection that her immune system had cleared. The HCV antibody test would still remain positive for her entire life despite clearing the infection. In that case, a negative HCV RNA result would have indicated that she was completely healthy. Unfortunately, the positive HCV RNA confirmed a chronic HCV infection.

What is your plan of treatment?

According to the guidelines set forth by the Department of Veterans Affairs (2006), every individual with HCV should be considered for antiviral therapy, which includes the drugs interferon and ribavirin. The dose, regimen, and prognosis of each therapy are determined by genotype and viral load. Treatment should be considered for those who have more than portal fibrosis determined by liver biopsy and those without contraindications to therapy. Contraindications to interferon include a platelet count <70,000 cells/uL, ANC <1500 cells/uL, uncontrolled autoimmune disorder, pregnancy, severe comorbidity, liver failure, inability to adhere to therapy or complete pretreatment requirements, uncontrolled psychiatric disease, ongoing injection drug use, and ongoing alcohol abuse. There are further contraindications to ribavirin, which can be found in the VA guidelines. If it's contraindicated, interferon monotherapy can be considered.

Before initiation of treatment, there are several evaluations needed. These include extensive history and screenings for depression and substance use. Pretreatment blood tests include ALT, bilirubin, albumin, INR, Hg/Hct, WBC with diff, serum creatinine, pregnancy test, TSH, HIV serology, HBV serology, HCV genotype, quantitative HCV RNA. A liver biopsy should also be done to determine degree of fibrosis (Yee, Currie, Darling, & Wright, 2006).

It should be noted that, unfortunately, genotype 1 is the least responsive to antiviral therapy. Approximately 50% of candidates respond to a 48-week treatment course of interferon and ribavirin. Genotypes 2 and 3 tend to respond better, with about 75% responding to only a 24-week therapy (Yee et al., 2006).

Once Jane has met the above pretreatment requirements, a therapy of interferon and ribavirin will be determined based on her weight. She will need continuous monitoring of various tests, with HCV RNA testing being specifically at weeks 4, 12, 24, end of therapy, and completion. The goal of her treatment will be an undetectable HCV RNA.

Side effects of interferon treatment include flu-like symptoms, fatigue, bone marrow suppression, autoimmune, pulmonary, cardiac/renal, and neuropsychological symptoms. Side effects of ribavirin treatment include anemia, teratogenicity, headache, rash, GI upset, irritability, and insomnia.

Are there any referrals needed?

If available, it would be wise to involve either an infectious-disease specialist or a gastroenterologist in Jane's care. It is within the scope of the generalist clinician to screen for and evaluate Jane's HCV infection, though treatment would likely be more comprehensive with the involvement of a specialist.

Are there standardized guidelines or resources that would help in this case?
The Veterans Adminsitration is an excellent resource for both the healthcare professional and the consumer. Information about HCV can be found online in easy to navigate quick notes and algorithms. http://www.hepatitis.va.gov.

The CDC also has a valuable web page for both healthcare professionals and consumers. http://www.cdc.gov/hepatitis/HCV/index.html.

REFERENCES AND RESOURCES

Alter, M. J., Kruszon-Moran, D., Nainan, O. V., McQuillan, G. M., Gao, F., Moyer, L. A., & Margolis, H. S. (1999). The prevalence of hepatitis C virus infection in the United States 1988 through 1994. *The New England Journal of Medicine*, *341*, 556–562.

Goroll, A. H., & Mulley, A. G. (2009). *Primary care medicine: Office evaluation and management of the adult patient*. Philadelphia, PA: Lippincott Williams & Wilkins.

Yee, H. S., Currie, S. L., Darling, J. M., & Wright, T. L. (2006). Management and treatment of hepatitis C viral infection: Recommendations from the Department of Veterans Affairs Hepatitis C Resource Center Program and the National Hepatitis C Program Office. *American Journal of Gastroenterology*, *101*, 2360–2378.

Case 8.19 Intractable Pain

By Geraldine F. Marrocco, EdD, APRN, CNS, ANP-BC

SUBJECTIVE

Roger, a 43-year-old male, presents to the primary care clinic with the chief complaint of intractable pain. One year ago, Roger was riding a motorcycle when he was hit by a car and thrown. His right leg was severed below the knee, and he had extreme facial injuries. At the hospital, leg reattachment surgery was unsuccessful; so an above-the-knee amputation was done. He was transferred to a level I trauma center, where he was intubated and trached during his 3-week hospitalization. He is now walking with crutches at home; he does not yet have prosthetics.

He complains of pain that is extremely severe and uncontrollable. He reports being "at his wit's end" because nothing is treating his pain. While in the hospital, he was prescribed Percocet for pain; but at the moment he is using over-the-counter analgesics with no effect.

Past medical and surgical history: Significant for esophageal fundoplication for severe GERD in 2001.

Family history: Both parents are alive and well, ages 70 (mother) and 75 (father). His mother has hypertension, and his father has dyslipidemia. He is an only child.

Social history: He reports drinking 2–3 beers weekly and 1 pack of cigarettes daily. He does not use any street drugs. He works as a parcel-delivery truck driver, but he is now on disability from work and collecting unemployment. He lives at home with his wife and 2 small children.

Medications: Ibuprofen, 600 mg every 4 hours for pain; Tylenol, 650 mg every 6 hours for pain.

Allergies: He has no known drug, food, or environmental allergies; and his immunizations are up to date.

OBJECTIVE

General: Trying to smile, but obviously in pain. Alert, with a child-like stoic look on his face. In no acute distress.

Vital signs: T: 97.8; P: 76; RR: 18; B/P: 120/84. His weight was not checked as he could not stand and be stable on the scale.

Clinical Case Studies for the Family Nurse Practitioner, First Edition. Edited by Leslie Neal-Boylan.
© 2011 John Wiley & Sons, Inc. Published 2011 by John Wiley & Sons, Inc.

Skin: Good color, no lesions.

HEENT: Obvious facial deformity with missing teeth. Fullness under right eye where plate was placed surgically. Nose is fractured. Severed palate is healing.

Neck: No lymphadenopathy. Thyroid nonpalpable. Tracheotomy wound healing.

Cardiovascular: Regular rate and rhythm. S1 and S2 are normal.

Respiratory: Chest is clear to auscultation.

Abdomen: Soft, nontender, and bowel sounds are present.

Musculoskeletal: Full range of motion in upper extremities. Stump is wrapped with an Ace bandage. Upon inspection, the incision is reddened but healing.

Genital: He has normal genitalia. There is no evidence of swelling. His testicular exam is normal, and there is appropriate hair growth.

CRITICAL THINKING

Which diagnostic or imaging studies should be considered to assist with or confirm the diagnosis?
___X-ray
___MRI
___CT scan
___CBC
___CMP

What is the most likely differential diagnosis and why?
___Phantom limb pain
___Neuropathic pain
___Chronic pain related to trauma

What is your plan of treatment?

Are there any referrals needed?

Are there standardized guidelines or resources that would help in this case?

NOTE: The author would like to recognize Amanda La Manna, RN, ANP for her contribution to the editing of this case.

RESOLUTION

Diagnostic tests: No testing is needed at this time.

What is the most likely differential diagnosis and why?
Phantom limb pain (PLP):
Complaints of pain can be a difficult and slippery slope for the clinician. When evaluating a chief complaint of pain, it is important to look at a detailed history to identify the possible source of the pain, if there is one. Roger's trauma history points strongly to PLP, as he describes pain in the limb that is no longer present. His description of pain is congruent with PLP, which is often described as tingling, burning, or pins and needles. PLP can be present in up to 80% of amputees and should always be part of the follow-up assessment. PLP has been studied and is felt some of the time in the majority of amputees, and most of the time in some amputees (Campbell et al., 2006).

Phantom pain is loosely defined as pain that is associated with nerve injury. This can refer to the phantom limb pain in up to 80% of amputees or to the neuropathic pain related to diabetes mellitus (Campbell et al., 2006). A more specific definition describes phantom pain as pain in a limb that is either no longer present due to trauma/amputation or completely numb due to major injury (Campbell et al., 2006). The source of PLP is unknown; discussion suggests it either derives from the peripheral nervous system activity or changes in the spinal/supraspinal body surface representations. The difficulty in knowing the source of the pain results in difficulty treating it.

There is reasonable evidence to suggest that PLP can be prevented preoperatively via a 72-hour epidural. Before amputation surgery, the patient is often in pain. This pain is thought to imprint a "pain path" on the brain, which causes pain postoperatively. Decreasing the preop pain via an epidural can significantly decrease postop PLP by reducing the pain messages that register with the brain before and during surgery (Larson, 2002). However, when a postoperative amputee newly presents to establish care and is in pain, there are several considerations to be made.

What is your plan of treatment?

While there is no single best therapy for the treatment of PLP, there are several different treatment modalities. There are strong recommendations for interventional therapy such as TENS (transcutaneous electrical nerve stimulation) and biofeedback, along with strong recommendations for pharmacotherapy. Current recommendations include a sequential or combined pharmacotherapy regimen from the following medication classes: NSAIDs, acetaminophen, temporary opioids, antiseizure medications (gabapentin, carbamazepine), tricyclic antidepressants (TCAs), and selective serotonin reuptake inhibitors (SSRIs).

NSAIDS, acetaminophen, and temporary opioids work as traditional analgesics. The antiseizure medications work by calming the nerves in the affected limb that may have become overactive following amputation. It is important to start low and go slow with these medications. TCAs and SSRIs, though antidepressants, can be especially helpful for many chronic pain conditions, including PLP. They work centrally on the brain by altering the chemical response to pain (Larson, 2002).

There are no definitive guidelines for the treatment of phantom limb pain; however, several sources outline the different options. The consensus seems to be to either treat with pharmacotherapy, combined with adjunct symptom management, or with the procedural options of TENS or biofeedback. If neither of those treatment modality pathways leads to alleviation of pain, specialty care should be sought out in or by a pain clinic, rehabilitation care, or an orthopedic specialist (Black, Pearsons, & Jamieson, 2009).

Several adjuvant therapy options should be considered, keeping in mind that some things may not work for all patients. They include acupuncture, hypnotherapy, magnetic therapy, mental relaxation, wrapping, heat, massage, pressure, and mirror box therapy. One of these methods that has been studied and shows considerable promise is mirror box therapy. This technique allows the amputee to perceive the missing limb through strategically placed mirrors. Focusing on the reflection of the limb can allow reconfiguration of the sensory cortex, thus leading to reduction in PLP (Black et al., 2009).

As outlined above, there are many different treatment options for phantom limb pain. An appropriate initial approach by the advanced practice nurse is to initiate pharmacotherapy. Since Roger's pain is severe and untouched by over-the-counter pain medications, it is appropriate to consider a combination of medications. Roger can start taking pregabalin (Lyrica), an anti-seizure medication used often for neuropathic pain. He should receive a prescription for 100 mg in the morning, 50 mg at noon, and 50 mg at bedtime. In addition, Roger can start a TCA, amitriptyline (Elavil), 50 mg at bedtime. Roger can also be started on oxycodone (Oxycontin) 20 mg twice daily for a temporary period of time, until his follow-up appointment, at which point the clinician should evaluate the effect of the other medications on his pain.

In adjunct to pharmacotherapy, Roger can consider the adjuvant therapies listed above, including hypnotherapy, mirror box therapy, and acupuncture. In the meantime, the clinician should tell Roger to try heat, massage, and pressure on the affected limb if he finds himself in pain between now and his follow-up visit.

In order to treat the healing stump and prevent infection, the clinician can start Roger on cephalexin (Keflex), 500 mg 3 times daily, and Bactroban ointment. Roger will be asked to follow up in 10 days, at which point his old records will be transferred and first assessments can be made regarding his pain control.

Are there any referrals needed?

At this time, it is appropriate to manage Roger's phantom pain in the primary care clinic setting. If pharmacotherapy does not work, or if he is interested in specific adjuvant or procedural therapies, referrals can be made to the appropriate specialist. If the therapies tried are unsuccessful, the patient should be referred to the pain clinic, orthopedics, or rehabilitation.

Are there standardized guidelines or resources that would help in this case?

There are no universal guidelines for the treatment of phantom limb pain. However, the Department of Veterans Affairs has a published set of guidelines that are widely referenced (Department of Veterans Affairs, 2007). Particularly insightful organizations include the Amputee Coalition of America and the Department of Pain Medicine & Palliative Care.

REFERENCES AND RESOURCES

Black, L. M., Pearsons, R. K., & Jamieson, B. (2009). What is the best way to manage phantom limb pain? *The Journal of Family Practice, 58*(3), 155–158.

Campbell, J. N., et al. (2006). *Emerging strategies for the treatment of neuropathic pain.* Seattle, WA: International Associate for the Study of Pain Press *amputation* (p. 00209).

Department of Pain Medicine & Palliative Care (2011). Phantom and stump pain. Retrieved from http://www.stoppain.org

Department of Veterans Affairs, Department of Defense (2007). *VA/DoD clinical practice guideline for rehabilitation of lower amputation* (p. 163). Washington, DC: Department of Veterans Affairs, Department of Defense.

Larson, A. (2002). Phantom pain: An update. *Newsletter for Amputee Support Group Leaders, Amputee Coalition of America, 3,* 1.

Section 9

The Older Adult

SUBJECTIVE

Mary is a 63-year-old female who presents with upper midback pain that began after lifting her 3 year old granddaughter 3 days ago. She says the pain began right after she lifted her granddaughter up over her head and then placed her into the high chair. Her granddaughter weight about 25 pounds. Mary says she has done this many times without any pain or problems in the past. Mary cares for her granddaughter during the day while her daughter is working. She describes the pain as sharp and notes that it radiates into her lower chest and around to her abdomen. Mary's pain is constant and heavy but does wane a little bit with rest (5–7 on a 1–10 scale). It is unaffected by non-steroidal antiinflammatory drugs (NSAIDs), acetaminophen, or topical rub, each of which she tried once. She feels slightly short of breath, described as "it is hard to take a full breath in, because it hurts." She found it difficult to put on a turtleneck shirt this morning.

Mary describes her overall health as "good." She says that she is enjoying retirement and caring for her granddaughter. She reports stable weight for the past 5–6 years; she had gained 5–10 pounds in the first 2–3 years after menopause. She identifies her usual weight as 120–125 pounds. She reports good energy and that she usually sleeps well but has not slept well since this pain began. She denies any substantive premenstrual syndrome (PMS) symptoms when she was having regular menses. She denies having had symptoms of Premenstrual Dysphoric Disorder (PMDD).

Mary reports her usual mood as "excellent!" Mary denies moodiness, nervousness, anxiety, irritability, or feeling quick to anger. She denies feeling depressed and says, "I laugh a lot. I have loads of fun caring for my granddaughter, and my husband is always quick with a joke." Mary denies anhedonia and says that she enjoys gardening, reading, and social activities with her husband, friends, and daughter and her family. Mary denies eating disorders. She says she has had to reduce her intake lately to keep her weight stable.

Mary denies problems with concentration, memory, or cognition. She says she uses a calendar to keep track of activities, especially appointments or play dates and preschool for her granddaughter. Mary reports no specific systemic complains. She denies general fatigue and says she did not have terrible hot flashes like her sister did with the change of life. She feels well.

Clinical Case Studies for the Family Nurse Practitioner, First Edition. Edited by Leslie Neal-Boylan.
© 2011 John Wiley & Sons, Inc. Published 2011 by John Wiley & Sons, Inc.

Review of systems

HEENT: Mary denies problems with headaches. She does have sinus headaches when her seasonal allergies are bothersome. Mary uses bifocals, which she has had for many ears. She has annual ophthalmologic exams with her optometrist. She denies changes in hearing, smell, taste, or swallowing. She reports some dry-eye symptoms and rarely needs to use eye lubricating drops. She has seasonal allergies that cause light rhinorrhea, sneezing, and itchy eyes in the fall.

Respiratory: Mary denies cough or wheeze. She describes a sensation of being short of breath since the pain began, saying, "It is not that I can't breathe; it is that I cannot take in a full, deep breath because it hurts."

Cardiovascular: Mary denies prior chest pain, palpitations, dyspnea on exertion (DOE), peripheral edema, or a history of blood clots. She says that the pain she has now radiates into her lower chest but is definitely coming from her upper midback area. She denies problems with cold hands and feet. She reports being diagnosed with high blood pressure about 8 years ago. She has been treated with HCTZ, which she tolerates well.

Breast: Mary reports that she does regular self–breast exams. She usually does them at the beginning of the month when she changes the calendar to the new month. She denies any concerns or recent breast changes. She denies any discharge, pain, or tingling. She did breast-feed her daughter.

Gastrointestinal: Mary denies heartburn or persistent abdominal pain. She reports daily regular bowel movements, without constipation or recent changes in color, consistency, or pattern of stools. Specifically, she denies seeing any blood or experiencing fecal incontinence. She describes some pain radiating into her abdomen but again states that it is definitely coming from her upper midback.

Genitourinary: Mary reports some urgency and occasional leakage of small amounts of urine, especially with coughing or laughing. She denies urinary frequency, history of recurrent urinary tract infections, pyelonephritis, renal stones, and urine dribbling or outright incontinence. She says she does not have dysuria. She reports occasional nocturia of once or twice at night. She says this is usual for her over many years and that she goes right back to sleep after using the toilet.

GYN: Mary reports no abnormal Pap smears or GYN surgeries. She denies vaginal or vulvar discharge, itching, irritation, soreness, burning, abnormal bleeding, or lesions. She denies pelvic pain or rash. She reports some vaginal dryness, especially noticed with sexual activity.

Pregnancy history: Mary has been pregnant twice. She is P2, G1, TAB 1 (for fetal demise at 11 weeks). Her daughter is healthy at age 32. Mary reports that she did breast-feed her daughter for 13 months.

Menstrual history: Mary reports that her LMP was 11 years ago. She reports that her menses were regular, lasting for 6–7 days with 2 days of light flow, followed by 3 days of heavier flow, and then 1–2 days of light flow again. She experienced menarche at 12 years of age; and after the first few years, she had very regular periods occurring about every 28 days. Her menses remained regular right up until her last period.

Menopause: Mary reports that her experience with the transition to postmenopause was fairly smooth. She had some hot flashes during the day and rarely at night. She did not experience drenching sweats. She never took hormone therapy or other medications for her symptoms. She has some vaginal dryness, and she and her husband do use lubricant when having sexual intercourse.

Contraception: Mary reports that she used oral contraceptive pills for contraception in the past. She stopped using oral contraceptive pills after her last pregnancy; she and her husband used either male condoms or withdrawal after that. She says that she would not have minded getting pregnant again, but it never happened.

Sexual: Mary reports that she is sexually active with her husband of 35 years. She is mostly satisfied, but she notes that it has become harder to get adequately lubricated and that it takes longer to achieve orgasm. She reports she has had 6 lifetime partners and has been monogamous with her husband for over 38 years. They have intercourse about once a week. She reports that her desire/libido is satisfactory but is less strong than it was when she was younger. She denies dyspareunia. She reports their usual sexual practices include initiation by her husband, cuddling and kissing, then foreplay that includes genital manipulation, and then vaginal intercourse with penile penetration. They regularly use over-the-counter (OTC) lubricants, due to her dryness. She says she feels good during sex and enjoys sex with her husband. She reports their relationship quality as "Wonderful. He is my partner and my best friend." She says that, due to the pain in her upper back, she did not engage in sex last night when her husband tried to initiate.

Musculoskeletal: Mary reports that she felt good up until 3 days ago. She has had rheumatoid arthritis (RA) for many years, and it is well controlled on her current DMARD (disease-modifying antirheumatic drug). She has used steroids for about the past 6 years (oral prednisone 5–10 mg daily depending on her symptoms) and then started DMARDs. She now takes a new DMARD, leflunomide; and she has not had a significant flare for a few years with this new medication. She does have some morning stiffness that is mostly relieved with a warm shower and movement. She gets regular exercise and is quite active in caring for her granddaughter with daily walks, often pushing the stroller, getting her in and out of the high chair, and playing with her on the swings at the park.

Endocrine: Mary denies polydipsia, polyuria, polyphagia, and symptoms of diabetes mellitus type 2.

Skin/hair: Mary denies any recent skin changes or lesions of concern. She has noticed some increased dryness and wrinkles and dry/thinning hair, especially on her head. She denies hirsutism or facial hair.

Hematologic: Mary denies any bleeding or bruising that doesn't correlate to a specific injury. She says she is a bit surprised that there is no bruising on her back as it feels like there should be something visible.

Neurologic: Mary denies numbness, tingling, fainting, dizziness (vertigo), feeling off balance, or difficulty walking. She had some numbness in her right shoulder-blade region the day after her pain began; that numbness has subsided.

Sleep: Mary's usual bedtime routine includes nighttime washing and tooth brushing followed by reading for about 20 minutes. She denies use of stimulants except for coffee each morning. She does wake every night to urinate and reports that she falls right back to sleep. Since her back pain began, she has had trouble sleeping. She does fall asleep OK but then awakens in pain and finds it very hard to get back to sleep because she cannot get comfortable. She usually goes to bed around 10 p.m. and falls asleep around 10:30 p.m. She gets up around 6:30 a.m. most days. She reports that she usually does feel refreshed when she wakes up but has not since her back pain began.

Past medical/surgical history: RA, well controlled at present; history of oral steroid use in the past 6 years; + hypertension, controlled; + seasonal allergies (fall). Wisdom teeth excisions at age 18; TAB at age 33.

Family history: Mother: deceased from breast cancer; father: DMT2, HTN, some dementia; sister: A+W.

Social history: Mary lives with her husband of 35 years and the family cat in a private home that they own. She is a retired elementary schoolteacher and currently provides day care for her granddaughter while her daughter works. She reports that she enjoys caring for her granddaughter very much and is thrilled that she can help her daughter and son-in-law by caring for her granddaughter. She reports no important recent life events; the most recent was her granddaughter's birth 3 years ago. She describes her usual day as follows: She awakes around 6:30 a.m., makes breakfast for herself and her husband, showers and dresses, greets her granddaughter and prepares her breakfast, reads a book with her granddaughter, and then they watch Sesame Street on TV. Some mornings they have a play date or go to the library for reading circle or music. She feeds her granddaughter lunch around noon and then settles her to nap from about 1–3 p.m. In the afternoons they might have a play date, go to the park, read, or play some games at home. Her daughter usually picks up the granddaughter around 5:30 p.m. Mary makes dinner most evenings and spends time in the evening with sewing, TV, playing cards with her husband, or doing household chores. She starts getting ready for bed around 10 p.m. She reports walking for about 1 mile most days with her granddaughter in the stroller. On the weekends she also goes to a water aerobics class. Her 24-hour diet recall reveals: cereal with 1% milk and coffee (black) for breakfast; tuna salad on toast for lunch; grilled chicken with garden salad for dinner; and carrot sticks for an afternoon snack. She reports that she eats out about once per week and enjoys dessert on occasion. She denies use of tobacco. She reports ETOH use as 1 glass of red wine most evenings. She denies use of recreational/illicit drugs. She reports feeling safe at home and with her husband and family. She denies ever having been hit, slapped, kicked, or otherwise physically hurt by someone (except her granddaughter who occasionally will "fight" when it is time to change clothes). She denies ever being forced to have sexual activities when she did not want to. She uses seatbelts and sun block regularly and has working smoke and carbon monoxide detectors at home. There are no guns in the home, and she denies any concerns for her granddaughter's or her personal safety. She denies having any current concerns about HIV.

Medications: OTC antihistamines for allergies PRN; nasal spray for allergies PRN; MVI daily; calcium (when she remembers); HCTZ, 25 mg daily; glucosamine sulfate with chondroitin, 1500 mg in divided dose daily; omega-3 supplements (fish oil), 2 g daily; leflunomide, 10 mg daily.

Allergies: NKDA, NKFA (but finds that too much yeast bothers her RA with increased AM stiffness and more joint swelling). Some "hayfever" in the fall.

OBJECTIVE

General: Appears well, but uncomfortable with slow careful movements and limited use of upper extremities; neatly dressed; appropriate affect.

Vital signs: BP: 130/78 (L) sitting; P: 74; RR: 10; weight: 130 lb; height 5 ft 5 inches; BMI 21.6.

Neck: Supple, w/o LAN. Thyroid NT, w/o palpable masses or enlargement. Carotids w/o bruits. Limited neck AROM, especially chin-to-chest, due to pain.

Respiratory: Clear to anterior and posterior; w/o wheezes, rales, rubs or rhonchi. Patient unwilling to take full inhalation due to pain.

Cardiovascular: RRR, normal S1 and S2 w/o murmurs, rubs, or gallops; +pain with manual compression to anterior and posterior chest wall. No cyanosis, edema, or clubbing; +2 pulses bilaterally.

Breasts: Without masses, skin changes, or discharge bilaterally. No lymphadenopathy.

Abdomen: Positive for bowel sounds x4 quadrants; soft, nondistended. NT with superficial or deep palpation; without HSM, masses, or bruits.

Spine: Good AROM at waist and for twisting with lower spine. Thoracic spine with limited AROM due to pain; +tenderness over T7 and T8.

Musculoskeletal: Positive for FAROM throughout; but limited upper spine mobility and upper extremities for full over-head movements, slight tenderness and swelling over MCP and PIP joints of BIL hands, joints w/o crepitus, no digital ulnar deviation, no swan neck or boutonniere deformities, no nodules. 5/5 motor strength, but with limited effort of bilateral upper extremities (BIL UEs).

Neurologic: CN II–XII grossly intact; gait even; DTRs 2+; Romberg negative.

CRITICAL THINKING

Which diagnostic or imaging studies should be considered to assist with or confirm the diagnosis?
___EKG
___CPKs
___Fasting lipid panel
___Fasting blood glucose
___Hemoglobin A1c (HgA1c)
___CBC
___ESR
___CRP
___LFTs
___BUN/creatinine
___eGFR
___Phosphorous
___TSH
___Fasting serum calcium
___24-hour urinary calcium
___Serum 25-OH-D (vitamin D)
___Spine films
___DXA with FRAX®

What is the most likely differential diagnosis and why?
___Back strain
___Atypical angina
___Costochondritis
___RA flare
___Extraarticular pulmonary RA manifestations
___Vertebral compression fracture

What is the most appropriate plan of treatment?

What additional patient education is important for Mary?

What is the plan for follow-up care?

Are any referrals needed?

Does Mary's psychosocial history affect her management plan?

What if Mary were under age 40?

What if Mary also had diabetes or hyperlipidemia?

What if Mary were a male?

Are there any standardized guidelines that the clinician will use to assess or treat Mary?

RESOLUTION

Diagnostic tests: Diagnostic testing is needed to diagnose both osteoporosis (OP) and vertebral compression fractures (VCFs).

1. EKG: Obtaining an EKG would be prudent for a 63-year-old woman who presented with typical or atypical angina symptoms. However, an EKG is not useful in verifying OP or VCFs.

2. CPKs: Obtaining CPKs would be prudent for a 63-year-old woman who presented with typical or atypical angina symptoms or who presented with myalgias such as are sometimes seen with statins. However, CPKs are not used to verify OP or VCFs.

3. Fasting lipid panel, fasting blood glucose, and hemoglobin A1C (HgA1c) level: While these tests would be useful to determine cardiovascular disease and diabetes risk profiles and might be appropriate if Mary has not been screened recently, these tests will not assist with verifying OP or VCFs.

4. CBC, ESR, and CRP: A CBC is drawn to evaluate the number and types of cells present in a serum sample. Anemia of chronic disease is a common finding with RA. A CBC is also useful to assess in patients suspected of having OP to rule out secondary causes of bone loss and to determine overall health status (Alexander & Lewiecki, 2008). ESR and CRP are nonspecific markers for inflammation and are indicative of disease activity with RA; however, they are not highly specific and will be elevated with other inflammatory processes as well (Colglazier & Sutej, 2005).

5. LFTs, BUN/creatinine, eGFR, phosphorous: These tests are often measured to assess general health and are appropriate to test in Mary to evaluate for secondary causes of OP. Knowing her liver and kidney function status may be important when determining whether to use pharmacotherapeutics to manage her OP and VCFs.

6. TSH: Obtaining a TSH level is appropriate to evaluate for secondary causes of OP despite the fact that Mary does not describe symptoms consistent with thyroid abnormality.

7. Fasting serum calcium, 24-hour urinary calcium, and serum 25-OH-D (vitamin D): These tests are done to identify calcium and vitamin D levels. This data is important for any patient suspected of OP, as low calcium levels may suggest underlying pathology or secondary OP, and must be rectified prior to starting any antiresorptive medication (Alexander & Lewiecki, 2008). Similarly, low vitamin D levels (below 30 ng/mL) need to be corrected (Dawson-Hughes, 2008). Adequate vitamin D is needed both for normal bone resorption processes and for calcium absorption.

8. Spine films: Spine films can be used to diagnose VCFs. In patients with greater than 30% bone loss, OP can be seen on radiological examination. However, X-ray is not used to diagnose OP. Patients with bone loss identified on X-ray are referred for diagnostic dual-energy X-ray absorptiometry (DXA).

9. DXA with FRAX®: DXA is considered the gold standard for diagnosis of OP (Dawson-Hughes, 2008; North American Menopause Society, 2010; US Department of Health and Human Services, 2004). Results are provided that include both T-scores and Z-scores; and, since early 2009, most reports also include the 10-year risk probability for hip and major OP fractures identified by the FRAX® algorithm. T-scores identify how the patient's bone density compares to that of a normal young adult of the same gender. The Z-score identifies how the patient's bone density compares to others of the same age and gender. Both T-scores and Z-scores are reported as standard deviations, with 0 meaning it is an exact match. Since they are standard deviations, a normal T-score is –1 to +1. Low bone mass, or osteopenia, is identified with T-scores of –1 to –2.5; and osteoporosis is identified with T-scores below –2.5. Severe OP is identified with T-scores below –2.5 in the presence of fragility fracture(s) (World Health Organization, 1994). Fragility fractures are those that occur with low trauma or a fall from standing height or less (US Department of Health and Human Services, 2004). FRAX® is an individualized algorithm that identifies the probability of fracture over the next 10 years based on the patient's height, weight, and bone density raw score and the presence or absence of 11 additional risk factors such as smoking, history of RA, steroid use, and parental history of hip fracture (World Health Organization, 2007a, 2007b). FRAX® is used to assist with determining whether a specific patient would benefit from the use of pharmacotherapeutics to prevent fracture and thus is used for patients who have not previously been treated with medication. Analyses were done on the US population to evaluate the cost of fracture and pharmacotherapy. These analyses revealed that it is cost effective to treat those with a 10-year risk of hip fracture of above 3% or a 10-year risk of major OP fracture of above 20% (Dawson-Hughes, 2008; Dawson-Hughes et al., 2008; Tosteson et al., 2008). It is important to note that a diagnosis of OP is not made based on DXA results alone. All patients, even those with a T-score of below –2.5, require a detailed history and physical examination with selected laboratory evalu-

ations to identify any secondary causes of OP that can be treated and to determine safety in using possible pharmacotherapeutic agents (Dawson-Hughes, 2008).

What is the most likely differential diagnosis and why?
Vertebral compression fracture (VCF):

A late midlife woman who presents with a chief complaint of acute onset upper midback pain that limits AROM and deep breathing and radiates to her lower chest and abdomen prompts the clinician to consider several differential diagnoses. The most common differential that accounts for this constellation of symptoms is vertebral compression fracture (VCF) due to osteoporosis (OP). This is a common presentation of OP as bone loss does not cause any pain or symptoms until a fracture occurs (Dawson-Hughes, 2008; North American Menopause Society, 2010). However, several other differentials may mimic some symptoms of VCFs or exacerbate these symptoms and must be carefully explored, such as back strain, atypical angina, and costochondritis. Less common differentials that the clinician will consider given Mary's history include an RA flare and extraarticular pulmonary RA manifestations.

VCFs commonly occur with usual activities when the spine is hyperextended or flexed as the vertebral bones are weakened due to bone loss and the anterior or posterior edges of the bones are crushed with the pressure of the flexion or extension of the spinal column. About two-thirds of patients who experience VCFs do not have significant pain. These patients may present with height loss or kyphosis. VCFs change the vertebral bone to a wedge shape instead of a square shape and lead to the classic forward-bent posture seen in patients with kyphosis of the spine. OP often presents with a fracture because there are no symptoms associated with bone loss until an actual fracture occurs (Dawson-Hughes, 2008; North American Menopause Society, 2010; US Department of Health and Human Services, 2004). This is why early screening is advocated (Dawson-Hughes, 2008; North American Menopause Society, 2010; US Department of Health and Human Services, 2004)

OP is diagnosed with a comprehensive history and physical exam, selected laboratory testing, and central bone density measurement such as DXA as discussed above. Mary's DXA revealed a T-score of −2.6 at her lower spine, −2.0 at her hip, and −1.7 for her combined hip. Her FRAX® 10-year fracture risk at the hip was reported as 3.0%; and for any major OP fracture, it was reported as 22.0%. Her physical examination findings are consistent with thoracic VCFs. Her laboratory testing revealed a normal fasting serum calcium and 24-hour urinary calcium and a serum 25-OH-D of 20 ng/mL, suggesting nutritional insufficiency. Finally, her spine films revealed stage 1 VCFs at T7 and T8 (20%–25% deformity).

The history and physical examination and laboratory tests are done to evaluate the possible presence of secondary OP. Secondary OP is present when a disease process or medication causes bone loss that results in OP. Mary is at risk for secondary OP because she has a high-risk disease (RA) and has needed to take high-risk medications (oral steroids) for many years in the past (Dawson-Hughes, 2008; North American Menopause Society, 2010; US Department of Health and Human Services, 2004). Since her need for daily steroids continued for many years, it is highly likely that her OP is secondary, at least in part, due to steroid use. The rate of bone loss also normally increases significantly in women during the early postmenopausal years (bone loss of up to 5% per year can occur); thus it is likely that Mary's OP is also partly primary and due to her postmenopausal status.

Musculoskeletal causes of back or chest-wall pain that are unrelated to OP must also be considered. Such differentials would include back strain and costochondritis. Her physical examination findings of pain upon movement and tenderness with chest-wall compression support each of these differentials. Back strain is the more likely of these differentials because of the history of physical activity that precipitated the onset of Mary's pain. Costochondritis is less likely as it tends to develop over time with overuse and inflammation as opposed to acute injury. However, neither of these differentials is supported by the physical examination finding of vertebral tenderness, this finding is more indicative of VCF.

Angina is an important differential that Mary's clinician cannot afford to miss. Mary is at increased risk for cardiovascular disease both due to her RA and to her age. Although cardiac manifestations of RA can occur; they are not common. RA is, however, associated with an increased risk for cardiovascular disease (Maradit-Kremers, Nicola, Crowson et al., 2005). Women are more likely to develop cardiovascular disease as they age, with postmenopausal women having an equal or greater risk for cardiovascular disease than men of the same age cohort (Mosca et al., 2007). While women do experience typical angina symptoms, angina often presents atypically among women with fatigue, neck pain, nausea, and shortness of breath. Women are less likely than men to present with acute infarction; rather, they have symptoms over a longer period of time and at rest. As women age, the likelihood that they will present with more typical angina symptoms increases (Jackson, 2005; Redberg & Shaw, 2003). In Mary's case, she has not described symptoms of atypical angina such as nausea or prolonged fatigue; rather, she stated that she usually awakes refreshed and well rested. Additionally, her pain is the posterior chest rather than the anterior chest, an acute onset related to a specific activity, radiates to her lower chest and abdomen, and is exacerbated with chest-wall palpation—all findings that suggest VCF more strongly than angina-related chest pain.

Given Mary's history of RA, her clinician would also likely consider an RA flare and extraarticular pulmonary RA manifestations as possible, yet less likely, causes of her pain. RA flares tend to present with increased symptoms in previously affected joints such as the metacarpal phalangeal (MCP) and proximal interphalangeal (PIP) joints in the hands. As the disease progresses, other joints may be affected such as the elbows or wrists; ankles, knees, or hips; shoulders; and cervical spine (such as C1 and C2) (Mies Richie & Francis, 2003). In Mary's presentation, she describes this pain as distinct from her usual morning stiffness associated with RA and does not associate it with the many RA flares that she has experienced in the past. Additionally, RA is not likely to affect other areas of the spine (Mies Richie & Francis, 2003); and Mary's symptoms are specifically centered in the T7–T8 region by both her history and her physical examination. Extraarticular pulmonary RA manifestations are even less likely. Pericardial effusions related to RA are normally asymptomatic. Pulmonary manifestations may include asymptomatic pleural effusions and are more commonly seen among men (Mies Richie & Francis, 2003). Similarly, lung nodules caused by RA are also more common in men. These pulmonary manifestations do not present with acute onset upper back pain.

What is the most appropriate plan of treatment?
Mary and her clinician need to address both of her diagnoses. She has documented VCFs identified by X-ray as well as OP identified by DXA. The plan for her pain management for the VCFs will be of a more short-term nature, while OP management will be long term.

Self-management lifestyle changes:
Mary will need to initially avoid activities that increase her pain. She needs to understand that it may take 3 months before she is fully healed and that a return to activity as soon as possible is important. It will be important for her to see the physical therapist for pain modalities early on, as well as for strengthening exercises for her upper midback and body mechanics retraining later to prevent further injury.

For OP management, she will need to adjust her activity and intake of vitamin D and calcium. Mary needs to increase her activity and ensure that it includes both resistance and weight bearing activities each day. These activities will serve to increase osteoblast activity and thus strengthen bone. Mary also needs to assure daily intake of vitamin D of 800–1000 IU and calcium of 1200 mg (Dawson-Hughes, 2008; North American Menopause Society, 2010; US Department of Health and Human Services, 2004). This level of vitamin D intake is enough to rectify her vitamin D deficiency within about a 3-month period (Dawson-Hughes, 2010). Since most people cannot achieve the recommended daily intake of vitamin D and calcium through diet alone, it is likely that Mary will require ongoing calcium and vitamin D supplementation), even after her vitamin D levels are normalized. Many different supplement brands and types are available. Calcium citrate is less constipating than calcium carbonate and can be taken with or without meals. Calcium carbonate must be taken with meals, as an acid environment is needed for it to be absorbed. Calcium carbonate would not be an appropriate option for Mary if she uses antacids of any kind. Both calcium carbonate and calcium citrate are also available as a combination tablet with vitamin D.

Mary also needs to implement a fall prevention program (Dawson-Hughes, 2008; North American Menopause Society, 2010; US Department of Health and Human Services, 2004). This is not because she is at a specifically increased risk for falls simply due to her OP; it is more that the likelihood of fracture from a fall is increased simply due to her OP. Mary's clinician will advise her to look around at home and remove any loose rugs or cords that she might fall or trip on. She will need to assure adequate lighting in case she needs to get up at night, again to lessen the risk of a fall. Similarly, she will need to ensure removal of snow, ice, or wet leaves and uncluttered walkways around her home to reduce the risk of a fall.

Complementary and alternative medicine therapies:

Mary may be interested in light massage therapy or acupuncture for pain management. While neither of these therapies will necessarily increase bone strength, each may help to reduce her pain while the VCFs are healing. Continuing with these therapies may increase her tolerance for exercise later as well. Other relaxation therapies that may be beneficial include yoga, aromatherapy, and meditation. Yoga should not be initiated until the VCFs have healed and will need to be modified to avoid any forward bending (flexion) of the spine.

Research results evaluating the use of soy to improve bone strength have been contradictory; some demonstrate a benefit, while others show none. A metaanalysis that reviewed randomized, controlled trials did not find overall support for the use of soy to prevent bone loss (Liu et al., 2009). While most soy products are available for purchase, OTC Fosteum Rx® is available via prescription (see Table 9.1.1).

Herbs that are marketed to increase bone strength are usually those that are thought to increase estrogen levels. These include herbs such as black cohosh, ginseng, cypress, sage, and licorice (Decker & Meyers, 2001).

Pharmacotherapeutics:

Pharmacotherapeutic agents for both Mary's VCF pain and management of her OP are reasonable. Her pain may be adequately managed by consistent use of acetaminophen, dosed at 1000 mg by mouth every 6 hours, or in combination with a nonsteroidal antiinflammatory drug (NSAID). If an NSAID is used, she must be cautioned to take it with food to reduce the likelihood of developing gastrointestinal irritation as a side effect, and especially if she is prescribed a bisphosphonate for her OP. If acetaminophen or a combination of acetaminophen and NSAIDs is ineffective, then acetaminophen combined with a narcotic analgesic, such as acetaminophen with codeine, may be tried. A return to usual activity as soon as possible is the goal.

Mary meets the criteria established by both the National Osteoporosis Foundation (NOF) and the North American Menopause Society (NAMS) for pharmacotherapeutic treatment of her OP. Both organizations recommend initiating medication therapy in individuals with documented OP, which Mary has. In fact, Mary meets the diagnostic criteria established by the World Health Organization (WHO) for severe osteoporosis, because she has a spine T-score of −2.5 on DXA plus fragility or low-trauma fractures (VCFs) (World Health Organization, 1994). Even if Mary's DXA scores had not indicated OP and she did not have VCFs, her clinician would still consider pharmacotherapeutic therapy for her as her FRAX® 10-year risk for major OP fracture was above the cutoff of 20.0%. This suggests that it would be cost effective, based on US population calculations, to treat Mary with medications for OP (Dawson-Hughes et al., 2008; Tosteson et al., 2008).

The purpose of pharmacotherapy for OP is to reduce fracture incidence and its related sequelae. Several different effective medications for OP management are currently available in the US and approved by the FDA including bisphosphonates, calcitonin, estrogen agonist/antagonists, hormone therapy (estrogen or estrogen-progestin therapy), a RANK-ligand inhibitor, and parathyroid hormone (see Table 9.1.1). These medications can be categorized into two groups: antiresorptive or anabolic. Antiresorptive agents increase bone strength by inhibiting the function of the osteoclasts and include bisphosphonates, calcitonin, estrogen agonist/antagonists (which were previously known as selective estrogen receptor modulators [SERMs]), and hormone therapy (HT, estrogen or estrogen-progestin therapy). Denosumab is also in this category and increases bone density by binding with RANK-ligand, which ultimately inhibits osteoclast formation and function. Anabolic agents stimulate bone formation by increasing osteoblast activity and include one agent—teriparatide. The prescription medical food, Fosteum Rx®, meets FDA GRAS criteria for "generally regarded as safe" and is also available by prescription.

For Mary, selecting an agent will focus on identifying an effective therapy that is acceptable to her, does not interfere with her current medications, and has a reasonable side-effect profile. Because she

TABLE 9.1.1. Prescription Agents for Osteoporosis Management.

Medication	FDA Approved Use and Dose	Considerations
Alendronate (Fosamax)	PMO Prevention—5 mg by mouth daily or 35 mg by mouth weekly. SIO—5 mg by mouth daily or 10 mg by mouth daily if postmenopausal and off estrogen. PMO and MOP Treatment—10 mg by mouth daily or 70 mg by mouth weekly.	Take oral doses first thing in the morning on an empty stomach with 8-oz glass of plain water; remain upright and take no other food or drink for at least 30 minutes. Take oral doses 2 hours before antacids/calcium. Caution with oral forms if upper gastrointestinal disease, clinical association with dysphagia, esophagitis, or ulceration. Beneficial effects may last for years after medication is discontinued.
Alendronate + cholecalciferol (Fosamax plus D)	PMO and MOP Treatment—70 mg plus 2800 IU Vitamin D_3 or 70 mg plus 5600 IU vitamin D_3 in combined tablet by mouth weekly.	Fosamax plus D—combined bisphosphonate and vitamin D_3 in a single tablet taken weekly. Actonel with Calcium—blister pack for 28-day use, provides Actonel in 1 tablet taken on day 1 and calcium in other 6 tablets taken days 2–7, repeated sequence over 4 weeks.
Risedronate (Actonel)	PMO prevention or treatment—5 mg by mouth daily, 35 mg by mouth weekly, 75 mg by mouth 2 consecutive days each month, or 150 mg by mouth monthly. SIO—5 mg by mouth daily. MOP—35 mg by mouth weekly.	IV ibandronate and zoledronic acid are not associated with gastrointestinal side effects or limitations on timing dose around food, water, calcium, or medication intake. Hypocalcemia must be corrected prior to use.
Risedronate + calcium carbonate (Actonel with calcium)	PMO prevention or treatment—35 mg risedronate day 1, 1250 mg (500 mg elemental) calcium carbonate days 2–7.	Osteonecrosis of the jaw (ONJ), exposed bone in the mouth for >3 months with nonhealing lesions, has been associated with high dose IV bisphosphonate therapy among individuals with cancer-related bone disease (2%–10%); cancer patients with dental problems, gum injury, oral bony abnormalities, or taking medications that interfere with healing; and, in very rare cases, healthy individuals with similar risk factors who are on bisphosphonates for osteoporosis (incidence estimated at 0.001%–0.002%). Consider stopping therapy for 2–3 months if invasive dental procedures are required and resume after healing is complete. Encourage usual dental care (e.g., cleaning, fillings, crown work).
Ibandronate (Boniva)	PMO prevention or treatment—2.5 mg by mouth daily or 150 mg by mouth monthly. PMO treatment—3 mg IV every 3 months.	
Zoledronic acid (Reclast)	PMO prevention—5 mg IV every 2 years. PMO, MOP, and SIO treatment—5 mg IV yearly.	Subtrochanteric fracture is an extremely rare event that has been associated with bisphosphonate use. Advise patients that the risk of this extremely rare event is far less than the risks associated with hip fracture and encourage them to take their prescribed bisphosphonates consistently.
Calcitonin (Miacalcin, Fortical NS)	PMO treatment—200 IU intranasal spray daily (Miacalcin or Fortical NS) or 100 IU subcutaneously 3 times each week (Miacalcin).	Usually administered as nasal spray. Alternate nares for nasal spray. Most often used for analgesic effect on acute pain due to vertebral compression fractures.
Denosumab (Prolia)	PMO treatment—60 mg injection (subcutaneous) every 6 months.	Denosumab is for those with multiple risks for fracture, with osteoporotic fracture history, and who have not responded to other treatments. Requires administration by a health care professional. Use may be associated with ONJ, oversuppression of bone turnover, skin infections, and dermatologic conditions. Individuals with latex allergy should not handle grey needle cover. Hypocalcemia must be corrected prior to use.

TABLE 9.1.1. *Continued*

Medication	FDA Approved Use and Dose	Considerations
Estrogen (i.e., Alora, Climara, Estrace, Estraderm, Menest, Menostar, Premarin, Vivelle, Vivelle Dot)	PMO prevention—doses and routes vary.	Also effective in alleviating most symptoms related to menopause (even Menostar, which has a very low dose and was shown to effectively reduce severity and frequency of hot flashes).
Estrogen-Progestin combination products (i.e., Activella, Climara Pro, Femhrt, Prefest, Premphase, Prempro)	PMO prevention—doses and routes vary.	Available in several forms (e.g., pills, patch, ring, cream, gel). Use for 2–3 years immediately following menopause may provide some beneficial effects on bone health after discontinuation.
Genistein + citrated zinc + cholecalciferol (Fosteum Rx®)	Prevention—1 capsule twice daily (each capsule contains 27 mg genistein, 20 mg citrated zinc, 200 IU cholecalciferol).	Medical food. Meets FDA standards for GRAS (generally recognized as safe). Not recommended if taking HT, estrogen agonist-antagonists.
Raloxifene (Evista)	PMO prevention or treatment—60 mg by mouth daily.	May cause hot flashes. Not recommended if taking ET or EPT. Also approved for prevention of breast cancer in women at high risk for invasive breast cancer.
Teriparatide [recombinant human PTH 1–34] (Forteo)	PMO, MOP, and SIO treatment (high fracture risk)—20 mcg subcutaneously daily. (A teriparatide patch for osteoporosis is under investigation.)	Reserved for use after failure of first-line agents Most effective when used sequentially following bisphosphonate.

PMO = postmenopausal osteoporosis; SIO = steroid-induced osteoporosis; MOP = male osteoporosis.

Table (adapted slightly in use column) is from Alexander, IM. (In press, 2011). Menopause and Midlife Women's Health (chapter). In *Comprehensive Women's Health Care*, Alexander, Johnson-Mallard, Kostas-Polston, and Leary eds. Philadelphia, PA: Elsevier Mosby.

Data from: US Department of Health and Human Services. *Bone health and osteoporosis: A report of the Surgeon General.* Rockville, MD: US Department of Health and Human Services, Office of the Surgeon General; 2004; Dawson-Hughes B. A revised clinician's guide to the prevention and treatment of osteoporosis. *J Clin Endocrinol Metab* Jul 2008; 93(7):2463–2465; Micromedex. Available to subscribers at: http://www.thomsonhc.com/hcs/librarian. Accessed January 27, 2010; ePocrates. Computerized pharmacology and prescribing reference. Updated daily. Available at: www.epocrates.com. Accessed January 27, 2010; North American Menopause Society. Management of osteoporosis in postmenopausal women: 2010 position statement of The North American Menopause Society. *Menopause.* Jan–Feb 2010; 17(1):25–54; Fosteum Prescribing Information. Available at: www.fosteum.com. Accessed February 27, 2008; North American Menopause Society. Government-Approved Postmenopausal Osteoporosis Drugs in the United States and Canada. *North American Menopause Society.* June 2009. Available for members at: http://www.menopause.org/otcharts.pdf. Accessed February 2, 2010; Novartis Pharmaceuticals. Reclast Prescribing Information. *Novartis Pharmaceuticals.* August, 2007. Accessed October 26, 2007; Roche Laboratories. Boniva Tablet Prescribing Information. *Roche Laboratories.* August, 2006. Available at: http://www.rocheusa.com/products/Boniva/PI.pdf. Accessed October 26, 2007; Roche Laboratories. Boniva Injectable Prescribing Information. *Roche Laboratories.* February, 2007. Accessed October 26, 2007. Available at: http://www.rocheusa.com/products/Boniva/Injection_PI.pdf; Bachmann GA, Schaefers M, Uddin A, Utian WH. Lowest effective transdermal 17beta-estradiol dose for relief of hot flushes in postmenopausal women: a randomized controlled trial. *Obstet Gynecol* Oct 2007; 110(4):771–779; Maggon, L. Denosumab (Prolia, Amgen) FDA review and approval. Available at: http://knol.google.com/k/denosumab-prolia-amgen-fda-review-approval#. Accessed January 27, 2010; Cosman F, Lane NE, Bolognese MA, et al. Effect of transdermal teriparatide administration on bone mineral density in postmenopausal women. *J Clin Endocrinol Metab.* Jan 2010; 95(1):151–158; Rizzoli R, Burlet N, Cahall D, Delmas PD, Eriksen EF, Felsenberg D, et al. Osteonecrosis of the jaw and bisphosphonate treatment for osteoporosis. Bone 2008; 42(5):841–7; McClung MR. Osteonecrosis of the Jaw. Menopause e-Consult 2007; 3(2); American Association of Oral and Maxillofacial Surgeons. AAOMS position paper on bisphosphonate related osteonecrosis of the jaw. In: American Association of Oral and Maxillofacial Surgeons; 2006; Shane E, Goldring S, Christakos S, Drezner M, Eisman J, Silverman S, et al. Osteonecrosis of the jaw: more research needed. J Bone Miner Res 2006; 21(10):1503–5; Bilezikian JP. Osteonecrosis of the jaw—Do bisphosphonates pose a risk? N Engl J Med 2006;355(22):2278–81; Bolland M, Hay D, Grey A, Reid I, Cundy T. Osteonecrosis of the jaw and bisphosphonates—Putting the risk in perspective. N Z Med J 2006;119(1246):U2339; Bagger YZ, Tanko LB, Alexandersen P, Hansen HB, Mollgaard A, Ravn P, et al. Two to three years of hormone replacement treatment in healthy women have long-term preventive effects on bone mass and osteoporotic fractures: the PERF study. Bone 2004; 34(4):728–35; Black DM, Kelly MP, Genant HK, et al. Bisphosphonates and Fractures of the Subtrochanteric or Diaphyseal Femur. N Engl J Med 2010; 10.1056/NEJMoa1001086, nejm.org, accessed November 2, 2010; Prolia Prescribing Information, available at: http://pi.amgen.com/united_states/prolia/prolia_pi.pdf, accessed March 8, 2011. Adapted from Alexander, I. M., & Andrist, L. A. (2005). Menopause (Ch. 11, pp. 249–289). In F. Likis & K. Shuiling (Eds.), *Women's Gynecologic Health.* Sudbury, MA: Jones and Bartlett.

has established OP, she needs a medication that is approved for OP treatment. This means that hormone therapy is not an appropriate option. If Mary had osteopenia and was also experiencing significant menopause-related symptoms, then HT might be a good option (North American Menopause Society, 2010). Bisphosphonates are frequently identified as first line options for OP. Several different medications are now available in this class with varied frequency of dosing and also varied routes of administration. Some are also available in generic formulation, which can significantly reduce cost. A precise procedure for taking oral bisphosphonates must be followed to reduce the risk of esophageal irritation. Other rare side effects are also possible (see Table 9.1.1). If Mary starts with a bisphosphonate and is unable to follow the oral medication regimen or has a low bone-density response, she might have better adherence with an injectable bisphosphonate or denosumab. If Mary was at high risk for breast cancer, raloxifene might be a better option for her. Calcitonin is sometimes used for the pain associated with VCFs and might be considered for Mary. However, other OP medications have better fracture prevention data and Mary's pain will likely be well managed with analgesics instead. Teriparatide is an unlikely option for Mary as it is generally reserved for use in patients that do not respond to first-line medication options. Poor adherence to OP medication is well documented (Gold, Alexander, & Ettinger, 2006). Therefore, it is important that Mary is an active participant in deciding which medication to use. She is much more likely to continue with the medication if it is taken on a schedule that works for her life. This may mean daily or nondaily oral medications, or possibly infrequent office visits for injectable medications. Ensuring insurance coverage of her selection is also crucial.

What additional patient education is important for Mary?
While OP is not wholly reversible, slowing bone loss with the described self-management strategies is crucial to reducing the impact of the disease and preventing future fractures. It is important for Mary to understand that she has a lifelong challenge ahead of her to retain her current bone strength and hopefully build upon it. This can only be successful with a combined management plan that includes self-management lifestyle strategies—such as regular exercise, adequate calcium and vitamin D intake, and careful monitoring of her RA—and consistent use of her OP medications.

What is the plan for follow-up care?
In addition to reevaluating Mary's ability to follow the management plan including both medications and self-management strategies at every visit, a followup DXA scan will be ordered for about 1–2 years to evaluate the efficacy of Mary's management strategies (Dawson-Hughes, 2008). It will be repeated every 1–2 years until her results are stable. If her T-scores do not improve after a few years, her clinician might consider changing the pharmacotherapeutic agent to an alternate class or consider referral to an OP specialist.

Are any referrals needed?
Referral to physical therapy initially for pain modalities and later for strengthening exercises and body mechanics training is appropriate. If Mary does not respond to routine pain management strategies or if her DXA T-scores continue to fall, then referral to a specialist may be indicated. Consultation with an OP specialist may be warranted if she is not responding to therapy. A pain specialist or ongoing physical therapy may help to alleviate her pain. Some patients with VCFs require referral for surgical intervention, such as kyphoplasty or vertebroplasty, to relieve pain and preserve function. Kyphoplasty (a balloon is inserted into the vertebral space, is inflated to straighten the vertebral bones, and is then replaced with a cement-like substance) is performed under local anesthesia so pain and function can be monitored throughout the procedure. Vertebroplasty is similar and was the precursor to kyphoplasty. Vertebroplasty is usually performed by interventional radiologists and involves injection of a cement-like substance into the fractured vertebrae. If effective, pain relief is almost immediate after either procedure.

Does Mary's psychosocial history affect her management plan?
Consideration of Mary's psychosocial history is important when developing a management plan with her. Consideration of Mary's healthcare insurance coverage of medications, physical therapy, and DXA evaluations is important. Many insurance companies dictate which pharmacotherapeutic agents are covered. Similarly, most companies have rules governing the frequency of covered DXA testing

and the length of physical therapy treatments. These issues are taken into account when deciding on a management plan with Mary so that financial barriers to the cost of medications, follow-up DXA testing, or PT do not become barriers to her ability to follow the agreed upon plan.

What if Mary were under age 40?

If Mary were under 40, a more aggressive search for other secondary causes of OP would be appropriate. Any conditions identified would then need to be managed to reduce bone loss. Additionally, most of the medications available for OP treatment and prevention do not carry FDA approval for use in premenopausal women, so agent selection options would be narrowed (see Table 9.1.1).

What if Mary also had diabetes or hyperlipidemia?

The disease processes themselves would not alter Mary's plan of care. However, pharmacotherapeutic agent selection for managing diabetes and hyperlipidemia would potentially be altered. Statins (e.g., Lipitor, Mevacor) have been demonstrated to improve bone health, though not enough to be used as OP agents, and might be a preferred class of agent for Mary if she also had hyperlipidemia (US Department of Health and Human Services, 2004). Conversely, thiazolidinediones (TZDs; e.g., Actos, Avandia) have been identified as potentially increasing risk for bone loss and may need to be avoided if Mary also had diabetes (Dawson-Hughes, 2008). Incidentally, hydrochlorothiazide diuretics have been identified as bone-preserving medications (US Department of Health and Human Services, 2004); thus the fact that Mary's hypertension is treated with HCTZ is optimal with regard to her OP.

What if Mary were a male?

Several of the medications available for OP treatment and prevention only carry FDA approval for use in postmenopausal women, so agent selection options would be narrowed (see Table 9.1.1).

Are there any standardized guidelines that the clinician will use to assess or treat Mary?

The US Surgeon General's 2004 report *Bone Health and Osteoporosis* helped to raise awareness about the importance of bone loss and its consequences (US Department of Health and Human Services, 2004). Since that report, the NOF has published at least 2 sets of guidelines for clinicians about managing OP and osteopenia, the most recent of which was published in 2008 (Dawson-Hughes, 2008). In 2010, the NAMS also published guidelines for OP and osteopenia management in their updated position statement; these are specifically geared to the postmenopausal woman (North American Menopause Society, 2010).

REFERENCES AND RESOURCES

Alexander, I. M., & Lewiecki, E. M. (2008). Prevention, identification and treatment of postmenopausal osteoporosis (online CME/CE program). Medscape, available at: http://www.medscape.com/viewprogram/17528

Colglazier, C. L., & Sutej, P. G. (2005). Laboratory testing in the rheumatic diseases: A practical review. *South Medicine Journal*, 98(2), 185–191.

Dawson-Hughes, B. (2008). A revised clinician's guide to the prevention and treatment of osteoporosis. *The Journal of Clinical Endocrinology and Metabolism*, 93(7), 2463–2465.

Dawson-Hughes, B. (2010). Treatment of vitamin D deficient states. Up-To-Dare, available to subscribers at: http://www.uptodate.com/online/content/topic.do?topicKey=bone_dis/11247&selectedTitle=1%7E139&source=search_result. Accessed November 1, 2010.

Dawson-Hughes, B., Tosteson, A. N., Melton, L. J. 3rd, Baim, S., Favus, M. J., Khosla, S., et al. (2008). Implications of absolute fracture risk assessment for osteoporosis practice guidelines in the USA. *Osteoporosis International*, 19(4), 449–458.

Decker, G. M., & Meyers, J. (2001). Commonly used herbs: Implications for clinical practice. *Clinical Journal of Oncology Nursing*, March/April; 15(2), 13. Pullout insert.

Gold, D. T., Alexander, I. M., & Ettinger, M. P. (2006). How can osteoporosis patients benefit more from their therapy? Adherence issues with bisphosphonate therapy. *The Annals of Pharmacotherapy*, 40(6), 1143–1150.

Jackson, G. (2005). Stable angina pectoris (recognition and management). In N. K. Wenger, & P. Collins (Eds.), *Women and heart disease* (2nd ed., pp. 195–204). London: Taylor & Francis Group.

Liu, J., Ho, S. C., Su, Y. X., Chen, W. Q., Zhang, C. X., & Chen, Y. M. (2009). Effect of long-term intervention of soy isoflavones on bone mineral density in women: A meta-analysis of randomized controlled trials. *Bone*, *44*(5), 948–953.

Maradit-Kremers, H., Nicola, P. J., Crowson, C. S., et al (2005). Cardiovascular death in rheumatoid arthritis: A population-based study. *Arthritis Rheum*, *52*(3), 722–732.

Mies Richie, A., & Francis, M. L. (2003). Diagnostic approach to polyarticular joint pain. *American Family Physician*, *68*(6), 1151–1160.

Mosca, L., Banka, C. L., Benjamin, E. J., Berra, K., Bushnell, C., Dolor, R. J., et al. (2007). Evidence-based guidelines for cardiovascular disease prevention in women: 2007 update. *Journal of the American College of Cardiology*, *49*(11), 1230–1250.

North American Menopause Society (2010). Management of osteoporosis in postmenopausal women: 2010 position statement of The North American Menopause Society. *Menopause*, *17*(1), 25–54, quiz 55–26.

Redberg, R. F., & Shaw, L. J. (2003). Diagnosis of coronary artery disease in women. *Progress in Cardiovascular Diseases*, *46*, 239–258.

Tosteson, A. N., Melton, L. J. 3rd, Dawson-Hughes, B., Baim, S., Favus, M. J., Khosla, S., et al. (2008). Cost-effective osteoporosis treatment thresholds: The United States perspective. *Osteoporosis International*, *19*(4), 437–447.

US Department of Health and Human Services (2004). *Bone health and osteoporosis: A report of the Surgeon General*. Rockville, MD: US Department of Health and Human Services, Office of the Surgeon General.

World Health Organization (1994). *Assessment of fracture risk and its application to screening for postmenopausal osteoporosis. Technical report series*. Geneva: WHO.

World Health Organization (2007a). WHO FRAX Technical Report. Retrieved June 6, 2008, from http://www.shef.ac.uk/FRAX/

World Health Organization (2007b). *WHO scientific group on the assessment of osteoporosis at primary health care level: Summary meeting report*. Brussels, Belgium: WHO Press, Geneva, Switzerland.

Case 9.2 Just Not Feeling Right

By Shelley Yerger Hawkins, DSN, APRN-BC, FNP, GNP, FAAN

SUBJECTIVE

Tom, a 70-year-old white male who lives alone, presents to the family practice with a chief complaint of "just not feeling right for 2–3 days." Last week he had lunch with his daughter and granddaughter, who had an upper respiratory infection. He developed a cold last week that was treated with Mucinex DM. He did not seek health care, since the medication was helpful; and he thought that it was resolved. He admits to increasing fatigue and found it difficult to "get started with his usual routine this morning." The fatigue initially started with a lack of energy; he has been unable to take his daily short walk and did not want to get out of bed this morning. Yesterday, he forgot a lunch scheduled with his daughter and forgot to take his medications.

He denies changes in vision or hearing. He denies headaches and myalgias. He denies fever, but admits to "some" shortness of breath with exertion. He denies cough, chest pain, or palpitations, but admits to feeling congested and having tightness in his chest at intervals, especially with exertion. He denies rhinorrhea, dysphagia, otalgia, sputum production, fever, or chills. He denies anorexia, abdominal pain, and changes in his bowel habits. He denies changes in urinary habits. He has had no falls. He admits to being lonely but verbalizes no suicidal ideations.

Past medical and surgical history: Hypertension: 10 years; osteoarthritis: 5 years; hearing aid and glasses: 5 years. Influenza and H1N1 vaccinations this year. Pneumovacc 4 years ago. Chest X-ray (CXR) 2 years ago was negative. PPD 2 years ago was negative. Dental and eye exams 1.5 years ago. Appendectomy 30 years ago.

Medications: Zestoretic 10/25 mg; Aleve PRN.

Allergies: Penicillin; Latex.

Family history: Father died at age 66 years from a myocardial infarction (MI), and mother died at age 75 from an MI. One sibling age 72 with hypertension and type 2 diabetes mellitus; a 45-year-old daughter divorced with hypertension; one 5-year-old healthy grandchild; and a 40-year-old married son, alive and well.

Social history: Retired accountant who continues to live in a one-level home that he and his wife resided in for 40 years. He has a weekly housekeeper who cooks some meals; otherwise, he eats many pre-packaged foods. He has good retirement benefits and adequate savings with health insurance. Smoked cigarettes for 15 years, has smoked none for the last 20 years. Drinks 4–6 oz wine daily, for

Clinical Case Studies for the Family Nurse Practitioner, First Edition. Edited by Leslie Neal-Boylan.
© 2011 John Wiley & Sons, Inc. Published 2011 by John Wiley & Sons, Inc.

30+ years. Difficult transition without wife; usually refuses socialization with friends. Drives car. Spends day watching television; reading history; and interacting with Eddie, his 9-year-old dachshund.

OBJECTIVE

General: Well nourished; appropriately dressed for season and setting; in no apparent distress. Skin: healthy color, with elastic recoil.

HEENT: Normocephalic; no dentures, mild plaque noted on teeth; mild AV nicking, sinuses nontender; TMs pearly gray; nares patent with small amount of yellow drainage; pharynx pink, no lymphadenopathy, thyroid nontender.

Cardiovascular: No JVD or anterior chest pulsations noted; carotids palpable and without bruits; S1 and S2 noted with regular rhythm; 2/6 systolic ejection murmur. No edema, 2+ pulses of upper extremities. Pedal pulses are 1+.

Respiratory: AP/transverse diameter is ½; equal and symmetrical chest expansion; no fremitus; mild dullness to percussion in right lower lobe; basilar crackles and expiratory wheezes in right lung; no extra lung sounds.

Abdomen: No pulsations noted; bowel sounds noted in all quadrants; nontender to palpation; no organomegaly.

Neurologic: Alert and oriented x4; follows commands appropriately; thought processes intact but somewhat slow in responses; gait steady, but slightly unsteady on feet.

CRITICAL THINKING

Which diagnostic or imaging studies should be considered to assist with or confirm the diagnosis?
___Anterior/posterior and lateral CXR
___CBC
___Metabolic panel
___Albumin
___Blood cultures
___Arterial blood gases
___Sputum culture and gram stain
___Urine specimen
___Pulse oximetry
___Pulmonary function tests

What is most likely differential diagnosis and why?
___Pneumonia
___Acute bronchitis
___Influenza
___Exacerbation of chronic bronchitis due to influenza
___Anemia
___Lung cancer

What is the plan of treatment?

Are any referrals needed at this time?

Does Tom's psychosocial history have implications on the plan?

How would treatment differ if Tom were already hospitalized when he presented with these symptoms?

How would management differ if he were in a nursing home?

What if he had accessibility and availability issues to health care since he lived in a rural setting and had limited transportation?

RESOLUTION

Diagnostic tests: An anterior/posterior and lateral chest X-ray showed minor emphysematous changes and an almost complete right lower lobe infiltrate.

Complete blood count: WBC count of 12,700/mm^3 with 74% neutrophils and 12% bands; Hgb 14; HCT 45.

Metabolic panel: Na: 140; K: 4.2; glucose: 86; BUN: 10; creatinine: 1.2; albumin: 4.1.

Pulse oximetry: 95%.

Sputum specimen obtained following Albuterol nebulizer treatment: *Streptococcus pneumoniae*, greater than 25 WBCs, and fewer than 10 epithelial cells per high-power field on gram stain with encapsulated gram-positive diplococci.

Confirming a diagnosis of pneumonia in older adults usually depends on the chest X-ray (CXR), although an infiltrate may be obscured by pulmonary edema or not apparent until 24–48 hours after rehydration (Erber, 2009). This patient is in relatively good physical health and had no obvious rehydration issues. This was confirmed with normal electrolytes, hemoglobin, and hematocrit, along with good skin turgor for an older male. A normal or mildly elevated total WBC count accompanied by a left shift in the differential is characteristic but nonspecific, as is arterial hypoxemia. Arterial blood gases are frequently helpful in assessing the severity of illness, but they were not indicated in this patient. An elevated pCO2 may indicate that the patient's respiratory effort is fatiguing. An arterial pO2 level that is lower than expected, after allowing for age and comorbidities, helps determine whether the patient is to be monitored on an ambulatory basis or hospitalized (Erber, 2009).

Analysis of an adequate sputum specimen is extremely useful (fewer than 10 epithelial cells and greater than 25 WBCs per high-power field), although success in obtaining a specimen is the exception rather than the rule. For patients who cannot produce an expectorated specimen and who are immunocompromised, not responding to therapy, or relapsing after an initial response, collection of a specimen by transtracheal aspiration or bronchoscopy may be indicated. Blood cultures have a diagnostic yield of 10%–20%, depending on the organism (Ebersole, Hess, Touhy, & Jett, 2005).

What is most likely differential diagnosis and why?
Pneumonia:
This patient presents with a fairly classic presentation for an older adult. He has no fever, chills, dyspnea, or productive cough that is typical for other age groups. He does have tachypnea, mild hypotension, fatigue, chest tightness, along with adventitious breath sounds and a confirming CXR. These findings are significant indicators of a diagnosis of pneumonia in an older adult (Eliopoulos, 2009).

The presentation of pneumonia in the older adult is frequently nonspecific, without the expected classic findings of productive cough, fever, chills, and pleuritic chest pain found in the rapid-onset lobar pneumonia typical of younger adults. Instead, the older adult may report poor appetite and weakness or appear to suffer from exacerbation of an underlying chronic illness. This slower, more insidious onset is frequently seen in older adults and does not necessarily imply an atypical cause as would such a presentation in younger adults (Gradon, 2006).

Physical examination findings in the older patient with pneumonia usually reveal tachypnea and tachycardia, both the most-sensitive and least-specific signs of illness (Saxon, Etten, & Perkins, 2009). A respiratory rate above 28 is probably the earliest clue. Mortality rates increase among patients with a severe vital sign abnormality. Fever may be blunted or absent in a significant proportion of patients even in the presence of bacteremia. Shallow respiration and crepitations in the lung bases are common findings in normal older adults because of decreased pulmonary compliance. Because of these non-specific features, pneumonia may be difficult to distinguish from acute bronchitis. Pneumonia should be suspected when the patient appears to have significant dyspnea or functional impairment (Mody, Sun, & Bradley, 2006).

Mental status changes such as the recent forgetfulness seen in this patient are due to a gradually changing oxygenation status associated with aging since overall lung function becomes less efficient. Acute mental status changes occur much more often in older adults versus younger patients. There is a much higher incidence of mortality when acute mental status changes have occurred (Naito et al., 2006).

Eighty to ninety percent of older adults with pneumonia have one or more concomitant illnesses such as cardiovascular disease, diabetes mellitus, or COPD which lower host defense mechanisms by several routes, most notably through impairment of alveolar macrophage activity. Under such circumstances, bacteria may reach the lower bronchial tree by inhalation, inoculation, aspiration, and direct spread from contiguous sites. Colonization of the oropharynx with potentially pathogenic bacteria such as gram-negative bacilli occurs frequently in older persons. Additional risk factors include the inability to walk without assistance, urinary incontinence, and difficulty in performing activities of daily living (Reuben et al., 2010). The increased incidence of colonization, combined with known decline in aging host defenses, places older adults at far greater risk for infection and adverse outcomes. The organisms that most commonly cause pneumonia vary depending on the patient's setting and functional status. In the community, *S. pneumoniae* is still most frequently recovered followed by *H. influenza* (Torres et al., 2004).

In most age groups influenza usually comes on suddenly and is often accompanied by one or more of the following: fever, headache, fatigue, dry cough, dysphagia, nasal congestion, and myalgias. Older adults often have an atypical presentation. They may present with confusion and absence of fever, making influenza a possible differential diagnosis (Erber, 2009). However, a thorough respiratory examination and diagnostic testing will usually confirm a diagnosis of pneumonia.

Similarly, older adults over age 70 with acute bronchitis may be relatively asymptomatic since they do not tend to mount an inflammatory response. Even though the main symptom of acute bronchitis is coughing, older adults may have minimal coughing and typically are afebrile. Acute bronchitis, like influenza, will typically be excluded with diagnostic testing.

What is the plan of treatment?

Bacterial pneumonia is frequently managed with aggressive, empirical treatment in the initial stages of illness, and the antibiotic must be chosen according to the organisms most likely to be present in the community and according to the patient's functional status (Gotfried, 2004). Overall, Tom is a healthy ambulatory patient who does not smoke and will therefore be treated on an outpatient basis. At this point, intravenous or intensive oxygen therapy is not warranted.

1. Antibiotic-azithromycin, 500 mg/daily by mouth for 2 weeks. Encourage him to take the complete prescription.
2. Rest and limit all activities and avoid going out of the home.
3. Encourage him in appropriate hydration—2 qt of fluid daily.
4. Encourage proper nutrition—3 meals daily.
5. Encourage frequent, proper handwashing.
6. Discuss the possibility of his daughter following up with him daily.
7. Have the patient return to the clinic in 3–5 days for followup.
8. Have the patient or family notify the clinic if symptoms worsen, such as fever, dyspnea, or productive cough.
9. Tylenol 325, 650 mg every 6–8 hours as needed.

Are any referrals needed at this time?

Given that Tom conveys sadness, continues to be grief-stricken about his wife's death, and has limited interpersonal interactions, it is important that he obtain counseling and possibly take an antidepressant. A referral to a psychologist, psychiatrist, or psychiatric mental health nurse practitioner would be appropriate.

Since Tom has not had dental care for 1.5 years and has noticeable buildup of plaque (increased oral bacteria predisposes to pneumonia and other infections), it is important that he has a dental cleaning with subsequent twice-yearly appointments.

Does Tom's psychosocial study have implications on the plan?

Given that Tom experiences depression due to his wife's death, frequent followup by family and/or friends would ensure that he is improving. The nurse practitioner will ask the patient's permission to discuss his current health with his daughter and explore his eligibility for a visiting nurse and/or food services.

How would treatment differ if Tom were already hospitalized when he presented with these symptoms?

Patients in the hospital are almost always immunocompromised and require much more aggressive antibiotic treatment because of the severity of the most likely organisms in the hospital setting.

How would management differ if Tom were in a nursing home?

There are two distinct groups in the nursing home—those who are reasonably healthy and those who are frail. Older adults with less functional impairment and few comorbid illnesses are often safely treated in the facility, depending on adequate nursing care. Frail, often immunocompromised older adults should be hospitalized. Patients with causative organisms such as staphylococci, gram-negative bacilli, aspiration, or postobstruction are considered high-risk and carry a substantially higher mortality rate than patients with other causes (Coleman, 2004).

What if he had accessibility and availability issues to health care since he lived in a rural setting and had limited transportation?

If telehealth is an option, followup could be done initially to ensure that he is compliant and that his condition is not worsening. This would offer opportunities for socialization, as well.

REFERENCES AND RESOURCES

Coleman, P. (2004). Pneumonia in the long-term care setting: Etiology, management, and evaluation. *Journal of Gerontological Nursing, 30*(4), 14–23.

Ebersole, P., Hess, P., Touhy, T. A., & Jett, K. F. (2005). *Gerontological nursing and healthy aging* (2nd ed.). St. Louis: Mosby.

Eliopoulos, C. (2009). *Gerontological nursing* (7th ed.). Lippincott, Williams, & Wilkins.

Erber, J. (2009). *Aging and older adulthood* (2nd ed.). Wiley & Sons.

Falk, G., & Fahey, T. (2009). C-reactive protein and community-acquired pneumonia in ambulatory care: Systematic review of diagnostic accuracy studies. *Family Practice, 26*, 10–21.

Ganz, F., et al. (2009). ICU nurses' oral care practices and the current best evidence. *Image: Journal of Nursing Scholarship, 41*(2), 132–138.

Gotfried, M. (2004). Appropriate outpatient macrolide use in community-acquired pneumonia. *Journal of American Academy of Nurse Practitioners, 16*(4), 146–156.

Gradon, J. (2006). Community-acquired pneumonia in the older patient. *Clinical Geriatrics, 14*, 39–45.

Marrie, T. (2000). Community-acquired pneumonia in the elderly. *Clinical Infectious Disease, 31*, 1066–1078.

Marrie, T., Lau, C., Wheeler, S., et al. (2000). Predictors of symptom resolution in patients with community-acquired pneumonia. *Clinical Infectious Disease, 31*, 1362–1367.

Mody, L., Sun, R., & Bradley, S. (2006). Assessment of pneumonia in older adults: Effect of functional status. *Journal of American Geriatrics Society, 54*, 1062–1067.

Naito, T., et al. (2006). A validation and potential modification of the Pneumonia Severity Index in elderly patients with community-acquired pneumonia. *Journal of American Geriatrics Society, 54*(8), 1212–1219.

Ooesterheert, J., et al. (2006). Effectiveness of early switch from intravenous to oral antibiotics in severe community-acquired pneumonia: Multicenter randomized trial. *British Medical Journal, 333*, 1193–1199.

Palacios-Cena, D., Alvarez-Lopez, C., Cachon-Perez, M., & Alonso-Blanco, C. (2009). Early detection of functional and cognitive decline after hospital discharge: The role of community nursing and multidisciplinary teams. *Journal of Gerontological Nursing*, 35(9), 41–47.

Ravago, T., Mosniam, J., & Alem, F. (2000). Evaluation of community acquired pneumonia guidelines. *Journal of Medical Systems*, 24, 280–296.

Redfern, S., & Ross, F. (2005). *Nursing older people* (3rd ed.). London: Churchill Livingstone.

Reuben, D., Herr, K., Pacala, J., Pollock, B., Potter, J., & Semla, T. (2010). *Geriatrics at your fingertips* (12th ed.). New York, NY: American Geriatrics Society.

Saxon, S., Etten, M., & Perkins, E. (2009). *Physical change and aging: A guide for the helping professions* (5th ed.). New York, NY: Springhouse.

Schermer, T., Leenders, J., Veen, H., van den Bosch, W., Wissink, A., Smeele, I., & Chavannes, N. (2009). Pulse oximetry in family practice: Indications and clinical observations in patients with COPD. *Family Practice*, 26, 524–531.

Torres, O., et al. (2004). Outcome predictors of pneumonia in elderly patients: Importance of functional assessment. *Journal of American Geriatrics Society*, 52, 1603–1609.

SUBJECTIVE

Allan is a 62-year-old white male. He comes in today with his wife after an incident last week at their house. The patient had attempted to light a stove burner that had a faulty ignition. He failed to smell the accumulating gas fumes. His wife, who was in an adjoining room, smelled the gas odor and ran into the kitchen to check the stove. The patient was surprised that his wife smelled the gas when he did not.

Upon further questioning, the patient admits to feeling a vague sense of fatigue for the past year and not being able to do his routine work around the house with as much energy and efficiency as he used to have. He attributes this to feeling "down" about having to take early retirement 9 months ago from the accounting firm with which he has worked for the past 30 years. Although he had planned to retire within the next 5 years, this "firing by early retirement" as he calls it was a serious financial setback for the couple; and he continues to seek various part-time jobs to supplement his wife's salary.

The patient's wife also mentioned that she has noticed over the past 3 months an occasional slight tremor in Allan's right hand that seems less noticeable when he reaches for his coffee cup; the patient, however, attributes this to too much caffeine and has recently cut back his usual 4–6 cups per day habit to 1 cup a day for the past month. He also jokingly added that his golf game has gotten worse, rather than better, since his "firing-retirement" last year and that this is his *real* reason for coming in today—he wants his usually-fluid golf swing back. Upon further questioning about his movement, he notes that he experiences initial stiffness in his right knee upon starting to walk, but that this sensation goes away after walking the length of 2 city blocks. This has been present for the past 6 months, but it does not bother or concern him.

The patient denies recent falls, serious illnesses, or recent nasal/sinus infections or surgery. He has worn glasses for reading for 8 years and has never had to wear glasses for distance until his last eye exam 3 months ago. When questioned about changes in behavior, the patient said he didn't think he had any, but his wife was of a different opinion. She mentioned that for the past year he has seemed less efficient than usual in his actions, easily losing his focus on what he is doing and unable to prioritize things he needs to do for the day.

Allan denies any chest pain, shortness of breath, joint pain or muscle aches, fever, nausea, vomiting, diarrhea, dysuria, hematuria, headaches, or back pain. He admits to recent problems with

Clinical Case Studies for the Family Nurse Practitioner, First Edition. Edited by Leslie Neal-Boylan.
© 2011 John Wiley & Sons, Inc. Published 2011 by John Wiley & Sons, Inc.

constipation for the last month, but he thinks that this is due to cutting back on the amount of caffeine he used to get from drinking 4–6 cups of coffee a day.

Past medical and surgical history: Negative for diabetes, cancer, hypertension, hyperlipidemia, respiratory disease, and neurological problems. Surgeries include tonsillectomy at age 9.

Family history: Father died of prostate cancer at age 73. Mother died of Alzheimer's-related complications at age 72. Brother (age 70) is alive and doing well following treatment 2 years ago for lung cancer. Sister (age 67) is alive and well.

Social history: Married to his high school sweetheart for 40 years. Works part-time out of his home as a tutor in math for local high school and college students. His wife works full time as a teacher. He has two children, both in graduate school and living away from home. He and his wife enjoy a glass of wine with dinner about 2–3 times per week, and he has a beer at the local pub once every weekend during the football season. He has never smoked. He states he enjoys playing bridge and joined a neighborhood bridge group 2 months ago as a social outlet. He does not notice any tremor in his right hand when he plays, but he says he cannot shuffle the cards as well as he used to.

Medications: Once daily OTC multivitamin tablet; as-needed ibuprofen for occasional elbow pain related to increased activity (golf).

Allergies: No known allergies (NKA).

OBJECTIVE

General: Older, white male appears stated age and in no distress.

Vital signs: HT: 69 inches; WT: 170 lb; BP: 130/70; HR: 72 and regular; temp: 97.6 F.

Skin: Warm, dry. Good skin turgor. No lesions, rashes, or pigment changes noted.

HEENT: Pupils equal, round, and reactive to light and accommodation (PERRLA); extraocular movements intact; funduscopic exam within normal limits: no vessel changes. Tympanic membranes clear bilaterally. Pharynx without erythema or postnasal drip.

Neck/lymph: Full range of motion of cervical spine without pain. No lymphadenopathy noted.

Lungs/thorax: Lungs clear to auscultation bilaterally. No masses or tenderness on palpation of the chest.

Heart: S1/S2 regular rate and rhythm. No murmurs noted. No S3 or S4.

Abdomen: Nontender, no masses noted on palpation. No hepatosplenomegaly.

Genitourinary/gynecological: Deferred. Routine prostate and genitourinary exam performed by primary care provider 6 months ago.

Musculoskeletal/extremities:

- Patient is right handed. Slight tremor in right hand observed at rest, which diminishes when patient is directed to reach for pen on the table in front of him. No tremor noted in the left hand.
- Relaxed right arm: Slight rigidity with passive range of motion (ROM), even when the patient is tapping left thumb to left index finger to distract his focus from the right arm.
- Relaxed right leg: Slight rigidity with passive ROM, even when the patient is tapping left foot to floor to distract his focus.
- Right foot: Unable to maintain rhythmic tapping of foot on floor after 7 taps.

- Left foot: No difficulty with ROM or tapping of foot on floor repeatedly.
- Gait: Steady but with decreased right arm swing. No dystonias noted.

Neurologic:

- Writing sample indicates beginning of small, cramped writing (micrographia) by word #5 in the following 10-word sentence: "I find it rewarding when I combine business with pleasure."
- Cranial nerves (CN) II–XII: intact; CN I: unable to identify peppermint oil by scent.
- Deep tendon reflexes (DTR): +2 bilaterally.
- Romberg: negative.
- Mini Mental Status Exam (MMSE): 30/30 score indicating basic cognitive functioning, such as orientation and short term memory.
- Center for Epidemiologic Studies—Depression scale (CES-D): 19, indicating mild depression. (Note: Scores range from 0 to 60, with higher scores indicating more symptoms of depression. CES-D scores of 16–26 are indicative of mild depression.).

CRITICAL THINKING

Which diagnostic or imaging studies should be considered to assist with or confirm the diagnosis?
___Electroencephalogram (EEG)
___Magnetic resonance imaging (MRI) of the brain
___Positron emission tomography (PET) scan of the brain
___Trial test with levodopa
___CBC with differential
___Comprehensive metabolic panel

What is the most likely differential diagnosis and why?
___Brain tumor
___Parkinson's disease
___Benign essential tremor
___CVA
___TIA
___Organic brain syndrome
___Alzheimer's disease

What is the plan of treatment and follow-up care?

Are any referrals needed at this time?

Does the patient's psychosocial history affect how you might treat this patient?

What if the patient were a postmenopausal female, age 50?

What if the patient were under age 40?

What if the patient also had diabetes or hypertension?

What if the patient lived in an isolated or rural area?

What if the patient did not live with a significant other, either related or unrelated?

What might an NP anticipate with regard to the long-term physical and psychological impact of the illness on the patient's life partner?

What resources are available to the patient?

Diagnostic testing:

1. Electroencephalogram (EEG)—This test usually would be obtained by the neurology practice and would be ordered to rule out problems indicated by abnormal changes in electrical patterns emitted by various areas of the resting brain.
2. Magnetic resonance imaging (MRI) of the brain—This test is a noninvasive test used to provide two-dimensional images of the structures of the body. The process uses intense magnetic fields to make images of the inside of the body and is frequently used to detect problems within the body or brain without surgery. It can identify abnormalities from outside the body.
3. Positron emission tomography (PET) scan of the brain—This test is an imaging test that can help reveal how tissues and organs are functioning. To show this chemical activity, a small amount of radioactive material is put into the body. The precise type of radioactive material and its delivery method depends on which organ or tissue is being studied by the PET scan. The radioactive material can be injected, swallowed, or inhaled. A PET scan is useful in evaluating a variety of conditions, including neurological problems, heart disease, and cancer, by showing areas of higher chemical activity.
4. Blood work—Complete blood count (CBC), comprehensive metabolic panel (CMP)—The CBC is one of the most commonly ordered blood tests. The complete blood count is the calculation of the cellular (formed) elements of blood. Primarily it is the measure of the concentration of the white blood cells, the red blood cells, and the platelets in the blood. The comprehensive metabolic panel (CMP) blood test is group of 14 blood tests that evaluate various organ functions and is commonly used to detect potential dysfunction of organs such as the kidneys, liver, and pancreas. The CMP screens for organ dysfunction by measuring glucose, calcium, prealbumin, albumin, electrolytes (sodium, CO_2, potassium, and chloride), blood urea nitrogen (BUN), creatinine, alkaline phosphatase (ALP), alanine amino transferase (ALT), aspartate amino transferase (AST), and bilirubin.
5. Trial test with levodopa—A one-dose trial of levodopa is usually performed by the neurologist and is a key indicator for the presence of Parkinson disease. If presenting symptoms are relieved or ameliorated by an increase in the level of levodopa in the system (a positive result), then Parkinson disease is suspected as the cause of the presenting symptoms.

Allan's test results:

1. EEG—Within normal limits (WNL).
2. MRI—Baseline established; WNL.
3. PET scan—Reduction in dopaminergic neural activity in left striatum.
4. Blood work—CBC, CMP—WNL.
5. Trial test with levodopa—Positive. Peak time for trial dosage of levodopa/carbidopa alleviated right arm swing and right knee stiffness.

What is the most likely differential diagnosis and why?
Idiopathic parkinson disease (PD):
Only the onset of idiopathic Parkinson disease accounts for all of the subjective and objective findings in this case scenario. The following findings and motor and non-motor symptoms support the diagnosis:

*   **Demographics:** White male, age 62 (Caucasians have a higher incidence; men have a higher incidence of PD than women; PD average age of onset is 60 years.)
*   **Subjective report:** Patient reports non-motor symptoms of reduced ability to smell obvious odors such as gas; increased sense of fatigue and inefficiency doing regular ADL and house maintenance routines; reduced executive functioning (focusing and prioritizing); and recent constipation problems for 1 month. Patient also reports motor symptoms of decreased fluidity of movement when

walking, playing golf, shuffling cards, as well as a resting tremor that diminishes when holding a cup of coffee. (Early non-motor symptoms of PD have been recently identified and include constipation, reduced olfactory sensory input, micrographia, and reduced executive functioning. Early motor symptoms include increased rigidity of the extremities, lack of arm swing when walking, and a resting tremor.)

- **Objective findings:** Normotensive (BP: 130/70); normal lipid levels/triglycerides; abnormal PET scan with diminished dopaminergic activity in left. Striatum; CN I, diminished olfactory sensory perception; resting tremor in right hand; writing sample evidences micrographia; rigidity during passive ROM with right arm and right leg, even when patient is distracted; reduced ability for repetitive motion on right side (foot tapping, finger tapping); walking without normal swinging of right arm; and positive response to trial dose of levodopa/carbidopa. (PD does not affect BP, blood chemistries, or hematologic tests. PET scan may show reduced functioning in the left or right striatum, depending on the affected side; and there is usually compromised olfactory sensation, passive ROM rigidity, and reduced ability for voluntary repetitive actions such as foot tapping.

Discussion of differential diagnoses:
Left-sided brain tumor:
Symptoms can vary by location of the tumor, but will present on the right side of the body. This diagnosis could account for the subjective and objective findings in the case study. However, there typically should be other key diagnostic manifestations for a brain tumor. The clinician would also expect to see headaches, vision problems, auras and/or seizures, and other signs of increased intracranial pressure such as elevated BP.

Benign essential tremor:
Benign essential tremor (BET) onset is usually about age 40, and there is frequently a family history of BET. It can affect almost any part of the body; but the trembling occurs most often in the hands, and sometimes the head and voice. The tremor is most noticeable when a person attempts to do simple tasks like reaching for an object or drinking a glass of water. Symptoms begin gradually, first affecting either one or both hands. Tremors also become worse with movement, emotional stress, fatigue, caffeine, or temperature extremes. While this diagnosis could explain the subjective findings of recent hand tremor, exacerbated by a reported history of excess caffeine intake, and unusual stress (job loss) experienced in the past 9–12 months, it is not supported by his age and lack of family history. It accounts for only the subjective and objective symptoms listed below and does not account for his other motor and non-motor symptoms.

What is the plan of treatment and follow-up care?
Briefly explain about PD, stressing high variability of symptoms and disease progression for each person with PD. Treatment will be primarily symptomatic. (Note: The nurse practitioner should be prepared to prescribe as-needed medications like stool softeners, suppositories, incontinence medications like VESIcare (solifenacin succinate) and Flomax (tamsulosin HCl), medications for decreasing salivary secretions/drooling, etc., if these symptoms arise.)

Address the patient about recent constipation by counseling the couple about the need to add more fiber to patient's daily diet and to drink 5–8 glasses of water each day. Provide written information and reliable websites for PD information such as NIH-NINDS, Northwest PD Foundation, American Parkinson Disease Association (APDA), and Parkinson Disease Foundation (PDF).

Assess the impact on ADL with the patient and his wife for possible referrals to occupational and physical therapy. Stress the importance of remaining as physically active as possible. Stress how far along medication treatment and surgical intervention for PD has come. Review the rationale for immediate "treatment," that is, not prescribing levodopa at the onset.

Stress the importance of having PD monitored by a neurologist who specializes in movement disorders, and provide several names of such neurologists. Counsel the couple as needed about maintaining clear and accurate verbal and nonverbal communication with one another, and together as a couple with the patient's health care providers.

The nurse practitioner should keep communication lines open, provide time for the patient and/or the couple to express concerns, and provide evidence-based information to guide the patient/couple as needed.

Patients should be seen every 6 months to monitor symptoms and watch for bradykinesia, tremors (both intentional and resting), and postural instability. It is important to be alert to other symptoms, such as excessive salivation, drooling, incontinence, constipation, hypomimia, flat affect, reduced executive functioning, depression, anxiety, social isolation, and withdrawal from couples' activities. The nurse practitioner should order medications for symptom treatment in conjunction with the PD medications ordered by the neurologist. The NP should make speech therapy (ST) and counseling referrals as needed.

There are potentially serious side effects to treatments to watch for and to ask the patient and spouse about, such as hypotension, compulsive behaviors like sexual fixation or hypersexuality, and gambling (especially with dopamine agonists like pramipexole [Mirapex] and ropinirole [Requip]), incontinence, constipation, dry mouth, nausea, hallucinations, somnolence, confusion and, rarely, liver failure (especially with COMT inhibitors like entacapone [Comtan] and tolcapone [Tasmar]). Consult with the patient's neurologist and coordinate medical treatment and counseling for these symptoms, as required. In addition to OT, PT, ST, and counseling, patients can be referred to PD support groups for social networking and personal information and insights regarding living with PD. A medical social worker can be beneficial to assist with financial counseling, health care benefits, the costs of PD medications (up to $1000+/month), and home care assistance.

Are there any referrals needed at this time?

A neurology referral—A neurologist would perform a comprehensive neurological exam, including all reflexes, as well as active and passive motor activity. Depending on the response to the various tests, this exam can evaluate what, if any, areas of the brain may be malfunctioning and can potentially narrow the diagnosis to a specific or several related processes or diseases. In Allan's case, all reflexes were +2; he demonstrated resting tremor in his right hand and lack of right arm swing and reduced right knee bending when walking. Micrographia was evident in his writing sample; he failed the scratch-and-sniff testing.

Ophthalmologic referral—An ophthalmologist will perform a thorough eye exam in order to assess for increased intracranial pressure by viewing the optic nerve fundi. In cases of brain tumors or stroke, intracranial pressure is usually increased, resulting in papilledema of the optic disc. Allan's ophthalmological exam was within normal limits.

Does the patient's psychosocial history impact how you might treat this patient?

Given the patient's current mild depression regarding recent job loss and the potential additive effects of the Parkinson disease diagnosis, he may benefit from counseling sooner, rather than later, in his progression. He does appear to have good family support and limited, but adequate financial support and resources. The couple may need guidance related to the patient's eventual reduced capacity to help maintain their home, to drive, and to remain independent in self-care. He is currently fairly active physically and socially, which should benefit him in terms of his Parkinson's and mild depression. Providers should note that, as PD progresses and dopamine levels are seriously compromised, depression often becomes a physiological part of the disease.

What if the patient were a postmenopausal female, age 50?

Recent epidemiological studies of women with PD, compared to matched non-PD women, indicate an association between lowered estrogen levels and development of PD. Additional studies on treatment of postmenopausal PD women with estrogen replacement therapy (ERT) indicates that ERT was related to reduced cognitive impairment and greater independence in ADL. However, it was also noted that the PD women using ERT were more likely to be depressed and using antidepressant medications. In addition to these challenges, women with PD face decreased ability for homemaking and for caring for their children; and, like PD men, they face the potential loss of a job if they work outside the home, the loss of driving ability, the loss of executive functioning, and the loss of the ability to make cogent financial and other decisions with their spouses. Also like men, women with PD must make adjustments to changes in roles, self-image, and appearance.

Unfortunately, western society's predilection toward stricter standards for women regarding their appearance and abilities to maintain a home and family may cause women with PD greater stress in these areas.

What if the patient were under age 40?

Usually people are in their mid 60s (range 50 onward) when diagnosed with Parkinson disease; but there is an increasing number of people under 50 diagnosed with it (called Young Onset PD). When people are in their 30s and 40s, this often results in additional difficulties related to having young children and/or teenagers who are still dependent on these parents. The responsibility for dependent children can magnify the stress of potential job loss, going on disability, the loss of driving skills, as well as reduced executive functioning and the ability to make cogent financial and home-maintenance decisions with the non-PD spouse. The overall treatment plan is determined based on individual progression and impact on quality of life, regardless of age.

What if the patient also had diabetes or hypertension?

Regarding diabetes, there is the potential that motor problems (especially tremors and rigidity) will increase the difficulty of giving oneself injections, doing daily testing of urine or blood, carrying out good foot and skin care, and similar recommended diabetes self care. Regarding hypertension, NPs must be aware that there are some PD medications (benztropine [Cogentin]; trihexyphenidyl [Artane]; levodopa/carbidopa; amantadine [Symmetrel]) that actually cause postural hypotension; antihypertensive medications may complicate this problem, as well as produce side effects of constipation and dry mouth.

What if the patient lived in an isolated or rural area?

Distance to adequate and appropriate resources would be a primary concern for the NP providing care for such a person. Finding a qualified movement disorder neurologist is imperative, as is excellent OT, PT, and ST; often such specialized services are not available or are not easily accessible in rural areas. In addition, keeping an adequate supply of PD medications on hand via the local pharmacist could be an important issue. A reasonable approach with PD patients would be to explore whether there are mail-in prescription services that can assist them in obtaining their refills in a timely manner, or whether their insurance plan covers such mail-in prescription services.

What if the patient did not live with a significant other, either related or unrelated?

When a person is diagnosed with PD and they live alone, without nearby family or close friends, maintaining their independence will be a paramount concern. At present there is no way to predict how rapidly PD will progress for a given individual or which PD symptoms will be experienced or when. The uncertainty of such a situation is a challenge for both the person with PD and his or her health care provider. Much will depend on the patient's financial resources. Living with other family members or with a very close friend might be an option. If a person has some financial resources, he or she may need to consult with a financial planner to plan for a time when living alone may no longer be an option. Assisted living facilities have varying costs and rules; some are prohibitively expensive. Some require that potential residents be totally independent when buying into the facility; only after residents have been living independently in the facility will they be eligible for the assisted living care. Most importantly, plans must be made while the person with PD is still independent and able to maintain his or her home or apartment.

What might an NP anticipate with regard to the long-term physical and psychological impact of the illness on the patient's life partner?

Research is increasing on the physical and psychosocial effects of providing informal care to a person with a chronic degenerative illness such as PD, Alzheimer disease, chronic heart disease, and rheumatoid and osteoarthritis. Findings indicate that informal caregivers and care partners have higher morbidity and mortality rates and are at greater risk for developing heart disease, hypertension, anxiety, and depression compared to age-matched, noncaregiving cohorts. Care partners of PD patients require attention to their own physical and emotional well-being. They may need to be reminded that keeping up their own health helps their partner with PD. They also may need encouragement to seek counseling to adjust to the changes in their roles and responsibilities created by their partner's progressing PD symptoms. Finally they may need advice as to resources in the community that can help address some of their issues, like financial concerns, home maintenance problems, making their home accessible for a person with limited mobility, and psychosocial support.

What resources are available to the patient?

Driving assessment: Area Agency on Aging website for information: http://www.agingcarefl.org/caregiver/fourStages/stageOne/section07.

PD information:

American Parkinson Disease Association (APDA): http://www.apdaparkinson.org/
Davis Phinney Foundation: http://www.davisphinneyfoundation.org
National Institute of Neurological Disorders and Stroke (NINDS): http://www.ninds.nih.gov/
National Parkinson Foundation: http://www.parkinson.org/
Northwest Parkinson Foundation: http://www.nwpf.org/
Parkinson Disease Foundation (PDF): http://www.pdf.org/
Veterans Affairs Healthcare System Parkinson's Disease Programs: http://www.parkinsons.va.gov/
We Move: http://www.wemove.org/

PD political action: Parkinson Action Network (PAN): http://www.parkinsonsaction.org/.

PD research: Michael J. Fox Foundation for Parkinson's Research: http://www.michaeljfox.org/.
Parkinson Alliance: http://www.parkinsonalliance.org/.
Videos and Books: http://www.michaeljfox.org/living_additionalResources_booksAndVideos.cfm.

REFERENCES AND RESOURCES

Archbold, P. G., Stewart, B. J., Greenlick, M. R., & Harvath, T. (1990). Mutuality and preparedness as predictors of caregiver role strain. *Research in Nursing & Health, 13,* 375–384.

Carter, J. H., Stewart, B. J., Archbold, P. G., Inoue, I., Jaglin, J., Lannon, M., et al. (1998). Living with a person who has Parkinson's disease: The spouse's perspective by stage of disease. *Movement Disorders, 13*(1), 20–28.

Fernandez, H. H., & Lapane, K. L. (2000). Estrogen use among nursing home residents with a diagnosis of Parkinson's disease. *Movement Disorders, 15*(6), 1119–1124.

Gilbert, D. A., & Hayes, E. (2009). Communication and outcomes of visits between older patients and nurse practitioners. *Nursing Research, 58*(4), 283–293.

Habermann, B., & Davis, L. L. (2005). Caring for family with Alzheimer's disease and Parkinson's disease: Needs, challenges, and satisfactions. *Journal of Gerontological Nursing, 31*(6), 49–54.

Jacopini, G. (2000). The experience of disease: Psychosocial aspects of movement disorders. *Journal of Neuroscience Nursing, 32*(5), 263–265.

Jaywant, A., & Pell, M. D. (2010). Listener impressions of speakers with Parkinson's disease. *Journal of the International Neuropsychological Society, 16,* 49–57.

Kaptein, A. A., Scharloo, M., Helder, D. I., Snoei, L., van Kempen, G. M., Weinman, J., et al. (2007). Quality of life in couples living with Huntington's disease: The role of patients' and partners' illness perceptions. *Quality of Life Research, 16,* 793–801.

Krack, P., Batir, A., Van Blercom, N., Chabardes, S., Fraix, V., Ardouin, C., et al. (2003). Five-year follow-up of bilateral stimulation of the subthalamic nucleus in advanced Parkinson's disease. *New England Journal of Medicine, 349*(20), 1925–1934.

Leiva-Santana, C., Monge-Argiles, J. A., & Galvan-Berenguer, B. (2007). A study of personality in Parkinson's disease: The influence of motor and non-motor factors. *Revista de Neurologia, 45*(1), 7–12.

Lombardi, W., Woolston, D., Roberts, J., & Gross, R. (2001). Cognitive deficits in patients with essential tremor. *Neurology, 57*(5), 785–790.

Martire, L. M., & Schulz, R. (2007). Involving family in psychosocial interventions for chronic illness. *Current Directions in Psychological Science, 16*(2), 90–94.

Rao, S. S., Hofmann, L. A., Shakil, A., Rao, S. S., Hofmann, L. A., & Shakil, A. (2006). Parkinson's disease: Diagnosis and treatment. *American Family Physician, 74*(12), 2046–2054.

Roland, K. P., Jenkins, M. E., & Johnson, A. M. (2009). An exploration of the burden experienced by spousal caregivers of individuals with Parkinson's disease. *Movement Disorders*, 25(2), 189–193. Retrieved from http://dx.doi.org/10.1002/mds.22939

Rothstein, T. L., & Olanow, C. W. (2008). The neglected side of Parkinson's. *American Scientist*, 96(3), 218–225.

Tickle-Degnen, L., & Lyons, K. D. (2004). Practitioners' impressions of patients with Parkinson's disease: The social ecology of the expressive mask. *Social Science and Medicine*, 58, 603–614.

Case 9.4 Visual Changes

By Sheila L. Molony, PhD, APRN, GNP-BC

SUBJECTIVE

Maureen is an 85-year-old woman who lives alone and comes to the office every 3–6 months for monitoring of hypertension and hyperlipidemia. Today she presents with a concern about vision changes. Maureen reports some vision changes including increased sensitivity to glare; increased difficulty with dark adaptation, with colors seeming not as vivid as they used to; and increased difficulty with reading. She states that she needs bright light to read comfortably. She isn't sure when these symptoms began, but they have become increasingly bothersome. She denies eye pain or discharge, diplopia, or halos. She has no history of eye trauma. Her last eye exam was 5 years ago. She denies any history of glaucoma but thinks she may have had some early cataracts on her last exam.

Past medical/surgical history: Hypertension; hyperlipidemia; peripheral arterial insufficiency; osteoporosis; generalized anxiety disorder; osteoarthritis; status post hip fracture with repair/pinning at age 82.

Family history: Mother: died at age 78, lung cancer; had age-related macular degeneration and migraines. Father: died at age 65, MI; had coronary artery disease, diabetes, and stroke.

Social history: She is widowed and lives alone in a one-bedroom, first-floor apartment with five steep stairs to enter the building. She is dating and attends ballroom dances at least once a week. She also gardens and walks a half mile on most days. She falls asleep without difficulty but awakens many times during the night and has difficulty falling back asleep. She is in bed for 8 hours but asleep for a total of 5.5 hours per night. She is sometimes sleepy during the day. She drinks 2 beers per night, 2–3 times per week. She quit smoking 25 years prior (smoked 1 pack of cigarettes per day for 40 years).

Diet: Maureen's typical diet includes toast with butter and jam for breakfast with black coffee; tomato soup and grilled-cheese sandwich with a glass of whole milk for lunch; roast beef, potatoes with gravy, and green beans with butter and salt for dinner; and no snacks. She eats out 2 or 3 nights per week and usually has some type of meat, potato or white rice, and a cooked vegetable. She does not drive (never has; uses public transportation). She is independent in all activities of daily living and instrumental activities of daily living.

Clinical Case Studies for the Family Nurse Practitioner, First Edition. Edited by Leslie Neal-Boylan.
© 2011 John Wiley & Sons, Inc. Published 2011 by John Wiley & Sons, Inc.

Medications: She has brought all of her medication bottles that include lisinopril, atorvastatin, citalopram, and alendronate. She has an expired prescription/bottle of hydroxyzine that she uses for "nerves." She also takes acetaminophen as needed for arthritis pain.

Allergies: Penicillin (causes rash).

Maureen admits to vision changes; difficulty hearing (mostly in crowded restaurants); postnasal drip; and occasional arthritis pain in her shoulders, fingers, hips, and knees. She admits to occasional leakage of urine when she has a cold/cough. She denies headache, falls, head trauma, cough, dyspnea, chest discomfort, abdominal pain, and change in appetite or weight, polyuria, polydipsia, polyphagia, weakness, numbness, and dizziness.

OBJECTIVE

Eyes: Visual acuity: 20/40 in both eyes (with eyeglasses). Latter one-third of eyebrows is absent. Slight ectropion bilaterally. Conjunctiva/sclera clear. No crescentic shadow. Positive for arcus senilis. PERRLA. EOMs intact with mild decrease in upward gaze; visual fields full. Positive for red reflex bilaterally; suboptimal retinal visualization.

The remainder of the physical examination is unchanged since her last visit.

CRITICAL THINKING

Which diagnostic or imaging studies should be considered to assist with or confirm the diagnosis?
___Amsler grid
___MacuFlow
___National Eye Institute Visual Functioning Questionnaire 25
___Ophthalmological referral for testing

Which differential diagnoses should be considered at this point?
___Macular degeneration
___Glaucoma
___CVA
___Cataracts

Which of the symptoms or signs related to Maureen's eyes or vision represent pathological changes versus normal aging?

What are the three most common diagnoses/conditions affecting vision in older adults? Are Maureen's signs and symptoms similar to the clinical presentations of these conditions?

What is your plan of care? Are any referrals needed?

What if Maureen were <65? Would that change your management plan?

What patient, family and caregiver education is important in this case?

A few weeks after the visit described above, you receive a phone call from Maureen telling you that she had an episode of slurred speech and she could not move her right arm for about 5 minutes. The symptoms occurred 30 minutes ago. She feels fine now but she is frightened. What advice do you give to Maureen and why?

What diagnostic evaluation will you complete?

What education is needed?

What is your management plan?

What are some of the most important domains of nursing assessment and management (physical, psychological) in the early post-stroke period?

RESOLUTION

Diagnostic testing: The history should include date of last eye exam, whether a retinal exam and glaucoma assessment was done, and a family history of eye disease. Assessment of the eye begins with measuring visual acuity. Acute vision loss or unexplained low vision warrants urgent referral (to an ophthalmologist or emergency room depending upon the clinical scenario (e.g., for risk factors for ocular or neurological disease, recent ocular injury, or foreign body). If foreign body or possible corneal scratch is suspected, fluorescein staining and Wood's lamp examination may be done.

If overall visual acuity is within the usual range, a screening test for macular degeneration should be done using an Amsler grid (Jager, Mieler, & Miller, 2008). A new Internet version of this test entitled MacuFlow is now available but has not been extensively tested (Frisén, 2009). Other helpful assessment tools include the National Eye Institute Visual Functioning Questionnaire 25 (NEV-VFQ-25) and the Pelli-Robson contrast sensitivity chart (Pelli, Robson, & Wilkins, 1988; Revicki, Rentz, Harnam, Thomas, & Lanzetta, 2010). There is no evidence that vision screening in asymptomatic older adults results in improved clinical outcomes, but these tests may help to detect hidden disease in persons at higher risk and also may assist the clinician in developing an individually tailored plan of care for older adults with visual impairment. Optimizing visual acuity is an important component of multicomponent interventions to prevent geriatric syndromes such as delirium (Chou, Dana, & Bougatsos, 2009; Inouye, Fearing, & Marcantonio, 2009).

Which of the symptoms or signs related to Maureen's eyes or vision represent pathological changes versus normal aging?

Maureen reports gradual, insidious changes in her vision. Her fear of blindness relates to her concern about having macular degeneration (like her mother). Normal aging changes in the eyes may result in an increased sensitivity to glare, difficulty with light/dark adaptation, decreased color discrimination, and loss of acuity in low-contrast and low-light conditions. Pupil size decreases. Visual processing time may also be decreased, potentially affecting reading and driving; but this may improve with training. While ectropion (outward turning of the lids) is not a normal aging change, it is a common, correctable condition (Duthie, 2007; Sterns & McCormick, 2007; Watson, 2009).

What are the three most common diagnoses/conditions affecting vision in older adults? Are Maureen's signs and symptoms similar to the clinical presentations of these conditions?

The three most common pathological conditions in older adults include cataracts (most common cause of low vision in the elderly), glaucoma, and macular degeneration. Diabetic retinopathy is also common in diabetics (Sterns & McCormick, 2007; Watson, 2009). Vision loss affects safety (driving, falls, identifying and dosing medicines), function (reading, television, work, recreation), and cognition (orienting cues, recognition, risk for delirium). Symptoms of cataracts include increased sensitivity to glare and/or to light, decreased contrast sensitivity and decreased blue-yellow color vision. Although glaucoma decreases peripheral vision, the loss is gradual and rarely noticed until severe. Macular degeneration results in blurred or distorted central vision or central vision loss. Unless hemorrhage occurs, changes are gradual and may not be noticed until moderate or severe. None of these conditions is painful. Pain in the eye suggests a serious condition that must be evaluated promptly. Sudden vision loss in part or all of the visual field in one or both eyes is an emergency and may represent ocular, neural, or vascular pathology (including stroke, retinal hemorrhage). Older adults are also at higher risk for a condition known as temporal arteritis (also called "giant cell arteritis") which may present with headache and sudden vision loss. Immediate evaluation and treatment are necessary to prevent permanent blindness and to differentiate this condition from acute stroke (Nakasato & Carnes, 2009; Sterns & McCormick, 2007).

What is your plan of care? Are any referrals needed?
A dilated retinal examination is needed to more thoroughly assess the health of the retina and macula. Maureen is referred to an ophthalmologist for this examination, as well as a measurement of eye pressure and peripheral vision testing.

What if Maureen were <65? Would that change your management plan?
These symptoms would be suspicious for ocular pathology in a younger person and comprehensive assessment and ophthalmology followup would be essential. Macular degeneration is almost exclusively found in persons over age 55 and cataracts in a younger person are usually secondary to other diseases/conditions.

Younger patients who present with TIA/stroke are more likely to have undiagnosed coagulopathies. If there are no vascular risk factors and no other apparent causes, diagnostics should be guided by history and physical exam and may include protein C, protein S, antithrombin III, activated protein C resistance/factor V Leiden, anticardiolipin antibody, lupus anticoagulant, and Von Willebrand factor (Easton et al., 2009). Younger patients have different risk/benefit ratios in terms of surgery and anticoagulation.

What patient, family, and caregiver education is important in this case?
Important topics for education include primary prevention (e.g., heart healthy diet, weight control, blood pressure control, no smoking and sun protection); the importance of eye exams (especially for persons with eye disease or risk factors); the benefits of contrasting colors; the importance of adequate lighting; strategies to avoid glare and shadow; and the availability of low-vision aids such as magnifiers, large print, computer enhancements, talking books, and watches. Vision rehabilitation is helpful for persons with visual loss that is affecting function or quality of life.

A few weeks after the visit described above, you receive a phone call from Maureen telling you that she had an episode of slurred speech and she could not move her right arm for about 5 minutes. The symptoms occurred 30 minutes ago. She feels fine now but she is frightened. What advice to you give to Maureen and why?
You advise Maureen to seek immediate evaluation in the emergency room. Her symptoms are consistent with a transient ischemic attack (TIA) but cannot be differentiated from a stroke without neurovascular imaging. The most common symptoms of brain ischemia include sudden weakness or numbness on one side (face, arm or leg), trouble speaking or slurred speech, trouble walking (due to sudden unexplained dizziness, loss of coordination or sudden "drop" attack and fall), or trouble seeing (sudden loss of visual field, sudden monocular or binocular vision loss, blurred vision or diplopia). Headaches, tinnitus and hearing loss may accompany vertebrobasilar insufficiency.

The ABCD^2 mnemonic is used to stratify the risk for subsequent stroke in patients with TIA symptoms. Points are given based on age, blood pressure, clinical presentation including site and duration of symptoms, and the presence or absence of diabetes. Persons with ≥3 points are considered high risk and should be evaluated in the hospital (Easton et al., 2009).

Older definitions characterized TIA as a focal neurologic deficit of acute onset that completely resolves within 24 hours. The American Heart Association/American Stroke Association (AHA/ASA) revised the definition in 2009 and provided updated guidelines for initial evaluation. Many patients with symptoms meeting the older definition of TIA were found to have magnetic resonance–detectable brain injury. Furthermore, the risk of stroke in the early post-TIA period was found to be higher than expected. Prompt workup and risk factor management may delay or prevent subsequent brain injury. The new definition of TIA is "a transient episode of neurological dysfunction caused by focal brain, spinal cord, or retinal ischemia, without acute infarction" (Adams et al., 2007; Easton et al., 2009; Hershey, 2007).

What diagnostic evaluation will you complete?
Along with stroke, the differential diagnosis of focal neurological deficits would include migraine aura, seizure, intracranial mass (e.g., tumor, hematoma), hypoglycemia, dissecting aortic aneurysm, and conditions leading to syncope or hyperventilation. If symptoms are confined to the face, Bell's palsy may be included; and if they primarily comprise of loss of vision, visual field, or acute vision

changes, ocular neuropathy or intraocular pathology may be included. Temporal arteritis (also known as giant cell arteritis) is a form of vasculitis that occurs almost exclusively in persons over age 50 and may present with temporal headache and/or sudden loss of vision. Permanent blindness may result unless this condition is diagnosed and treated promptly. Persons with rheumatoid arthritis are at higher risk for this disease.

If Maureen's clinical presentation had been less severe (a score of 1 or 2 on the ABCD^2) and she was considered low risk in the initial emergency department evaluation, she might be referred back to her primary care provider (same day visit) for further evaluation. Physician collaboration is recommended in planning and implementing a comprehensive and cost-effective workup that includes appropriate neurovascular imaging. The AHA/ASA guidelines recommend imaging within 24 hours of symptom onset, preferably with MRI, including diffusion-weighted imaging. If MRI is not available, a head CT is recommended. Doppler ultrasound, transcranial ultrasound, MR angiography, or CT angiography are used to detect carotid vascular pathology. An EKG should be done to detect atrial fibrillation, a common cause of thrombus formation; and lab work should include CBC, chemistry profile, and PT/PTT (to rule out hypoglycemia or other metabolic abnormalities, polycythemia vera, and hypercoagulopathy). If no other cause is found, a cardiac echo may be needed to rule out patent foramen ovale, valve disease, and other conditions associated with cardiogenic thrombus formation (Easton et al., 2009). The majority of strokes in the elderly are ischemic (often due to cardiac embolism or small vessel disease) versus hemorrhagic. Atherosclerosis of the carotid or atherosclerosis of the vertebral arteries are also potential causes (Hershey, 2007).

What education is needed?
Maureen and her family need to learn about the importance of stroke prevention strategies and immediate transfer to the emergency department for evaluation in the event of symptoms. *In the case of a stroke, it is important for the public to understand, "Time is brain," meaning that the longer emergency treatment is delayed, the greater the risk of brain cell damage and brain cell death, leading to permanent disability.* "Clot-busting" agents (if indicated) must be given within the first 3 hours after onset of symptoms for optimal effect (1 hour is optimal).

Patients and family members are taught to recognize the signs of a "brain attack" or stroke using the mnemonic "FAST."

- **F** (Face)—Ask the person to smile. Does one side of the face droop?
- **A** (Arms)—Ask the person to raise both arms. Does one arm drift downward?
- **S** (Speech)—Ask the person to repeat a simple sentence. Are the words slurred or is there difficulty repeating the sentence correctly?
- **T** (Time)—If the person has any one of these symptoms, they should activate EMS (call 911) and go to the hospital immediately. Emergency personnel will want to know the last known symptom-free time, since duration of symptoms is an important parameter in calculating the risk/benefit of various treatment options. A family member or friend should travel to the hospital, if possible, to provide information.

Other symptoms of stroke include trouble seeing in one or both eyes, trouble walking, dizziness, loss of balance or coordination, or sudden severe headache with no known cause.

What is your management plan?
Acute/initial inpatient management includes evaluation for tPA therapy, aspirin administration, skillful management of blood pressure, hydration and blood sugar, prevention of iatrogenic complications, comprehensive rehabilitation, and early discharge planning.

After stabilization and discharge, the nurse practitioner has a critical role in partnering with the patient to facilitate risk factor reduction, to reduce the likelihood of future strokes, disability, and possibly vascular dementia. It is important to optimize therapy for hypertension, smoking cessation, hyperlipidemia, diabetes mellitus, and atrial fibrillation. Antiplatelet therapy is used for secondary prevention of noncardioembolic, ischemic stroke (Adams et al., 2007). Anticoagulation (with warfarin) is used instead of antiplatelet therapy for patients with atrial fibrillation. Older adults are at higher risk of bleeding from antiplatelet and/or anticoagulation therapy, and the risk-to-benefit ratio needs to be evaluated for each patient, guided by the latest available evidence. Physician consultation and collaboration is recommended. Age alone is not a contraindication to anticoagulant therapy, and there is evidence of undertreatment in high-risk older adults (Adams et al., 2007). Patients with carotid stenosis >70% should be referred for surgical evaluation without delay. It is recommended that surgery be performed within 2 weeks of TIA symptoms in order to minimize morbidity and mortality (Adams et al., 2007; Easton et al., 2009).

If Maureen was admitted to the hospital with a CVA she would very likely be discharged to a rehabilitation hospital following her hospital course.

What are some of the most important domains of nursing assessment and management (physical, psychological) in the early post-stroke period?
Goals in the early post-stroke period are to restore maximal function and too assist with emotional and physical adjustment during the rehabilitation period. Skillful nursing assessment, care, education and monitoring are needed in collaboration with the interdisciplinary team, the patient and the family. The goals of care include maintaining or improving mobility, self-care, communication, swallowing, bladder control, bowel function, sexual function, emotional adjustment and family coping. Instructing formal and informal caregivers is an important nursing role in order to prevent injury (e.g., shoulder dislocation), avoidable complications (choking, aspiration, fecal impaction), and frustration related to unrealistic expectations and unmet needs for adaptive equipment, technologies or assistance. Systematic cognitive and psychosocial assessments are required to enable early intervention and management of complications such as anxiety, depression, and visuospatial neglect. Frequent consultation with physical, occupational, and speech therapy will facilitate appropriate tailoring of the rehabilitation plan; and social service involvement is critical to service planning and coordination across health care settings (Mauk & Hanson, 2010).

REFERENCES AND RESOURCES

Adams, H. P. Jr., Del Zoppo, G., Alberts, M. J., Bhatt, D. L., Brass, L., Furlan, A., . . . Wijdicks, E. F. M. (2007). Guidelines for the early management of adults with ischemic stroke: A guideline from the American Heart Association/American Stroke Association Stroke Council, Clinical Cardiology Council, Cardiovascular Radiology and Intervention Council, and the atherosclerotic peripheral vascular disease and quality of care outcomes in research interdisciplinary working groups. *Stroke, 38*(5), 1655–1711.

Chou, R., Dana, T., & Bougatsos, C. (2009). Screening older adults for impaired visual acuity: A review of the evidence for the U.S. preventive services task force. *Annals of Internal Medicine, 151*(1), 44–58.

Duthie, E. H. (2007). History and physical examination. In E. H. Duthie, P. R. Katz, & M. L. Malone (Eds.), *Practice of geriatrics* (4th ed., pp. 3–15). Philadelphia, PA: Elsevier.

Easton, J. D., Saver, J. L., Albers, G. W., Alberts, M. J., Chaturvedi, S., Feldmann, E., . . . Sacco, R. L. (2009). Definition and evaluation of transient ischemic attack: A scientific statement for healthcare professionals from the American Heart Association/American Stroke Association Stroke Council; Council on Cardiovascular Surgery and Anesthesia; Council on Cardiovascular Radiology and Intervention; Council on Cardiovascular Nursing; and The Interdisciplinary Council on Peripheral Vascular Disease. *Stroke, 40*(6), 2276–2293.

Frisén, L. (2009). The Amsler grid in modern clothes. *British Journal of Ophthalmology, 93*(6), 714–716.

Hershey, L. A. (2007). Cerebrovascular disease. In E. H. Duthie, P. R. Katz, & M. L. Malone (Eds.), *Practice of Geriatrics* (4th ed., pp. 373–380). Philadelphia, PA: Elsevier.

Inouye, S. K., Fearing, M. A., & Marcantonio, E. R. (2009). Delirium. In J. B. Halter, J. G. Ouslander, M. E. Tinetti, Studenski S., K. P. High, & S. Asthana (Eds.), *Hazzard's geriatric medicine and gerontology* (6th ed.). (Chapter 53). McGraw-Hill. Retrieved from: http://www.accessmedicine.com/content.aspx?aID=5119453

Jager, R. D., Mieler, W. F., & Miller, J. W. (2008). Age-related macular degeneration. *New England Journal of Medicine, 358*(24), 2606–2617.

Mauk, K. L., & Hanson, P. (2010). Management of common illnesses, diseases and health conditions: Poststroke rehabiliation. In K. L. Mauk (Ed.), *Gerontological nursing: Competencies for care* (2nd ed., pp. 395–402). Jones & Bartlett Publishers.

Nakasato, Y. R., & Carnes, A. (2009). Myopathy, polymyalgia rheumatica, and temporal arteritis. In J. B. Halter, J. G. Ouslander, M. E. Tinetti, S. Studenski, K. P. High, & S. Asthana (Eds.), *Hazzard's geriatric medicine and gerontology* (6th ed.). (Chapter 119). McGraw-Hill. Retrieved from: http://www.accessmedicine.com/content.aspx?aID=5135557

Pelli, D. G., Robson, J. G., & Wilkins, A. J. (1988). The design of a new letter chart for measuring contrast sensitivity. *Clinical Vision Sciences*, 2(3), 187–199.

Revicki, D. A., Rentz, A. M., Harnam, N., Thomas, V. S., & Lanzetta, P. (2010). Reliability and validity of the national eye institute visual function questionnaire-25 in patients with age-related macular degeneration. *Investigative Ophthalmology & Visual Science*, 51(2), 712–717.

Sterns, G. K., & McCormick, G. J. (2007). Ophhalmologic disorders. In E. H. Duthie, P. R. Katz, & M. L. Malone (Eds.), *Practice of geriatrics* (4th ed., pp. 301–316). Philadelphia, PA: Elsevier.

Watson, G. R. (2009). Assessment and rehabilitation of older adults with low vision. In J. B. Halter, J. G. Ouslander, M. E. Tinetti, S. Studenski, K. P. High, & S. Asthana (Eds.), *Hazzard's geriatric medicine and gerontology* (6th ed.). (Chapter 43). McGraw-Hill. Retrieved from: http://www.accessmedicine.com/content.aspx?aID=5116392

Case 9.5 Confusion

By Joanne DeSanto Iennaco, PhD, PMHCNS-BC, APRN

SUBJECTIVE

Ruth is a 70-year-old widowed female who is brought to your office by her daughter who reports she has not been herself lately. She does not take part in activities with her friends as often and seems not to pay as much attention to her hygiene or to caring for her home or surroundings as usual. Her daughter reports that she seems down and is not as interested in what is happening with the family. Ruth also frequently repeats the same stories or asks the same questions in social situations. She has been more forgetful than usual, having lost her house and car keys repeatedly in the past few months. An avid reader, Ruth has not attended her book club in several months; she states she can't concentrate enough to get through the stories. Her daughter wonders if her mother's vision is impaired, as she frequently finds things soiled in her mother's home. Ruth would miss stains on the counter or in the bathroom when cleaning, but she reports not seeing the stains. Ruth's daughter reports that Ruth stays at home most of the time, watching television. Ruth indicates that she is feeling "just fine" and that her daughter worries about her too much.

Past medical history: Ruth has a history of hypertension and high cholesterol since age 62.

Social history: She lost her husband of 45 years 2 years ago and suffered from depression that was successfully treated with sertraline.

Medications: Lisinopril, 10 mg PO QD; Simvastatin 20 mg PO QHS.

Allergies: None known.

OBJECTIVE

Vital signs: BP: 132/84; P: 68; R: 16; T: 98.4; height: 5 ft 4 inches; weight: 135 lb; BMI: 23.2.

Mental status exam: Ruth is alert and oriented to her environment; however, she is unsure of the month and day, despite knowing the year. Registration of objects was 3 of 3; but recall at 5 minutes was only 2 of 3. She was not able to complete serial 7s or to spell "world" backwards. MMSE: 24 out of 30.

Vision screening: Normal.

Clinical Case Studies for the Family Nurse Practitioner, First Edition. Edited by Leslie Neal-Boylan.
© 2011 John Wiley & Sons, Inc. Published 2011 by John Wiley & Sons, Inc.

Cardiovascular: Regular rate and rhythm, S1 and S2. Pulses without bruits. Carotids +2.

Respiratory: Lungs clear to auscultation bilaterally.

CRITICAL THINKING

Which diagnostic or imaging studies should be considered to assist with or confirm the diagnosis?
___MRI
___Neuropsychological testing
Labs:
___CBC
___Chem-7
___LFTs
___Calcium
___Magnesium
___B12
___Folate
___TSH
___ESR
___RPR

What is the most likely differential diagnosis and why?
___Dementia/type
___Delirium
___Major depressive disorder
___Mild cognitive impairment

What is your plan of treatment?

Are any referrals needed?

Does the patient's psychosocial history impact how you might treat this patient?

What if the patient were under the age of 65 years?

RESOLUTION

TABLE 9.5.1. Diagnostic Testing.

Thyroid Panel	CBC & Differential	Metabolic Panel
TSH: 1.9 uU/mL	WBC: $5.8 \times 10^3/mm^3$	Na: 135 mmol/L
T3: 1.0 ug/dL	RBC: $5.1 \times 106/mm^3$	K: 3.7 mEq/L
T4: 9 ug/dL	Hgb: 13.7 g/dL	Glucose: 97 mg/dL
	Hct: 37%	Ca: 9.8 mg/dL
	MCV: 90	Cl: 99 mEq/L
	MCH: 31	CO_2: 27 mEq/L
	MCHC: 35	BUN: 21 mg/dL
	Neutrophils: 50%	Creatinine: 0.8 mg/dL
	Lymphocytes: 40%	
	Monocytes: 6%	
	Eosinophils: 3%	
	Basophils: 0.8%	
	Thrombocytes: $225,000 \times 10^3/mm^3$	

What is the most likely differential diagnosis and why?
Dementia:
Dementia is the most likely diagnosis, particularly given the lack of other depressive symptoms (depressed mood, change in appetite, sleep, weight). There is impairment in activities, including poor hygiene compared to normal, not following through on bills, responsibilities, or activities.

The primary difficulties in memory and recall suggest the potential for a cognitive disorder like dementia. Forgetfulness, poor hygiene, lack of initiative, decreased activity and interest, as well as difficulty in concentration and attention, also fit the criteria for disturbances in executive functioning that are commonly present in dementia.

Ruth has a history of depression and is at risk for recurrence of depression. Her daughter identifies her as seeming "down," and the lack of interest in usual activities could be a manifestation of anhedonia. Problems with concentration are also frequently a symptom of depression.

Forgetfulness and memory problems are key criteria found in diagnosing mild cognitive impairment. This is a consideration if activities of daily living are intact but memory problems occur.

What is your plan of treatment?
Refer Ruth for the MRI to determine if there are any changes evident that would substantiate a diagnosis of dementia. Consider starting Ruth on medications including memantine (starting with a dose of 5 mg and titrating up to 10 mg 2 times per day) and donepezil (starting with a dose of 5 mg per day) to attempt to improve cognitive functioning.

Plan to see Ruth within 2 weeks to evaluate the effect of the new medications on her functioning. In addition, begin to discuss important planning for the future with Ruth and her daughter. Ruth's financial affairs may need more management; and Ruth would benefit from structured activity that might be available in a senior center, day program, or an assisted living setting. Ruth may need to move to a setting where others can assist her with her needs.

Are any referrals needed?
Refer Ruth to elder-care services to evaluate whether there are appropriate programs that would provide Ruth with structure and activity to optimize her functioning.

Does the patient's psychosocial history impact how you might treat this patient?
Given that Ruth is a widow and lives alone, the strategies for intervention may differ from those implemented if her spouse were still alive and able to provide some support with daily needs.

What if the patient were under the age of 65 years?
If the patient were under age 65, there would be greater need to evaluate for an Alzheimer's type dementia that can occur at much younger ages. In addition, it would be wise to evaluate for other types of dementia, such as Pick's or Wilson's.

REFERENCES AND RESOURCES

American Psychiatric Association (2000). *Diagnostic and statistical manual of mental disorders, fourth edition, text revision.* Washington, DC: American Psychiatric Association.

Sadock, B. J., Sadock, V. A., & Ruiz, P. (2009). *Kaplan & Sadock's comprehensive textbook of psychiatry* (9th ed.). Philadelphia: Lippincott, Williams & Wilkins.

Case 9.6 Itching and Soreness

By Sheila L. Molony, PhD, APRN, GNP-BC

SUBJECTIVE

Rosa is a 74-year-old woman who presents with a complaint of itching and soreness in her left side and upper back. She tells you that she has been gardening and that she thinks she may have a spider or bug bite, but she cannot see this area. She felt an "irritation" 2–3 days ago with intermittent itching. She took some OTC Benadryl© without benefit. She now complains of intermittent "shooting pain" and "tingling" sensations. She has been wearing a camisole instead of a bra for comfort. She denies itching in any other location on the body and has no other dermatological complaints. She is not aware of any tick bites, and she denies recent trauma to the chest or back. She denies use of new shampoos, lotions, laundry products, clothing, perfumes, or topical agents.

Past medical history: Positive for hypertension (HTN); osteoarthritis (OA, primarily of the knees and fingers); gout; osteoporosis, and polymyalgia rheumatica (PMR).

Medications: Zestoretic, 1 tablet qd; fosomax, 70 mg po, once per week; allopurinol, 200 mg po once per day; Prilosec, 20 mg po qd; and prednisone, 7.5 mg po qd. She has been taking these medicines for over 1 year (with varying prednisone dose adjustments).

Allergies: She denies any environmental, contact, or medication allergies.

OBJECTIVE

Head: Abundant, slightly dry hair in normal distribution with no alopecia or breaking. Head is normocephalic and atraumatic.

Lymph nodes: No palpable lymphadenopathy in head, neck, thorax, or axilla.

Skin: Pale with multiple scattered, small, bright-red, pinpoint papules over the chest and back, as well as several irregularly shaped, flat, light-brown macules. She has no visible rash, discoloration, or lesion in the affected area, and no obvious insect bite or entry wound. Her skin is very dry in all areas.

Clinical Case Studies for the Family Nurse Practitioner, First Edition. Edited by Leslie Neal-Boylan.
© 2011 John Wiley & Sons, Inc. Published 2011 by John Wiley & Sons, Inc.

Thorax: Exquisite tenderness on palpation in the left subscapular area, extending to the anterior axillary line, lateral to the left breast.

Her remaining physical examination is within normal limits.

CRITICAL THINKING

Which diagnostic or imaging studies should be considered to assist with or confirm the diagnosis?
__Erythrocyte sedimentation rate (ESR or "sed rate")
__Immunoglobin E titer
__Immunoglobin G titer for varicella zoster
__Metabolic (chemical) profile including LFTs, BUN/creatinine, electrolytes, and TSH
__Polymerase chain reaction testing
__Skin biopsy
__Skin scraping for microscopy

What is the most likely differential diagnosis and why?
__Bug bite
__Contact dermatitis
__Eczema
__Herpes zoster
__Infestation (lice or scabies)
__Medication-related adverse effects
__Polymyalgia rheumatica (exacerbation)
__Rib fracture
__Seborrheic dermatitis
__Systemic disease
__Xerosis (dry skin)

What is your management plan for Rosa?

Are any referrals appropriate at this time?

Which of the clinical findings are consistent with normal aging changes?

What are the most common causes of pruritus (itching) in older adults? What are the risks and benefits of antihistamine therapy for pruritus, such as diphenhydramine (Benadryl©)?

If new lesions continued to appear after 1 week, what additional considerations would you address?

Which specific vaccines' dates of administration should be included in immunization documentation for older adults?

List two additional questions the practitioner should consider to guide clinical care. These questions should be considered in your approach to <u>all</u> geriatric care, in tandem with the workup, diagnosis, and management of the presenting problem.

RESOLUTION

Diagnostic testing: Herpes zoster is a clinical diagnosis based on dermatomal-pattern vesicular rash with neurosensory symptoms. Diagnostic tests are not needed unless there is diagnostic uncertainty or possible disseminated disease in an immunocompromised individual. Viral identification by PCR or fluorescent antibody testing may be helpful in those cases. An ESR may be used to assess inflammation related to PMR, but it is not as useful in the context of an acute dermatologic condition. Chemistry profiles may identify systemic disease but are not warranted by dermatologic symptoms alone. Skin scrapings and microscopy are useful for scabies identification.

What is the most likely differential diagnosis and why?
Herpes zoster infection (shingles):

You suspect shingles based on the neurosensory symptoms in a dermatomal pattern. Your suspicions are confirmed when Rosa returns several days later with a weeping rash along the T5 dermatome associated with a sharp stinging sensation. You find a mixture of erythematous papules and vesicles. She has no prior history of a similar rash. She did have chickenpox in childhood and has no history of receiving the herpes zoster vaccine (Zostavax®). Risk factors for varicella zoster virus (VZV) reactivation include older age and immunosuppression. Stressful life events may also play a role.

Aside from cherry angiomas and seborrheic keratoses, Rosa has no visible entry wound or lesions. She has no papules, vesicles, urticaria, redness, or swelling in the affected area. The absence of a rash, lesion, or visible insect bite makes bug bites, contact dermatitis and seborrheic dermatitis unlikely. The initial small, red papule associated with scabies may be difficult to see; but it is often accompanied by small linear burrows that assist in diagnosis. Scabies often appears in areas such as the finger webs, axillary or subgluteal folds, and/or flexor (wrists) or extensor (elbows and knees) surfaces of the joints. This condition is intensely pruritic, especially at night. Rosa's irritation and tenderness are not consistent with scabies. Xerosis and systemic diseases may contribute to pruritus (as described earlier), but they do not explain the localized sensory symptoms.

Medication side effects should always be considered in the differential diagnosis of new symptoms in the elderly. Medications may precipitate changes in mental status, falls, or functional decline. Older adults experience adverse drug effects more often due to polypharmacy, drug interactions, and age-related changes in pharmacokinetics and pharmacodynamics. Dermatologic side effects of medicines may result in maculopapular rashes, photosensitivity, or desquamation. Toxic epidermal necrosis (TEN) and Stevens-Johnson Syndrome (SJS) are rare, life-threatening conditions that may appear within weeks to months of starting a new medicine. (There are also non-medication related causes.) These syndromes may present with skin pain, burning, or paresthesias prior to the typical, rapidly evolving dermatologic manifestations (Valeyrie-Allanore & Roujeau, 2008). Allopurinol is one of the medicines that may precipitate this reaction, but Rosa has been taking this medicine for some time. She has no suspicious eye or mucous-membrane findings and has not had any prodromal flu-like symptoms.

Musculoskeletal pain may also be associated with medications. Rosa is taking alendronate; cases of serious bone, joint, or muscle pain have been reported with the use of bisphosphonates (U.S. Food and Drug Administration [FDA], 2009). Pain begins days to months after beginning therapy and typically begins locally but spreads and may become severe, interfering with daily activities. Rosa's pattern of symptoms and her findings on examination suggest a distinctly different etiology for her discomfort, but it would not be unreasonable for the clinician to hold the next dose of alendronate pending confirmation of the diagnosis.

Rosa's history of osteoporosis suggests an increased risk of fracture. The nurse practitioner would know that thoracic discomfort and tenderness may be consistent with a rib fracture, which can occur with little or no trauma in older adults with osteoporosis. Fracture would be suspected if Rosa's pain was aggravated by inspiration or if point tenderness was found on palpation when she took a deep breath. Rosa's corticosteroid therapy increases her risk for osteoporosis, skin changes (thinning and easier bruising), high blood sugar, and other effects.

Rosa's history of polymyalgia rheumatica (PMR) may result in symptoms such as aching, stiffness (worse in the morning and late at night), and weakness in the upper arms, thighs, neck or lower back; but PMR is *not* associated with itching or significant tenderness on palpation. (NOTE: Older adults with PMR should be educated to notify their clinician immediately if they have vision changes or headache, since PMR can be associated with a serious condition in the elderly called giant cell arteritis (GCA), also known as temporal arteritis. Early recognition and treatment of GCA may prevent permanent blindness and other serious sequelae.

What is your management plan for Rosa?

The management plan has three main goals: to treat the presenting disease or condition, to prevent negative sequelae and excess disability, and to promote comfort. For persons over age 50 with herpes zoster confined to one dermatome, antiviral therapy is recommended within the first 72 hours after onset of the rash. While there is insufficient evidence to support benefit after 72 hours, this may still be considered if new lesions are still emerging or in cases of ophthalmic involvement. Early antiviral therapy inhibits viral replication and may accelerate healing and/or decrease acute pain. Antiviral therapy may reduce the risk of postherpetic neuralgia (PHN), a painful complication of shingles. The two greatest risk factors for PHN are older age and severity of acute symptoms (i.e., pain and rash). Acyclovir, famciclovir, and varaciclovir are the currently available antiviral agents. They differ in cost, dosing frequency, and efficacy in treating acute and postherpetic neuralgia. The most common side effects of these agents are nausea, vomiting, diarrhea, and headache.

Corticosteroids are sometimes prescribed with the antiviral agent, for healthy elderly patients with severe pain or facial paresis. Steroids are not routinely recommended because of potential side effects, particularly in persons with comorbid conditions such as diabetes, hypertension, or osteoporosis.

Patients with disseminated lesions and/or impaired immune competence (e.g., patients with HIV, and malignancies) should be referred to a physician or specialist. Facial lesions or paralysis should prompt an assessment of the ear canals for involvement. If the VZV affects the facial nerve (Ramsay Hunt syndrome), it may cause facial paralysis, intense ear pain, hearing loss, dizziness, tinnitus, or loss of balance. Patients with facial or trigeminal nerve involvement or lesions in the ears or near the eyes should be referred. Ocular zoster is an emergency that may result in permanent vision loss, and patients should be immediately referred to an ophthalmologist. A lesion on the tip or side of the nose suggests ocular nerve involvement and warrants referral.

The risk of secondary infection may be decreased by keeping the area clean and dry. Cleansing daily with mild soap and water is recommended. When vesicles and pustules are actively draining, Domeboro® soaks may be used. Baking soda, calamine lotion, or cornstarch may enhance comfort.

Persons who have already had chickenpox are not at risk for zoster infection from contact with the infected person. While herpes zoster is not spread from person to person, it is possible for persons who are not immune, to acquire chickenpox. It is possible that respiratory or droplet transmission of viral material could result in varicella infection in nonimmune individuals. Until all lesions are crusted over, the individual should avoid contact with pregnant women and persons who are not immune to chickenpox.

Pain management is a key component of care. Patients may avoid any touch or topical therapy because of exaggerated pain sensation in the affected area. Topical therapies, such as lidocaine patches, may be used to provide relief without systemic side effects. Aggressive pain management is indicated for PHN. The World Health Organization (WHO) guidelines for chronic pain management should be followed, with around-the-clock dosing and stepwise therapy; but it may need to be modified to avoid the many potential toxicities of NSAIDS in the older adult. Adjunctive therapies such as tricyclic antidepressants or gabapentin may be used in combination with other pain relief agents. Proactive measures to avoid constipation, falls, and oversedation are particularly important for the older adult.

Nonpharmacologic strategies for pain management include progressive muscle relaxation, meditation, guided imagery, deep breathing, physical exercise, and distraction. Nutritional assessment and counseling are key strategies to support immunologic competence. The Centers for Disease Control have specific nutritional recommendations in their "Shingles Self-management Kit" available at: http://www.healingwithnutrition.com/sdisease/shingles/pplan.html.

In geriatric patients, it is important to recognize that even well-intentioned medical therapies may produce iatrogenic harm (harm caused by a prescribed treatment). In order to prevent this harm, new medicines should be started slowly (start at a low dose and increase slowly); should be titrated to a specific, targeted beneficial effect or optimum dose; and prescribed after consulting references for special dosing instructions for the elderly. If clear therapeutic targets are not specified, it is likely that medicines will be used that offer little or no therapeutic benefit, yet contribute to potential drug interactions or cumulative hazards of polypharmacy. Many medicines are excreted by the kidneys and many older adults have reduced creatinine clearance.

Pain management may involve use of acetaminophen and/or opiates. Oral NSAIDS are not as useful in older adults due to their toxicity profile. The maximum daily dosage of acetaminophen in persons with normal liver function should not exceed 4000 mg, and some sources recommend a maximum of 2.6 gm as a maximum daily dose. It is important to educate patients and caregivers about the presence of acetaminophen in many over-the-counter and combination pain relievers, since additional "hidden" doses may exceed the maximum daily dose and potentiate liver toxicity. Excess alcohol intake may also potentiate acetaminophen toxicity.

NSAIDs pose greater risks for older adults; and if prescribed, should be used in the lowest dosage and for the shortest time necessary. NSAID-related sodium and fluid retention may decrease the effectiveness of diuretic and antihypertensive therapy and may complicate heart failure or renal disease. NSAIDs may acutely worsen renal function in persons with preexisting renal insufficiency. Gastrointestinal bleeding is a complication of NSAID therapy that occurs more often in the elderly, particularly in high-risk patients (persons with prior bleeding history or on anticoagulants or steroids, etc.). If NSAIDs are used in persons at risk, GI prophylaxis with high dose H2 receptor antagonists or proton pump inhibitors is recommended.

Frequent followup and evaluation of pain relief and psychosocial well-being are essential. Stress management techniques and psychosocial interventions may be indicated. PHN-related pain may decrease quality of life and may result in depression, decreased activity level, decreased appetite, impaired sleep, decreased function, and social isolation. Some older adults may use alcohol or other substances to obtain symptom relief.

Are any referrals appropriate at this time?

Referral to a mental health professional for assessment and counseling may be indicated. Referral to a pain specialist is indicated for severe or persistent pain. Cognitive-behavior modification, biofeedback, and relaxation training may be used, as well as nerve blocks.

Which of the clinical findings are consistent with normal aging changes?

Aging is associated with changes in cellular structure and function resulting in changes in skin function, vascularity, and elasticity (Gilchrest, 2007; Norman, 2008; Rabe, Mamelak, McElgunn, Morison, & Sauder, 2006; Rabe et al., 2006) Aging skin is more susceptible to wrinkling, uneven tearing, and purpura (purplish discolorations caused by extravasation of blood into the tissues after minor trauma). Decreases in sensory perception, sweating, injury repair, and vitamin D production have also been documented (Gilchrest, 2007; Norman, 2008; Rabe et al., 2006). Benign lesions such as seborrheic keratoses (yellow, light tan, brown, or brown-black scaly or waxy growths) and cherry angiomas (tiny, bright-red papules) are more common in older adults. Many skin changes are related to environmental factors including air quality and chronic sun exposure over the life course, contributing to accelerated skin aging, dryness, and increased risk for premalignant (e.g., actinic keratoses) or malignant skin growths (including basal cell and squamous cell carcinomas and malignant melanomas). Genetic factors and lifestyle habits contribute to heterogeneity in dermatologic changes in older adults. For example, smoking is associated with increased photoaging (Martires, Fu, Polster, Cooper, & Baron, 2009).

Some of Rosa's dermatologic findings may be attributed to normal, age-related interactions with genetic factors (e.g., the cherry angiomas and seborrheic keratoses); and her new complaint of pruritus (itching) may stem in part from xerosis (dry, cracked or rough skin, which occurs more commonly in cold, low-humidity environments and in older age); but neither aging nor xerosis provides a sufficient explanation for her sensory symptoms and tenderness to touch. The nurse practitioner needs to pursue a more comprehensive assessment and diagnostic approach.

What are the most common causes of pruritus (itching) in older adults? What are the risks and benefits of antihistamine therapy for pruritus, such as diphenhydramine (Benadryl©)?

Dry, rough skin with a "cracked porcelain" appearance (xerosis), especially over the lower legs, is a common skin finding in older adults. This condition may be associated with pruritus. Older adults may present with pruritus rather than rash due to a decrease in inflammatory response to common disorders including contact dermatitis, eczema, infestation, or medication sensitivity (Gilchrest, 2007). If these conditions have been ruled out but the pruritus persists, systemic or metabolic causes should also be considered. Systemic conditions associated with pruritus include renal disease, liver disease, thyroid disease, celiac disease, hematologic disease (including iron deficiency anemia, polycythemia vera), cholestasis, and cancer (Gilchrest, 2007; Norman, 2008). These conditions typically cause generalized, rather than limited, pruritus.

Dry skin is treated by avoiding or reducing exposure to aggravating agents (e.g., harsh detergents and soaps; chemicals including chlorine; and long, hot baths) and treating liberally with emollients such as Aquaphor, Vanicream, and Eucerin cream applied to moist skin, immediately after bathing, to seal in moisture. (Berger, 2010) Keratolytics such as ammonium lactate 12% lotion are used to reduce flaking, fissuring, and inflammation in severe cases. Cases complicated by dermatitis respond to topical steroids (Berger, 2010; Norman, 2008). Humidification of dry environments may be helpful.

Diphenhydramine is appropriate for emergency allergic reactions; but is not recommended for routine use in older adults as a hypnotic or antipruritic, due to the risk of confusion and sedation. Diphenhydramine is one of the medications listed in the Beers criteria list (Fick et al., 2003; Molony, 2004; Molony, 2004). The published Beers criteria include two lists of medications that may be inappropriate for older adults, based on the ratio of benefits to risks. The first list includes medicines that may be inappropriate regardless of diagnosis or condition, and the second list includes medicines that pose risk to older adults diagnosed with certain concomitant medical problems or conditions (e.g., the use of nonsteroidal antiinflammatory drugs (NSAIDS) in persons with renal insufficiency) (FDA, 2008).

If new lesions continued to appear after 1 week, what additional considerations would you address?

Patients with new lesions appearing after 1 week may have underlying conditions that impair immune function and should be referred for more extensive evaluation.

Which specific vaccines' dates of administration should be included in immunization documentation for older adults?

In addition to the standard recommendations for all adults, USPSTF recommendations for primary prevention for older adults (over age 65 unless otherwise specified) include herpes zoster immunization (a single dose for persons 60 years and over, even if they have had prior herpes zoster infection), influenza immunization (yearly), tetanus immunization (Td every 10 years), and pneumococcal polysaccharide vaccination (1 dose in all unvaccinated persons age 65 and over; revaccinate if 5 years or more have elapsed since first dose given at age < 65 years or in persons with functional or anatomic asplenia, or conditions associated with immunocompromise) (Immunization Action Coalition [IAC], 2010).

When an older adult presents with new symptoms, accurate diagnosis facilitates appropriate treatment to prevent further health and functional decline. List two additional questions the practitioner should consider to guide clinical care. These questions should be considered in your approach to *all* geriatric care, in tandem with the workup, diagnosis, and management of the presenting problem.

What are possible sequelae of the symptoms or health condition? How can these sequelae be prevented or detected at an early stage?

While diagnostic tests are carried out to inform the differential diagnosis of chronic diarrhea, measures must be taken to assess and manage any resulting hypokalemia, orthostatic hypotension, or dehydration. While the causes or contributors to dizziness are being evaluated, measures must be taken to mitigate fall risk.

How can comfort be enhanced (physical, psychosocial, and spiritual), beginning immediately? How can suffering be reduced?

By correcting any myths or unfounded fears, using nonpharmacologic or pharmacologic comfort measures, alleviating uncertainty, enhancing a sense of control and participation in self-care, and providing reassurance.

REFERENCE AND RESOURCES

Berger, T. G. (2010). Dermatologic disorders (Chapter 6). In S. J. McPhee, M. A. Papadakis, & L. M. J. Tierney (Eds.), *Current medical diagnosis & treatment*. McGraw-Hill.

FDA, 2008 available at: http://www.fda.gov/Drugs/DrugSafety/PostmarketDrugSafetyInformationforPatientsandProviders/ucm124165.htm.

Fick, D. M., Cooper, J. W., Wade, W. E., Waller, J. L., Maclean, J. R., & Beers, M. H. (2003). Updating the Beers criteria for potentially inappropriate medication use in older adults: Results of a US consensus panel of experts. *Archives of Internal Medicine, 163*(22), 2716–2724.

Gilchrest, B. A. (2007). Skin disorders. In E. H. Dulthie, P. R. Katz, & M. L. Malone (Eds.), *Practice of geriatrics* (4th ed., pp. 531–546). Philadelphia, PA: Saunders-Elsevier.

Immunization Action Coalition [IAC] (2010). Recommendations for adult immunization. Retrieved 07/13, 2010, from http://www.immunize.org/catg.d/p2011.pdf

Martires, K. J., Fu, P., Polster, A. M., Cooper, K. D., & Baron, E. D. (2009). Factors that affect skin aging: A cohort-based survey on twins. *Archives of Dermatology, 145*(12), 1375–1379.

McCarberg, B. (2003). Managing the comorbidities of postherpetic neuralgia. *Journal of the American Academy of Nurse Practitioners, 15*(12 Suppl), 16–21, quiz 22.

Molony, S. (2004). Try this: Best practices in nursing care to older adults Beers' criteria for potentially inappropriate medication use in the elderly. *Dermatology Nursing, 16*(6), 547–548.

Nicholson, B. D. (2003). Diagnosis and management of neuropathic pain: A balanced approach to treatment. *Journal of the American Academy of Nurse Practitioners, 15*(12 Suppl), 3–9.

Norman, R. A. (2008). Common skin conditions in geriatric dermatology. *Annals of Long-Term Care, 16*(6), 40–45.

Novatnack, E., & Schweon, S. (2007). Shingles: What you should know. *RN, 70*(6), 27–31, quiz 32.

Rabe, J. H., Mamelak, A. J., McElgunn, P. J. S., Morison, W. L., & Sauder, D. N. (2006). Photoaging: Mechanisms and repair. *Journal of the American Academy of Dermatology, 55*(1), 1–19.

Schmader, H. (2003). Herpes Zoster, p. 1043–1056. In Cassel, C. K., Cohen, H. J. and Larson, E. B. (Eds.), *Geriatric medicine: An evidence-based approach*. Secaucus, NJ, USA: Springer-Verlag New York, Incorporated.

U.S. Food and Drug Administration (FDA) (2009). Information for healthcare professionals: Bisphosphonates (marketed as actonel, actonel+Ca, aredia, boniva, didronel, fosamax, fosamax+D, reclast, skelid, and zometa). Retrieved 07/13, 2010, from http://www.fda.gov/Drugs/DrugSafety/PostmarketDrugSafetyInformationforPatientsandProviders/ucm124165.htm

Valeyrie-Allanore, L., & Roujeau, J.-C. (2008). Epidermal necrolysis (stevens-johnson syndrome and toxic epidermal necrolysis). In K. Wolff, L. Goldsmith, S. Katz, B. Gilchrest, A. S. Paller, & D. J. Leffell (Eds.), *Fitzpatrick's dermatology in general medicine* (7th ed., p. 85). McGraw-Hill.

Wright, W. L. (2003). Diagnosis and treatment of herpes zoster: Role of the nurse practitioner. *Journal of the American Academy of Nurse Practitioners, 15*(12 Suppl), 10–15.

Case 9.7 Knee Pain

By Leslie Neal-Boylan, PhD, CRRN, APRN-BC, FNP

SUBJECTIVE

Sharon, a 68-year-old obese woman, presents with bilateral knee pain described as "aching pain around the knee." The pain is worse going down stairs, with activity, and at night. She denies any recent trauma other than kneeling activities. She denies hearing any popping sounds or experiencing any locking or giving way of the knee. She denies being bitten by a tick, although she does occasionally work in her garden. She denies fever or chills or general malaise or confusion. She is the mother of 4 adult children and 3 young grandchildren and stays very busy babysitting and helping in the children's households. However, the knee pain has recently limited her activities. When she was a young woman, she was athletic and participated in sports; but, since her children grew up, she has been in a sedentary office job and rarely exercises. She has felt well and has not seen a health care provider for 5 years. She does still get occasional hot flushes but has not had a period for 16 years. She does experience vaginal dryness and states that she does not participate in sexual activity, as she is a widow.

Past medical/surgical history: Sharon had surgery for carpal tunnel syndrome bilaterally 20 years ago. She also has had several suspicious skin lesions removed that have been benign. She had one episode of nephrolithiasis at age 35. Two of her children were born by cesarean section, and two were born via vaginal childbirth. There were no complications with any of the births.

Family medical history: Her mother had rheumatoid arthritis and died of complications at age 55.

Social history: Sharon is a nonsmoker, drinks "socially" (one glass of red wine when she goes to a restaurant once each week), and has never used recreational drugs. Sharon lives alone but has her family and many friends to keep her busy. She feels safe at home and is generally happy with her life but a little tired from all of the babysitting and housework she has been doing.

Medications: Her medications include a multivitamin and occasional aspirin or acetaminophen for "aches and pains." These medicines have relieved her knee pain somewhat but not to her satisfaction. Sharon is not allergic to any medications.

Clinical Case Studies for the Family Nurse Practitioner, First Edition. Edited by Leslie Neal-Boylan.
© 2011 John Wiley & Sons, Inc. Published 2011 by John Wiley & Sons, Inc.

OBJECTIVE

Vital signs: Sharon is afebrile. Her blood pressure is 160/90; HR is regular and 84; respiratory rate is regular at 14. Her weight is 210 lb.

Cardiac: Regular rate and rhythm with no murmurs, clicks, gallops, or rubs.

Respiratory: Lungs are clear bilaterally.

Abdomen: Obese and soft without organomegaly or bruits.

Musculoskeletal: Sharon's knees are mildly swollen without erythema or warmth. There is no tenderness to palpation. Drawer, McMurray, and Lachman tests are negative. The bulge and ballottement signs are also negative. There is mild nonpitting ankle edema.

Skin: Without any current suspicious lesions, any rashes or ulcers.

CRITICAL THINKING

Which diagnostic or imaging studies should be considered to assist with or confirm the diagnosis?
__Lyme titer
__CBC
__CMP
__Lipids
__TSH
__Colonoscopy
__Mammogram
__Pelvic exam
__ESR
__Rheumatoid factor
__CCP
__DEXA scan
__Vitamin D level

What is the most likely differential diagnosis and why?
__Ligament strain or tear
__Bursitis
__Osteoporosis
__Osteoarthritis
__Patellofemoral syndrome
__Gout
__Pseudogout
__Lyme disease
__Rheumatoid arthritis

What should be the plan of treatment?

What should be the plan for health maintenance testing for this patient?

Does she need gynecological care and treatment at this time?

Are any referrals needed?

RESOLUTION

Diagnostic testing: A rheumatoid factor, Lyme titer, and a CCP as well as an ESR should be included in the lab work for Sharon. Further, Sharon may be osteoporotic and should therefore receive a DEXA scan if she hasn't had one in the last year or 2. Sharon should have X-rays of the knees if these have not previously been done or if they have not been done for a long time. In addition to lab work this visit (Lyme titer, rheumatoid factor, CCP, ESR), Sharon should have a CBC, CMP, and TSH as her blood pressure is elevated and she is fatigued. These tests could be delayed, for reimbursement purposes, until she returns to the office for a complete physical. At that time, the clinician should order a mammogram, colonoscopy, and DEXA scan, and also should include a pelvic exam with Pap smear as part of the physical.

What is the most likely differential diagnosis and why?
Osteoarthritis (OA):
Obesity, age, and a previous history of an active lifestyle can contribute to OA. People with OA usually have symptoms that occur with activity or shortly after embarking on activity. Stairs can present a particular problem. OA is most often unilateral but can be polyarticular and symmetric. Sharon did not experience any popping, twisting, clicking, or giving way; so ligamental strains and tears are less likely. She denies experiencing a tick bite, but it is important to remember that one does not always remember a bite or being outdoors and may still have Lyme disease. However, Lyme disease typically presents with unilateral knee pain and swelling. A Lyme titer might be a good test to include in the diagnostics for this case just to rule out the possibility. However, current tests for Lyme disease are not sufficiently specific and sensitive to confirm a diagnosis. History and clinical presentation are more reliable. Gout and pseudogout typically include acute onset of severe pain accompanied by erythema and warmth. They are most often unilateral.

Patellofemoral syndrome is most common in teens and young adults. Anterior knee pain is the most common complaint. Difficulty with stairs is a symptom with difficulty going down stairs typically more severe than going up stairs. Sitting for prolonged periods causes pain that is relieved with walking, and a sense of joint locking instability is common (McPhee & Papadakis, 2010). Rheumatoid arthritis (RA) is typically symmetric and may appear in later life; so Sharon should be questioned regarding morning stiffness, other joint pain and swelling, and fatigue, especially since she has a positive family history for RA. If Sharon experienced unilateral knee pain with an acute onset specific to the area just inferior and medial to the patella (classic location), she would most likely have anserine bursitis.

What should be the plan of treatment?
Clearly, Sharon needs a physical to determine her overall health status and to evaluate her health maintenance. She should be advised to lose weight, exercise, and begin taking calcium and vitamin D. If she is determined to be osteoporotic, her vitamin D levels should be tested. While the clinician can order this test without a DEXA scan, it may not be reimbursed without a clear cause for doing the test.

In addition, Sharon should decrease weight bearing while her knees are causing her pain. Swimming in a heated pool is a good alternative. She should avoid kneeling and try to do less housework, if possible. Plan to see Sharon back to discuss the X-ray and lab results and to perform her physical and pelvic exams.

What should be the plan for health maintenance testing for this patient?
Sharon should see the dermatologist annually to assess and treat any suspicious skin lesions. If the primary care clinician observes any suspicious lesions between these annual visits, the patient should see the dermatologist sooner. Sharon should also have a colonoscopy if she has not had one or if the last one was 5 or more years ago depending on the findings at that time. She should also have annual mammograms. Sharon should have a DXA scan to look for osteoporosis or osteopenia (National Osteoporosis Foundation, (2008). In addition, she should have basic laboratory screening including CBC, LFTs, CMP, and a lipid panel.

Does she need gynecological care and treatment at this time?

Even though Sharon is a widow and is not engaged in sexual activity, it is important that she have a pelvic exam to check for abnormalities. The vaginal dryness is probably due to atrophy and should be examined. Sharon may want and/or require treatment. The American Cancer Society recommends Pap test screening until age 70 years for a healthy patient (Smith, Cokkinides, & Brawley, 2008).

Are there any referrals needed?

No referrals are needed at this time. However, if treatment fails, then an orthopedic and/or a rheumatologic referral should be considered. Sharon can be treated with NSAIDs to begin with, and diclofenac gel can be used to rub into her knees. Alternation of ice and heat may also help. If swelling increases and limits her mobility, corticoid injections into the knee should be considered. Synvisc injections are also possible treatments. Finally, total knee replacements may need to be considered in the future if her symptoms worsen.

REFERENCES AND RESOURCES

Bockenstedt, L. K. (2007). Lyme disease. In J. Imboden, D. Hellmann, & J. Stone (Eds.), *Current diagnosis & treatment: Rheumatology* (2nd ed., pp. 372–382). New York: McGraw Hill-Lange.

Fauci, A. S., Braunwald, E., Kasper, D. L., Hauser, S. L., Longo, D. L., Jameson, J. L., & Loscalzo, J. (2009). Gout, pseudogout, and related diseases. In A. S. Fauci, E. Braunwald, D. L. Kasper, S. L. Hauser, D. L. Longo, J. L. Jameson, & J. Loscalzo (Eds.), *Harrison's manual of medicine* (17th ed., pp. 903–907). New York: McGraw Medical.

McPhee, S. J. & Papadakis, M. A. (2010). *Current medical diagnosis & treatment* (49th ed). McGraw Hill Lange.

National Osteoporosis Foundation (2008). *Clinician's guide to prevention and treatment of osteoporosis*. Washington, DC: National Osteoporosis Foundation.

O'Dell, J. R. (2007). Rheumatoid arthritis: The disease—diagnosis and clinical features. In J. Imboden, D. Hellmann, & J. Stone (Eds.), *Current diagnosis & treatment: Rheumatology* (2nd ed., pp. 161–169). New York: McGraw Hill-Lange.

Smith, R. A., Cokkinides, V., & Brawley, O. W. (2008). Cancer screening in the United States, 2008: A review of current American Cancer Society guidelines and cancer screening issues. *CA Cancer Journal of Clinical, 58*(3), 161–179.

Wilke, W. S., & Carey, J. (2009). Osteoarthritis. In W. Carey (Ed.), *Cleveland clinic current clinical medicine* (pp. 1187–1189). Philadelphia: Saunders.

Case 9.8 Delirium

By Sheila L. Molony, PhD, APRN, GNP-BC

SUBJECTIVE

Antonio is an 84-year-old male resident of a continuing care retirement community (CCRC). The residential director admitted him to the nursing home respite care wing last evening due to behavior changes including agitation, disorientation, and wandering outside without appropriate clothing. The director brings him to the on-site clinic the next morning. She reports that the clinician on call last evening ordered 1 mg of IM haloperidol, which was given soon after the resident came to the unit. The residential director reports that Antonio had a poor appetite for a few days before this and was found napping in the lounge, which is not unusual. He fell on his way to the dining room on the previous morning, but he sustained no apparent injury. During his last annual health maintenance visit 3 months prior, he scored 26/30 on the Mini-Mental State Examination (MMSE) and 22/30 on the Montreal Cognitive Assessment (MoCA) and was diagnosed with "mild cognitive impairment (MCI)." He is usually alert and oriented to season, year, place, and person and has no difficulty navigating inside and outside his residence.

His only complaint today is a new complaint of frequent heartburn that he has been treating with over-the-counter (OTC) pills (he can't remember the name). He denies pain, cough, shortness of breath, or changes in bladder/bowel habits.

Past medical history: Coronary artery disease (CAD) with angioplasty/stent placement x2, hypertension (HTN), benign prostatic hypertrophy (BPH), asthma, hyperlipidemia (HLD), heart failure with normal ejection fraction (HFNEF), mild cognitive impairment (MCI), osteopenia, and osteoarthritis (OA). He had a motorcycle accident in his youth with a left leg injury.

Psychosocial history: Antonio moved to the CCRC one year ago with his wife, who died 4 months prior. He cared for her until she died, then stayed in his apartment, complaining of anxiety and difficulty sleeping. He recently became more involved in community activities and has been making friendships in the building. He has been attending two meals per day in the communal dining room, until this week, and has been independent in bathing, dressing, grooming, walking, transferring, eating, and toileting. He does not climb stairs due to poor endurance but is able to walk on level ground over modest distances without fatigue. Before his wife died, he would take the community van to local shops twice a month. He has a daughter-in-law and two nieces who live within 50 miles, call weekly, and visit once or twice a month.

Medications: Advair 2 inhaler x; Simvastatin, 40 mg qd; atenolol, 100 mg qd; losartan, 50 mg qd; furosemide, 20 mg qd; K-dur, 10 mEq qd; isosorbide mononitrate ER (Imdur), 30 mg qd; alendronate, 70 mg q week; multivitamin (MVI) with iron, 1 qd; vitamin C, 500 mg bid; docusate sodium succinate, 1 qd; OTC medication of unknown name for heartburn.

Allergies: NKDA.

Health maintenance: Td vaccine 2007. Never had the flu vaccine, Pneumovax, or Zostavax (received education/information on last visit and stated he would "think about" it).

OBJECTIVE

Vital signs: Temperature: 100.0°F; pulse: 58 (irreg.); respirations: 28; blood pressure: 168/58; weight: 161 (164 last month); height: 72 inches.

NOTE: His usual vital signs are: Temperature: 97.4°F; pulse: 70–80 (reg.); blood pressure: 130–140/60–70).

General: Today Antonio appears sleepy, disheveled, restless and vague. He is able to walk to the examination room but is unsteady and needs assistance getting undressed for the physical examination. He is unable to fully cooperate with the exam. His skin is dry, especially over the lower extremities.

Mental status: Speech is slow but clear; thought processes are slow and disorganized; irritable mood; distractible; decreased ability to focus. MMSE 19/30.

Head: Normocephalic without obvious lesions, masses, depressions, or tenderness. No temporal bruits.

Eyes: Visual acuity 20/40 bilaterally with glasses. Eyelids are symmetrical with no ptosis, but slight ectropion bilaterally. PERRLA. Conjunctiva and sclera clear with slight arcus senilis. EOMs and visual fields WNL with slight decrease in upward gaze bilaterally. He has a few beats of horizontal nystagmus on extreme lateral gaze. Red reflexes intact but incomplete visualization of retinas due to difficulty cooperating with exam and frequent eye closing/sleepiness.

Ears: Unable to cooperate with hearing acuity screen. External ears are without lesions or tenderness. Canals are obstructed with dark cerumen bilaterally. Unable to visualize TMs.

Nose/sinuses: Nares patent with pink mucosa; no lesions, deviations, or discharge. No frontal or maxillary sinus tenderness.

Mouth/throat: Oral mucosa dry and intact. Tongue and uvula midline, and tongue movement is symmetrical. Pharynx clear. No lesions, masses, cavities, or bleeding.

Neck: Supple; no carotid bruits or thyromegaly. No cervical lymphadenopathy.

Chest: No skin lesions, deformities, tenderness, crepitus, axillary lymphadenopathy, or breast masses. No rubs or thrills. PMI nonpalpable.

Heart: Regular rhythm with frequent pauses. No murmurs or obvious gallops.

Lungs: Symmetrical chest wall expansion. Resonance on percussion throughout all fields. Fremitus palpable and symmetrical. Fine crackles at left base, and coarse inspiratory crackles and expiratory rhonchi over right lower lung field. No egophony, bronchophony, or whispered pectoriloquy.

Abdomen: Soft, nontender, with quiet bowel sounds in all quadrants; No palpable masses, organomegaly, or bruits. Soft stool in rectum; hemoccult negative. Slightly enlarged prostate, symmetrical. No palpable masses.

Neurologic: Gait shuffling with small steps. Slightly unsteady, leaning to one side. Unable to stand with feet together without swaying. No pronator drift. No postural or intention tremor. CNs II–XII grossly intact. Reflexes 3+ and symmetrical in both upper extremities. Lower extremities: 2+ patellar reflex, 1+ Achilles reflex. Plantar reflex ↓. Able to detect pain in all extremities, but unable to cooperate with full sensory or coordination testing.

Musculoskeletal: Muscle strength 4/5 in upper and lower extremities bilaterally.

Peripheral vascular: Bounding radial and brachial pulses: 2+. Femoral and popliteal: 2+. Pedal: 1+. Unable to detect posterior tibial pulse. Ankle edema bilaterally with left > right: 2-3+.

CRITICAL THINKING

Which diagnostic or imaging studies should be considered to assist with or confirm the diagnosis?
___CT scan of the brain
___Chest X-ray
___Urinalysis
___EKG
___CBC with diff, chemistries including BUN/Creatinine, electrolytes, glucose
___Arterial blood gas or pulse oximetry
___TSH, free T4, T3
___Orthostatic blood pressure
___Depression screening (e.g., with Geriatric Depression Scale [GDS], Patient Health Questionnaire—9 item version [PHQ-9], or other screening tool)
___RPR
___B12/folate
___Lumbar puncture
___Electroencephalogram (EEG)

Which differential diagnoses should be considered at this point?
__Dementia
__Depression
__Delirium

What is the treatment plan for Antonio?

Are any referrals needed?

What aspects of the health history require special emphasis in older adults?

What if Antonio were under age 65? Would that change the management plan?

What patient, family, and/or caregiver education is important in this case?

Are there any standardized guidelines that you should use to assess or treat this case?

What are some of the possible contributors to Antonio's hypotension? Are any referrals needed? What management strategies should be considered?

RESOLUTION

Diagnostic testing: The choice of diagnostic tests should be guided by the list of likely differential diagnoses. Many factors guide the choice of diagnostics including urgency of the clinical condition, sensitivity and specificity of the diagnostic test, availability of the test, burden to the patient (cost, invasiveness, and transportation), and, most importantly, the goals of care. The clinician should consider whether the results of the specific diagnostic test will change the treatment plan in any way. If the answer is no, the diagnostic test should be reconsidered.

In this case, laboratory and diagnostic studies should be used to detect common conditions such as infection, metabolic imbalance, or nutritional imbalance; and they usually include serum electrolytes, creatinine, glucose, calcium, complete blood count, liver enzymes, and urinalysis/culture. EKG, CXR and ABGs may be ordered in persons with cardiac or respiratory diseases or symptoms. Subacute cognitive changes also warrant assessment of vitamin B12, folate, and TSH (Inouye, Fearing, & Marcantonio, 2009; Sendelbach & Guthrie, 2009).

Therapeutic drug levels should be ordered, if appropriate (e.g., digoxin, lithium). A toxic screen for ingested substances, an ammonia level, and/or syphilis serologies may be appropriate, based upon the individual's risk profile and/or assessment findings. (Ham, 2007; Inouye et al., 2009; Rudolph & Marcantonio, 2007). Brain imaging (such as CT or MRI) is indicated in patients suspected of having a brain lesion (e.g., stroke, bleed, or tumor) and/or patients without other identifiable causes of delirium. Patients with delirium and recent unexplained falls or symptoms of NPH (triad of gait changes, memory disturbance, and urinary incontinence) should also be referred for brain imaging. Brain imaging is definitely indicated if focal neurological abnormalities are found on physical examination. Additional diagnostic tests should be based on the patient's clinical presentation (Inouye et al., 2009).

For Antonio, the additional studies would include an EKG because of his history of coronary artery disease with assessment findings of bradycardia and irregular rhythm. His new complaint of heartburn may also be cardiac in origin. Pulse oximetry should be done to provide a quick, noninvasive assessment of oxygen saturation. Antonio's recent fall and his gait and balance difficulties are suspicious, and a head CT should be ordered. If head trauma had been sustained or if he was taking warfarin (an anticoagulant), intracranial bleeding would be high on the list of differential diagnoses.

A standardized depression screen using the GDS or PHQ-9 may be useful because depression can mimic dementia, coexist with delirium and dementia, and/or mimic hypoactive delirium. Standardized screening tools identify individuals needing further assessment and provide indicators of responses to treatment over time. Depression screening may not be feasible in the acutely delirious person, due to impaired attention and/or more urgent clinical symptoms. Antonio has difficulty staying focused, so this assessment should be deferred.

Taking orthostatic vital signs (blood pressure and pulse in both lying and standing positions) is useful to obtain a baseline in all geriatric patients. Orthostatic blood pressure and pulse measurement are essential in patients with a history of falls, symptoms of lightheadedness, or weakness with position changes. Older adults are more likely to experience orthostatic drops in blood pressure due to changes in baroreceptor sensitivity in the carotid sinus. Orthostasis is more likely in patients on antihypertensives and/or diuretics and in patients who are dehydrated. Orthostatic hypotension is unlikely to be a sole cause of persistent delirium, but it may be one indicator of hypovolemia (e.g., due to dehydration and/or anemia) that may impair brain perfusion and precipitate delirium (Inouye et al., 2009; Rudolph & Marcantonio, 2007).

If the initial workup does not reveal a cause, physician and/or neurology consultation is recommended. Patients with fever or other features suggesting possible meningitis or encephalitis require a lumbar puncture (after brain imaging). An EEG may be ordered to rule out seizure activity in patients with altered level of consciousness (Inouye et al., 2009; Rudolph & Marcantonio, 2007).

Which differential diagnoses should be considered at this point?
Delirium:
Antonio's clinical presentation is consistent with delirium. He has predisposing vulnerabilities or risk factors including age, severity of illness (acute infection and possible dehydration), and pre-existing cognitive impairment (MCI). Antonio had an acute onset of symptoms, including inattention, disorganized thinking, and an altered level of consciousness. (Symptom fluctuation pattern is unclear and may be complicated by antipsychotic administration).

Delirium is a change in cognition or perceptual disturbance that develops over a short period of time (usually hours to days) and tends to fluctuate over the course of the day (increasing and decreasing in severity). It is also characterized by a reduced ability to focus and/or distractibility. Persons with delirium also have either a change in level of consciousness (lethargic or hyperalert or alternating from one to the other) or have disorganized thinking, a confusing flow of ideas, incomprehensible conversation, and/or unpredictable switches in topic (DSM-IV) (American Psychiatric Association, 2000).

The Confusion Assessment Method (CAM) is a standardized, efficient assessment tool to assist clinicians in recognizing delirium and differentiating it from dementia or depression. It is usually completed after cognitive assessment using the Folstein Mini-Mental State Examination (MMSE) and/or other cognitive assessments such as trail-making, digit span or reciting months of the year, days of the week or words (such as "world") backward (Inouye et al., 2009). These tasks specifically challenge attention span and focus, and help to distinguish delirium from dementia and depression (Folstein, Folstein, & McHugh, 1975; Inouye et al., 1990; Waszynski, 2007).

Dementia is more subtle in onset (months to years) and slowly progressive, with problems in memory and executive function (planning, sequencing, and performing goal-directed activities). Attention processes are normal until later stages, and level of consciousness is not impaired. Lewy body dementia may be difficult to distinguish from delirium since patients with this disease may experience hallucinations and/or fluctuating cognition as part of the dementia. The coexistence of Parkinson-like features of Lewy body dementia and the less acute onset may help distinguish between the diagnoses. Persons with preexisting dementia or other types of brain disease are vulnerable to developing superimposed delirium; and therefore any sudden, significant deviations from usual cognition, behavior, or function should be assumed to be delirium until it is ruled out (Fick, Hodo, Lawrence, & Inouye, 2007). Medical causes of delirium should also be ruled out prior to attributing symptoms to psychiatric disease. Antonio has no apparent symptoms of psychosis (paranoia, hallucinations, delusions, or thought disorder) and no past psychiatric history. A new onset of primary psychiatric disease is possible, but less likely in this case.

Depression may slow mental processing and impair cognitive performance on mental status tests. The depressed patient may make a poor effort on cognitive testing or answer questions with "I don't know," or "I can't." Antonio has recently experienced grief and associated anxiety and sleep disturbance, but he was beginning to improve in activity and social engagement. His irritability may be a sign of depression; but his distractibility, impaired attention, and acute behavior changes are classic symptoms of delirium, rather than depression or dementia. His mood and mental status should both be reassessed after infection or other acute contributors to delirium are treated.

Delirium is a syndrome or cluster of symptoms, rather than a diagnosis. It reflects a condition in which precipitants or "insults" overwhelm individual capacities due to underlying predisposing factors or "vulnerabilities" (Inouye et al., 2007). If delirium is suspected, a prompt, systematic search for reversible contributors should be conducted. The mnemonic "MIND ESCAPE" is useful in remembering potential reversible contributors to changes in mental status in the elderly (adapted from: Molony, 1999, p. 78).

Metabolic changes (e.g., dehydration, electrolyte imbalance, hypercalcemia, liver, kidney, or thyroid disease, hypo- or hyperglycemia, hypoxia, and hypercarbia).

Infection (acute or chronic)/impaction/inability to void.

Nutrition (B12/folate deficiencies; overall malnutrition)/neoplasm/NPH.

Drugs/drug withdrawal (medication effects, including prescription and OTC or street medications).

Environmental toxins/environmental changes.

Sleep deprivation/sensory overload or sensory deprivation.

Cardiovascular/cerebrovascular (stroke, hypoxia, shock, heart failure, myocardial infarction, arrhythmia).

Alcohol or alcohol withdrawal/aknemia.

Pain.

Emotional or mental illness.

After reviewing Antonio's history and exam findings, infection, metabolic disturbance, nutritional deficiency, drug effects, and cardiac problems are identified as the most likely precipitants of delirium, with sensory deprivation (poor vision and hearing) and possibly sleep deprivation as contributing factors.

Older adults often have atypical presentations of disease (Ham, 2007). This is particularly true in advanced age and in persons with multiple chronic conditions or frailty. For example, older adults may have serious infections (including sepsis) with only a low-grade fever and minimal elevation in the white blood cell count. Myocardial infarctions may present without chest pain ("silent" or atypical symptoms such as sudden shortness of breath, hypotension, dyspnea, mental status change, or gastrointestinal symptoms). Hyperthyroidism may present with apathetic lethargy and constipation. Depression may present with irritability and feelings of worthlessness or helplessness instead of sadness. Older adults with acute intraabdominal conditions (e.g., appendicitis, ruptured diverticulum, mesenteric thrombosis) may present without severe pain, guarding, or rebound tenderness. Poor appetite, declining physical function, new urinary incontinence, falls, and mental status changes are often the heralds of geriatric clinical distress. These symptoms signal a need for skilled assessment and management (Amella, 2004; Ham, 2007).

Antonio's temperature is >2.4°F above his baseline, a sensitive threshold for possible infectious disease (High et al., 2009), and his lung findings suggest a possible pneumonia. The urinalysis and chest X-ray will help to identify a source of infection and guide treatment.

Antonio's bradycardia and irregular rhythm suggest possible heart block or other dysrhythmia that may affect cardiac output and perfusion. Older adults with hypertensive heart disease and left ventricular hypertrophy are more likely to have heart failure with preserved systolic function (i.e., normal ejection fraction). Ventricular filling during diastole is affected, and they are very sensitive to any changes in rate, rhythm, or volume that impairs filling time, preload, or cardiac output (CO). The EKG and CBC will identify rhythm changes or anemia that may impair CO and perfusion.

Antonio is taking furosemide, a loop diuretic. Thiazide and loop diuretics may contribute to hypokalemia, hyponatremia, hyperglycemia, and azotemia, which are metabolic conditions that may affect mental status. He is on a low dose of diuretic, but his poor oral intake may increase the risk of fluid and electrolyte imbalance. Antonio's dry lower extremity skin is common with aging, but his dry oral mucous membranes suggest poor hydration. Poor renal perfusion may contribute to renal insufficiency. Laboratory studies will detect these conditions.

Adverse drug effects are common contributors to delirium. A comprehensive medication list that includes prescription, over-the-counter (OTC), and nutritional/herbal supplements is an important part of clinical assessment in all health visits with older adults. Older adults have changes in body composition, liver enzyme systems, and renal function that affect drug distribution, activity, and clearance (Cusack, 2004). They are also more likely to experience drug-drug, drug-food, and drug-disease interactions, due to the number of medicines prescribed, the presence of multiple concurrent diagnoses, and the use of inappropriate doses (based on half-life, renal function, etc.). Older adults may also be more sensitive to drugs that cross the blood-brain barrier. While some medicines have been identified as potentially inappropriate for older adults due to risks that outweigh benefits, it is essential for the clinician to review all medicines as possible contributors to delirium (Fick, Mion, Beers, & Waller, 2008; Molony, 2003; Molony, 2009). Pharmacist consultation is recommended, if available.

Antonio received Haldol, an antipsychotic medication with extrapyramidal side effects including dystonias (prolonged unintentional muscular contractions), Parkinson-like symptoms (i.e., tremor, rigidity and bradykinesia) and akathisia (restlessness, often exhibited as pacing or rocking). Akathisia is often mistaken for worsening agitation and treated with additional doses of the offending antipsychotic agent. Haldol also has anticholinergic properties (including confusion, dry mouth, urinary retention, constipation). Anticholinergic effects of different drugs may accumulate and contribute to delirium, and/or may also lead to urinary retention in patients with BPH. Antonio reported using some type of OTC product for heartburn. Omeprazole (Prilosec®) and cimetidine (Tagamet®) are both available OTC. Cimetidine may precipitate delirium, particularly in higher doses, and may also interact with other medicines, through effects on cytochrome P450 enzyme systems in the liver (Drugs in the Elderly, 2006; Drugs That May Cause Psychiatric Symptoms, 2008; Cusack, 2004; Lindblad et al., 2006).

Constipation is common in older adults if they take insufficient fluid or fiber; are inactive; are immobile; and/or take constipating medicines such as iron, calcium, and/or opioids. Prevention, assessment, and management of constipation are important aspects of geriatric care. Adequate fluid intake, fiber, and mobilization are important prevention strategies. Fecal impaction or bowel obstruction may contribute to delirium, but these have been ruled out for Antonio.

Primary neurologic diseases such as Parkinson disease (PD), normal pressure hydrocephalus (NPH), and cerebrovascular accident (CVA) are less likely diagnoses for Antonio. PD is sometimes misdiagnosed in patients with drug-induced parkinsonism. Antonio's small, shuffling steps could be consistent with parkinsonism, particularly if they appeared only after he received antipsychotic medication; but his gait may also reflect generalized imbalance, fear of falling, and chronic changes. His gait should be monitored during follow-up visits. He does not display cogwheel rigidity, resting tremor, or bradykinesia, which are the cardinal signs of PD (Bunting-Perry & Vernon, 2007). His slight decrease in upward gaze is consistent with normal aging. Persons with normal pressure hydrocephalus (NPH) typically have a wide-based gait with difficulty taking steps (sometimes described as a magnetic gait). In NPH, urinary incontinence and memory loss cluster together with gait changes to form a diagnostic triad typical of the disease. A cerebrovascular accident (ischemic, thrombotic, or hemorrhagic) is possible in view of Antonio's cardiovascular risk factors; but his examination revealed no focal neurological deficits. Small infarcts may still be present, and brain imaging has been ordered to rule this out. If his EKG demonstrated new onset atrial fibrillation (a-fib), a common condition in older adults, the clinical suspicion for CVA would be much higher, since a-fib increases the risk of thrombotic stroke.

What is the treatment plan for Antonio?

Antonio's chest X-ray and WBC findings are consistent with pneumonia. His BUN is elevated and his BUN:creatinine ratio is 26:1(usually 14:1). His higher-than-normal BUN:creatinine ratio suggests impaired renal perfusion, most likely due to hypovolemia/dehydration (other possible causes include acute hypotension, heart failure, or renal ischemia due to artery stenosis).

The first priority is to decide whether to treat Antonio's pneumonia in the hospital. By preventing unnecessary hospitalization, iatrogenic risks that may worsen cognitive function (e.g., changes in medication, sleep patterns, diet, sensory stimulation and/or environment; antibiotic-resistant infections; and/or immobility) may be avoided. On the other hand, older adults are at higher risk for serious complications of pneumonia, including sepsis or respiratory failure; and hospitalization is indicated for high-risk groups and/or worrisome clinical presentations.

Otherwise-healthy older adults with community-acquired pneumonia may be treated as outpatients with appropriate followup. The decision to treat in the community relies in part on the clinician's assessment of the patient's (or caregiver's) ability to follow through with the treatment plan, the ability to monitor clinical status, and the ability to contact the clinician if symptoms persist or worsen. The severity of the delirium, the ability to deliver needed fluids and medication, and the availability of around-the-clock support until mental status improves will also be factored into the decision. The CURB-65 guideline is used to assist with decision making regarding site of care for older adults with community-acquired pneumonia (Mandell et al., 2007; Mills, Graham, Winslow, & Springer, 2009). Antonio's age, BUN, and confusion give him a score of 3, and his pulse oximetry reading is declining. The decision to hospitalize him should be made.

Antonio's delirium should improve with appropriate diagnosis and treatment of reversible contributors and with the provision of supportive care, but some cases of delirium linger for weeks or months (Kiely et al., 2009). Skillful nursing care is needed to minimize polypharmacy and optimize nutrition and hydration, oxygenation, electrolyte balance, comfort, bowel and bladder function, sleep, and activity. Regular reassessment of function and care needs is important to prevent negative sequelae (Sendelbach & Guthrie, 2009).

Are any referrals needed?

Pneumonia, dehydration, and delirium are the top three concerns, and physician involvement is advisable. Cardiology consultation is recommended due to the recent changes in his beta-blocker therapy and episode of pulmonary edema.

What aspects of the health history require special emphasis in older adults?

One of the most important components of geriatric assessment is the functional assessment. It is essential to assess and document the degree to which an older adult can independently complete activities of daily living (feeding, toileting, bathing, turning in bed, moving from bed to standing or bed to chair, and walking) and the amount of supervision or assistance needed. Older adults in independent living should also be assessed for the ability to perform instrumental activities of daily living (cooking, housecleaning, laundry, managing medications, using a telephone, managing finances, shopping, and use of transportation).

When assessing the health of older adults, the clinician should recognize that many conditions and symptoms are underreported in older adults. The geriatric review of systems and physical examination should therefore specifically include assessment for the following: cognitive impairment, dental/oral health, falls, foot problems, gait or balance problems, hearing loss, vision loss, incontinence, nutrition, pressure ulcers, mental health issues (including depression, anxiety, and grief), sexual history, and sleep problems.

What if Mr. A. were <65? Would that change the management plan?

An otherwise-healthy younger adult with community-acquired pneumonia is likely to be treated as an outpatient. Treatment of pneumonia in younger adults would include consideration of appropriate prescribing practices for possibly pregnant or breast-feeding women.

What patient, family, and/or caregiver education is important in this case?

Patient and family education should focus on prevention and early detection. If the patient is treated in the community, the importance of taking all medicine as prescribed must be emphasized. Education on prevention includes counseling to promote pneumonia and influenza vaccine, smoking cessation, and information about hand and cough hygiene. After hospital discharge, Antonio should be encouraged to continue cough and deep-breathing exercises to clear mucus and to maintain adequate fluid intake. Oxygen safety principles should be reviewed if he is discharged on oxygen. Antonio (and/or his caregivers) should be educated regarding symptoms that require a call to the clinician, such as difficulty breathing, fever, or becoming more confused or very sleepy.

It is essential that nursing assistants and personal care assistants benefit from the clinical education given to patients and family members. They are often the first ones to notice clinically important changes and are the most influential determinants in whether follow-up care or self-care strategies are maintained.

Are there any standardized guidelines that you should use to assess or treat this case?

The 2007 Infectious Diseases Society of America/American Thoracic Society consensus guidelines on the management of community-acquired pneumonia in adults and the 2009 update are key references (Lim et al., 2009; Mandell et al., 2007).

Lower respiratory infections (LRI) often result in avoidable hospitalizations in nursing home residents. A program to reduce avoidable hospitalization due to LRI or other causes may be found at: **http://interact.geriu.org/**.

Followup: Antonio is admitted to the hospital, started on intravenous (IV) fluids and moxifloxacin 400 mg IV × 7 days. His atenolol is switched to labetalol in response to elevated blood pressure readings. On day 3 of treatment, he develops acute pulmonary edema treated with IV diuretics followed by an increase in his oral diuretic dose.

The next day he develops watery diarrhea, which continues for days. Donnatal is ordered to treat the diarrhea. A C-difficile titer is sent, and he is started on metronidazole (which is discontinued after negative titers x2). On day 6 of his admission, he develops acute urinary retention; and a Foley catheter is inserted. He is started on tamsulosin and finasteride. The diarrhea slows and the Foley catheter is removed. An episode of hypotension on the day before hospital discharge results in discontinuation of the labetalol. Antonio's lungs are clear, but he is weak and has no appetite. He is alert and oriented, and his mental status is back to baseline. He is discharged to the rehabilitation facility for physical therapy to improve strength, balance, and endurance.

His primary care provider is asked to see him because he had a "fainting spell" the day after admission, after walking 50 feet in physical therapy. His blood pressure at the time was 80 systolic (palpable). His medications now include: Losartan, 50 mg po qd; furosemide, 40 mg po qd; K-dur, 20 mEq po qd; isosorbide mononitrate ER (Imdur), 30 mg po qd; simvastatin, 40 mg po qd; and Advair 2 puffs qd. His temperature, pulse, and respiratory rate are normal. His weight is 157 lb. His color is good, and his MMSE score is 25/30. His affect is mildly depressed. Oral mucous membranes and tongue are dry. His heart rate is 88 and regular with occasional pauses. His lungs are clear, and he has 1–2+ ankle edema (L > R). He has mildly hyperactive bowel sounds; no aortic, renal or femoral bruits. His abdomen is soft and nontender; no palpable masses; no hepatosplenomegaly. His blood pressure in both arms, while sitting, is 98/60 and drops to 84/50 upon standing. He is "woozy" after walking a few feet from the chair to the bed. His neurologic exam is unchanged from the previous exam.

What are some of the possible contributors to Antonio's hypotension? Are any referrals needed? What management strategies should be considered?

Age-related changes in baroreceptor function increase the risk of orthostatic hypotension in the elderly. Medications, hypovolemia, and electrolyte imbalances may contribute to orthostasis. Autonomic nervous system disease or neuropathies are other common causes. Unexplained hypotension (with or without position change) may be an early sign of shock or cardiac pathology. Antonio is dehydrated and is taking several medicines that may contribute to hypotension, including Tamsulosin. In addition to ordering elastic support stockings, teaching Antonio to perform ankle exercises before standing, and increasing his oral fluid intake, it should be recommended that he discontinue the Tamsulosin with instructions to monitor for urinary retention. While liberalizing sodium is an option in some cases or orthostatic hypotension, Antonio's history of heart failure warrants caution. His recent weight loss may represent fluid and nutritional losses, and further assessment of his intake is needed.

REFERENCES AND RESOURCES

Abramowicz, M. (2006). Drugs in the elderly. *The Medical Letter on Drugs and Therapeutics, 48*(1226), 6–7.

Abramowicz, M. (2008). Drugs that may cause psychiatric symptoms. *The Medical Letter on Drugs and Therapeutics, 50*, 1301–1302.

Amella, E. J. (2004). Presentation of illness in older adults. *American Journal of Nursing, 104*(10), 40–52.

American Psychiatric Association (2000). *Diagnostic and statistical manual of mental disorders, fourth edition, text revision (DSM-IV-TR)*. Arlington, VA: American Psychiatric Association. doi:10.1176/appi.books.9780890423349.

Bunting-Perry, L., & Vernon, G. (2007). *Comprehensive nursing care for parkinson's disease*. New York: Springer Publishing Company, Inc.

Cusack, B. J. (2004). Pharmacokinetics in older persons. *American Journal Geriatric Pharmacotherapy, 2*(4), 274–302.

Fick, D. M., Hodo, D. M., Lawrence, F., & Inouye, S. K. (2007). Recognizing delirium superimposed on dementia: Assessing nurses' knowledge using care vignettes. *Journal of Gerontological Nursing, 33*(2), 40–47.

Fick, D. M., Mion, L. C., Beers, M. H., & Waller, J. L. (2008). Health outcomes associated with potentially inappropriate medication use in older adults. *Research in Nursing and Health, 31*(1), 42–51.

Folstein, M. F., Folstein, S. E., & McHugh, P. R. (1975). 'Mini mental state'. A practical method for grading the cognitive state of patients for the clinician. *Journal of Psychiatric Research, 12*(3), 189–198.

Ham, R. J. (2007). Illness and aging. In R. J. Ham, P. D. Sloane, G. A. Warshaw, M. A. Bernard, & E. Flaherty (Eds.), *Primary care geriatrics: A case-based approach* (5th ed., pp. 25–49). Philadelphia, PA: Mosby Elsevier.

High, K. P., Bradley, S. F., Gravenstein, S., Mehr, D. R., Quagliarello, V. J., Richards, C., & Yoshikawa, T. T. (2009). Clinical practice guideline for the evaluation of fever and infection in older adult residents of long-term care facilities: 2008 update by the Infectious Diseases Society of America. *Journal of the American Geriatrics Society, 57*(3), 375–394.

Inouye, S. K., Fearing, M. A., & Marcantonio, E. R. (2009). Chapter 53. delirium (chapter). In J. B. Halter, J. G. Ouslander, M. E. Tinetti, S. Studenski, K. P. High, & S. Asthana (Eds.), *Hazzard's geriatric medicine and gerontology* (6th ed.). McGraw-Hill.

Inouye, S. K., Van Dyck, C. H., Alessi, C. A., Balkin, S., Siegal, A. P., & Horwitz, R. I. (1990). Clarifying confusion: The confusion assessment method: A new method for detection of delirium. *Annals of Internal Medicine, 113*(12), 941–948.

Inouye, S. K., Zhang, Y., Jones, R. N., Kiely, D. K., Yang, F., & Marcantonio, E. R. (2007). Risk factors for delirium at discharge: Development and validation of a predictive model. *Archives of Internal Medicine, 167*(13), 1406–1413.

Kiely, D. K., Marcantonio, E. R., Inouye, S. K., Shaffer, M. L., Bergmann, M. A., Yang, F. M., . . . Jones, R. N. (2009). Persistent delirium predicts greater mortality. *Journal of the American Geriatrics Society, 57*(1), 55–61.

Lim, W. S., Baudouin, S. V., George, R. C., Hill, A. T., Jamieson, C., Le Jeune, I., . . . Woodhead, M. A. (2009). BTS guidelines for the management of community acquired pneumonia in adults: Update 2009. *Thorax, 64*(Suppl. 3), iii1–ii55.

Lindblad, C. I., Hanlon, J. T., Gross, C. R., Sloane, R. J., Pieper, C. F., Hajjar, E. R., . . . Schmader, K. E. (2006). Clinically important drug-disease interactions and their prevalence in older adults. *Clinical Therapeutics, 28*(8), 1133–1143.

Mandell, L. A., Wunderink, R. G., Anzueto, A., Bartlett, J. G., Campbell, G. D., Dean, N. C., . . . Whitney, C. G. Infectious Diseases Society of, A., & American Thoracic, S (2007). Infectious diseases society of America/American thoracic society consensus guidelines on the management of community-acquired pneumonia in adults. *Clinical Infectious Diseases, 44*(Suppl. 2), S27–S72. Retrieved from http://ovidsp.ovid.com/ovidweb.cgi?T=JS&NEWS=N&PAGE=fulltext&D=medl&AN=17278083

Mills, K., Graham, A. C., Winslow, B. T., & Springer, K. L. (2009). Treatment of nursing home-acquired pneumonia. *American Family Physician, 79*(11), 976–982.

Molony, S. L. (1999). Mnemonic for reversible causes of confusion. In S. L. Molony, C. M. Waszynski, & C. H. Lyder (Eds.), *Gerontological nursing: An advanced practice approach* (p. 78). Stamford, CT: Prentice Hall.

Molony, S. L. (2003). Beers' criteria for potentially inappropriate medication use in the elderly. *Journal of Gerontological Nursing, 29*(11), 6.

Molony, S. L. (2009). How to try this: Monitoring medication use in older adults. *American Journal of Nursing, 109*(1), 68–78.

Rudolph, J. L., & Marcantonio, E. R. (2007). *Delirium* (4th ed., pp. 335–344). Philadelphia, PA: Elsevier.

Sendelbach, S., & Guthrie, P. (2009). Evidence-based practice guideline: Acute confusion/delirium. Iowa City: University of Iowa Gerontological Nursing Interventions Research Center, Research Translation and Dissemination Core.

Waszynski, C. M. (2007). How to try this: Detecting delirium. *The American Journal of Nursing, 107*(12), 50–59, quiz 60.

Index

Clinical Case Studies for the Family Nurse Practitioner, First Edition. Edited by Leslie Neal-Boylan.
© 2011 John Wiley & Sons, Inc. Published 2011 by John Wiley & Sons, Inc.

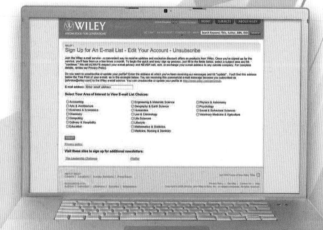
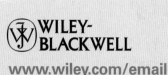